T0201328

Overactive Bladder

Practical Management

Overactive Bladder

Practical Management

EDITED BY

Jacques Corcos MD, FRCS(S)

Professor of Urology
Department of Urology
McGill University
Montreal, QC, Canada

Scott MacDiarmid MD, FRCPSC

Director
Bladder Control and Pelvic Pain Center
Alliance Urology Specialists
Greensboro, NC, USA

John Heesakkers MD, PhD

Urologist
Department of Urology
Radboud University Medical Center
Nijmegen, The Netherlands

WILEY Blackwell

This edition first published 2015 © 2015 by John Wiley & Sons, Ltd.

Registered Office

John Wiley & Sons, Ltd, The Atrium, Southern Gate, Chichester, West Sussex, PO19 8SQ, UK

Editorial Offices

9600 Garsington Road, Oxford, OX4 2DQ, UK

The Atrium, Southern Gate, Chichester, West Sussex, PO19 8SQ, UK

111 River Street, Hoboken, NJ 07030-5774, USA

For details of our global editorial offices, for customer services and for information about how to apply for permission to reuse the copyright material in this book please see our website at www.wiley.com/wiley-blackwell

Library of Congress Cataloging-in-Publication Data

Overactive bladder (Corcos)

  Overactive bladder : practical management / edited by Jacques Corcos, Scott MacDiarmid, John Heesakkers.
    p. ; cm.
  Includes bibliographical references and index.
  ISBN 978-1-118-64061-6 (cloth)
I. Corcos, Jacques, editor. II. MacDiarmid, Scott A., editor. III. Heesakkers, John, editor. IV. Title.
  [DNLM: 1. Urinary Bladder, Overactive–therapy. WJ 500]
  RC919
  616.6′2–dc23
                       2015004410

A catalogue record for this book is available from the British Library.

Cover credit: ©iStock.com/serknor

Wiley also publishes its books in a variety of electronic formats. Some content that appears in print may not be available in electronic books.

Set in 9.5/13pt Meridien by SPi Publisher Services, Pondicherry, India

Printed and bound in Malaysia by Vivar Printing Sdn Bhd

1 2015

Contents

Contributors

Karl-Erik Andersson, MD, PhD
Faculty of Health, Institute for Clinical Medicine
University of Arhus
Arhus, Denmark

Apostolos Apostolidis, MD, PhD, FEBU
Assistant Professor of Urology-Neurourology
Second Department of Urology,
Papageorgiou General Hospital, Aristotle
University of Thessaloniki
Thessaloniki, Greece

Kari Bø, PhD
Professor of Exercise Science
Norwegian School of Sport Sciences,
Department of Sports Medicine
Oslo, Norway

Mathieu Boudes, PhD
Laboratory of Experimental Urology
Department of Development and Regeneration
KU Leuven, Leuven, Belgium

**Christopher R. Chapple, BSc, MD,
FRCS (Urol), FEBU**
Consultant Urological Surgeon, Department
of Urology, Royal Hallamshire Hospital
Honorary Senior Lecturer of Urology,
University of Sheffield
Visiting Professor of Urology
Sheffield Hallam University
Sheffield, UK

Jacques Corcos, MD, FRCS(S)
Professor of Urology
Department of Urology
McGill University
Montreal, QC, Canada

Jill Danford, MD
Vanderbilt University
Medical Center, Nashville, USA

G.W. Davila, MD
Cleveland Clinic Florida
Weston/Fort Lauderdale, FL, USA

Dirk De Ridder, MD, PhD, FEBU
Laboratory of Experimental Urology
Department of Development
and Regeneration
KU Leuven
Leuven, Belgium

Roger Dmochowski, MD, FACS
Professor of Urology / Gynecology
Vanderbilt University Medical Center
Nashville, TN, USA

Jerzy B. Gajewski, MD, FRCSC
Professor of Urology & Pharmacology
Dalhousie University
Halifax, NS, Canada

Lara C. Gerbrandy-Schreuders, MD
Department of Urology
AMC University Hospital
Amsterdam, The Netherlands

Barry G. Hallner Jr, MD
Female Pelvic Medicine and
Reconstructive Surgery
Department of Obstetrics & Gynecology
Louisiana State University Health
Sciences Center
New Orleans, LA, USA

John Heesakkers, MD, PhD
Department of Urology
Radboud University Medical Center
Nijmegen, The Netherlands

Sender Herschorn, BSc, MD, FRCSC
Sunnybrook Health Sciences Centre
University of Toronto
Toronto, ON, Canada.

Jack C. Hou, MD
UT Southwestern Medical Center
Dallas, TX, USA

Vik Khullar, BSc, FRCOG, MD, AKC
Consultant Urogynaecologist
St. Mary's Hospital, NHS Trust
Imperial College London
London, UK

Ryan M. Krlin, MD
Assistant Professor of Urology
Department of Urology
Louisiana State University School of Medicine
New Orleans, LA, USA

Scott MacDiarmid, MD, FRCPSC
Director
Bladder Control and Pelvic Pain Center
Alliance Urology Specialists
Greensboro, NC, USA

Geneviève Nadeau, MD, M.Sc, FRCSC
Division of Urology
Centre Hospitalier de l'Université de Québec
Québec, QC, Canada.

Diane K. Newman, DNP, ANP-BC, FAAN
Research Investigator Senior and Adjunct
Associate Professor of Urology in Surgery
Perelman School of Medicine, University
of Pennsylvania
Co-Director of the Penn Center for Continence
and Pelvic Health
Division of Urology, University of Pennsylvania
Medical Center, Philadelphia, PA, USA

Nadir I. Osman, MBChB (hons), MRCS
Department of Urology
Royal Hallamshire Hospital
Sheffield, UK

L.N. Plowright, MD
Cleveland Clinic Florida
Weston/Fort Lauderdale, FL, USA

Fadi Sawaqed, MD
Dalhousie University
Halifax, Canada

Anand Singh, MBBS, BSc
Specialist Trainee in Obstetrics and
Gynaecology
Clinical Research Fellow in Urogynaecology
St. Mary's Hospital, NHS Trust
Imperial College London
London, UK

Adrian Wagg, MBBS, FRCP, FRCP (E), FHEA
Research Chair in Healthy Ageing
Department of Medicine,
University of Alberta
Edmonton, AB, Canada

Hessel Wijkstra, MSc, PhD
Department of Urology
AMC University Hospital
Amsterdam, The Netherlands

J. Christian Winters, MD, FACS
Professor and Chairman, Department
of Urology
Louisiana State University Health Sciences
Center
New Orleans, LA, USA

Philippe E. Zimmern, MD
UT Southwestern Medical Center
Dallas, TX, USA

Foreword

I had the chance to witness the conception of Overactive Bladder Syndrome as a product of two bright and leading brains as Paul Abrams and Alan Wein, with their ability to involve and ignite the experts network and coagulate their knowledge and expertise. I must admit – despite my reservations – that this has been a major advance in the communication with non-experts in functional urology and a tremendous instrument to raise the awareness of the clinical relevance of urinary urgency and related lower urinary symptoms. It has been a remarkable fruit of a magic period in which major revisions of lower urinary tract related terminology have been undertaken. Noticeably, while to describe the occurrence of urgency with/without frequency with/without urinary incontinence the wording target has been the bladder (OABs), almost simultaneously an organ-related wording such as prostatism or prostatic symptoms has been abandoned in preference of a more descriptive terminology that has became extremely popular and efficacious (Lower Urinary Tract Symptoms: LUTS). The continuously progressing knowledge about the physio-pathology of badder dysfunctions by means of functional CNS imaging and basic research shows, with increased evidence, that in most instances the etiopathogenesis of bladder-related symptom syndromes relies on alterations of bladder control outside the target organ. Consequently I am convinced that a term such as "Altered Bladder Control" will be more adherent to our present knowledge, more open to future interpretations, and equally easy to understand for a non-expert. Others will witness a second magic period with bright changes of terminology such as those cleverly introduced with the wording of Overactive Bladder.

Walter Artibani
Professor and Chair of Urology
at the University of Verona
General Secretary of the International
Continence Society (2005–2007)

Foreword: The impact of Overactive Bladder on Urogynecology

As providers of care to women with urogynecologic problems, our practice patterns have largely been determined by two main variables: (i) the identification and impact assessment of quality of life problems related to pelvic floor dysfunction, and (ii) development of new technology and innovations aimed at reducing the burden of these conditions. Overactive bladder certainly fits within this paradigm. That overactive bladder has a significant QOL impact on its sufferers is certain. A multiplicity of instruments have been developed to better quantify individual impact, and we – as clinicians – have developed disease classification schemes (and terminology) designed at better understanding the condition. In parallel, researchers and industry have developed innovative therapeutic modalities, from pharmacotherapy to rehabilitative and neuromodulation modalities. As a result, our patients have received significant benefit, and we can tell each OAB patient with certainty that we will be able to "make you better."

In my various roles within the International Urogynecological Association (IUGA), I have been witness to this evolution of the role of OAB in our field. IUGA, like other large professional associations focused on pelvic floor dysfunction, has been able to better fulfill its mission in large part due to the expanded role of OAB within our field. Those of us who have been in practice more than 20 years will recall times when our annual meeting presentations and industry booths were largely focused on epidemiology, urodynamics techniques, and basic prolapse repair techniques. Our only OAB treatment modalities, besides physiotherapy, were anticholinergic meds that had been available for many years and were thus not actively marketed. The involvement of industry in our field led to the massive expansion in clinical and research activity we have recently witnessed. I can identify two main turning points responsible for the phenomenon: the launch of tolterodine by Pharmacia, and the launch of suburethral sling kits such as TVT by Gynecare and other companies. Industry involvement allowed IUGA to increase funding for educational programs, expand the scope and size of the annual meeting, and fund the organizational infrastructure required to maintain the association's engine running. It has been a very exciting ride. The future brings about yet more technology and expanded therapeutic options. Will a neuromodulation or chemomodulation company be our next Pharmacia? Will stem cells or tissue modulation technology open doors to other novel therapeutic approaches? One thing is certain: we will have new options to offer our OAB and urogynecologic patients. And, that will continue to fuel our research, education, and organizational efforts.

As our knowledge on pelvic floor problems expands, this book on Overactive Bladder provides the reader with an up-to-date source of data and information that will allow him/her to better care for OAB patients. Congratulations and thanks to Jacques Corcos, Scott MacDiamid, and John Heesakers for this very timely text.

G. Willy Davila, MD
President, International Urogynecological
Association (IUGA)

Foreword

Overactive bladder syndrome remains an enigma that significantly affects the health and wellbeing of 12–17% of adult men and women throughout the world. The development of this term to describe the symptom complex of urgency, frequency, and nocturia with or without urgency urinary incontinence became a necessity 16 years ago with the introduction of the first new medication to treat this constellation of symptoms in over two decades. North American trials of tolterodine failed to show that it worked better than placebo to reduce urinary incontinence episodes, and thus it could not be marketed to treat urgency urinary incontinence. This seemingly bad news for a pharmaceutical company turned out to be a bonanza for all parties involved. Admitting to having urgency urinary incontinence was a marked deterrent to patients seeking care for these symptoms. However, patients had far less embarrassment in seeking care for their overactive bladder syndrome. The direct to consumer marketing efforts for tolterodine and the seven branded products that followed in the next decade have dramatically increased the number of patients willing to seek care for their overactive bladders from about 1 in 13, 15 years ago, to 1 in 5 more recently. Along with this has come increased attention from the industry and the investment community, which has helped to dramatically increase funding and research into new technologies and compounds to address the treatment of overactive bladder syndrome and related conditions over the last decade. This financial bounty has also spilled over into supporting the activities of our professional societies and increased grant funding for young investigators. While I and many academicians resented the introduction of this term, it has greatly benefitted all involved in the care of these men and women; but mostly it has benefitted our patients. This has also served as an excellent model of how industry and the academic community can work together to help promote our mutual goals and to help further the care of our patients.

What does the future hold for the treatment of overactive bladder syndrome? With changes in healthcare delivery systems and funding in North America will we see continued innovation and spending on new therapies for our patients with overactive bladder syndrome? These questions remain to be answered, but as this excellent textbook attests, there are still great minds that remain dedicated to answering the important questions that remain for those affected by overactive bladder syndrome. The editors have assembled a great group of authors who represent some of the best minds in our field. Hopefully, reading this text will inspire other young investigators to take on the challenge of innovating and seeking out the important answers that will lead to a complete understanding of the pathophysiology of the overactive bladder syndrome and its cure.

Peter K. Sand, MD
Professor of Obstetrics & Gynecology
Director, Evanston Continence Center
NorthShore University HealthSystem
University of Chicago, Pritzker School of
Medicine

Preface

Two years ago, the publisher approached me with the suggestion that I become the editor of a textbook about OAB. Initially, I was reluctant to accept this invitation because I was starting my editorial duties for the third edition of the *Textbook of the Neurogenic Bladder*. While considering my options, it became apparent that there was a crucial need for such a book, due to recent developments in the understanding of this specific topic. General interest in a non-life-threatening disease is directly proportional to the interest shown by the pharmaceuticals industry. OAB is a good example of this equation. Industry supported research has allowed us to produce good epidemiological studies and well-developed basic research to better understand the pathophysiology as well as new molecules and techniques to treat the condition. The sum of this recent knowledge serves as the foundation of this book.

My co-editors are two individuals with advanced expertise in the field: one living and practicing in North America and one living and practicing in Europe. Each continent has its own particularities in the practice of medicine, resulting in a diverse variety of approaches. Scott and John bring different perspectives as co-editors, which allows for thorough reviews of each chapter.

Together, we have designed the table of contents, trying to be as didactic as possible in the divisions of our book. After a short introduction to the topic, there is a review of current knowledge on pathophysiology. The book continues with chapters about evaluation practices, including the timing of evaluation, which may vary for each patient depending on where the medical practice is located. The interview and physical examination are considered, including questionnaires, which are extremely useful in the initial assessment of OAB cases. Urodynamics is essential in the evaluation of neurogenic detrusor overactivity but has become optional in primary OAB evaluation.

Treatment chapters follow, divided into first-line, second-line, and third-line therapies, as well as surgery. Behavioral and lifestyle modifications are extremely important in primary and secondary OAB treatments and a significant addition to any other form of treatment. Physiotherapy is another treatment option for OAB, although it is not widely used for this purpose in North America at the present time. A review of the currently available and potential future medications is an important part of this book, considering that most of our patients use at least one drug to control symptoms at varying stages of the disease. Co-medication is the focus of an entire chapter because we think that it is under-used. Other forms of non-invasive, frequently forgotten techniques are the basis of the next chapter, which reviews knowledge on bladder training, acupuncture, naturopathic and herbal remedies, magnetic stimulation, catheters, and tissue engineering. Three other important chapters cover the role of two neuromodulation modalities and botulinum toxin injections, approaches in which significant progress has been made over the last decade. It is important to note that these approaches can be employed differently, one before the other one, depending on physician experience and place of practice. Finally, the surgical approach, used frequently in neurogenic conditions, completes the treatment section of the book. The last part of the book addresses important considerations regarding special populations: older people and men with outlet obstruction. In conclusion, a synthesis chapter provides a practical clinical summary of the principal themes of the book.

The contributor selection process was exceedingly difficult, since we have so many highly competent colleagues and friends with expertise in OAB. We apologize to those who are not participating in this venture and congratulate all the authors for the high quality of their work and for their efforts in (almost) respecting the deadlines. We are proud of the end result of this collaboration and we believe that this book will be very useful for learners at all stages: medical students, residents, and established physicians. This book will be practical for other healthcare professionals, with first-hand involvement in treating the potentially debilitating symptoms of OAB. Additionally, members of the industry can gain a better understanding of the condition and an overview of what their peers can offer to treat OAB.

May this book provide inspiration to present and future medical professionals in this field!

Jacques Corcos MD

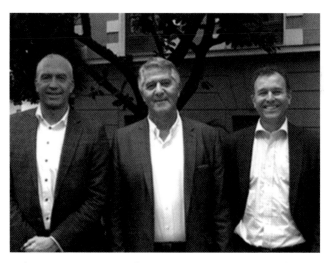

Left to right: Dr. Scott MacDiarmid, Dr. Jacques Corcos, and Dr. John Heesakkers

SECTION 1
Introduction

CHAPTER 1

Overactive bladder: terminology and problem spectrum

John Heesakkers

Department of Urology, Radboud University Medical Center, Nijmegen, The Netherlands

---

KEY POINTS

- The key symptom in the OAB syndrome is urgency, which can be interpreted in many different ways.
- Urgency is difficult to appreciate by patients and caregivers.
- Therefore incidence and prevalence data have to be looked at with caution.

It is a challenge to really appreciate the exact terminology introduced to describe the symptoms and suffering from overactive bladder complaints.

In the last part of the 20th century the term urge incontinence was used frequently to describe the situation in which there is a strong sensation to go to the toilet and void or lose urine and when someone is in the process of getting there in time. However there were also patients who complained of frequent voiding and the feeling of needing to void who were often not incontinent. The compelling sensation was particularly regarded as abnormal. In 1988 Paul Abrams called this sensation "urgency," defined as: a strong desire to void accompanied by fear of leakage or fear of pain (1988). [1] Although anyone could more or less understood which group of patients was meant, it was not easy to test this definition: not every patient had a fear of leakage or fear of pain. In 2002 this was further specified and explained as: the complaint of a sudden compelling desire to pass urine, which is difficult to defer. [2] Again, it was not easy to define what was sudden, compelling, *and* difficult to defer.

In 2002 the ICS defined overactive bladder complaints as: a medical condition referring to the symptom of urgency with or without urge incontinence, usually with frequency and nocturia. Other pathology like a urinary tract infection should be ruled out or treated. Urgency is the most important symptom here. It is a sensory sensation that makes you go to the toilet often (=frequency). If you have to do that at night it is called nocturia and if you do not get in time to the toilet it causes incontinence. It also means that urgency alone constitutes the OAB symptom syndrome. It is felt to be important to distinguish

---

Overactive Bladder: Practical Management, First Edition. Edited by Jacques Corcos, Scott MacDiarmid and John Heesakkers.
© 2015 John Wiley & Sons, Ltd. Published 2015 by John Wiley & Sons, Ltd.

urgency, which is regarded as pathological, from urge which is the normal, healthy strong sensation to go to the toilet. This is difficult to understand for non–native English speakers because the translation of urgency or urge to another language is very often exactly the same. However, many contributions have been made by key experts on OAB in the past in order to explain the difference and also its pathophysiological mechanism. Chris Chapple contributed in 2005 to the discussion with the following. "It is important to differentiate between *'urge'* which is a normal physiologic sensation, and *urgency* which we consider pathological. Central to this distinction is the debate over whether urgency is merely an extreme form of 'urge.' If this was a continuum, then normal people could experience urgency, but in the model we propose, urgency is always abnormal. "[3] Michel and Chapple postulated that urgency originates in pathology while urge does not. "The mechanisms of *urgency* differ from those involved in the symptom of *urge*, which occurs during a physiologic bladder filling (C-fibers supposed to convey *urgency* and A-delta-fibers supposed to convey *urge*)." [4] Jerry Blaivas noted that: "Urgency is comprised of at least two different sensations. One is an intensification of the normal urge to void and the other is a different sensation. The implications of this distinction are important insofar as they may have different etiologies and respond differently to treatment." [5]

So this all means that urge is a healthy sensation and urgency a not-healthy sensation, the latter based on pathology, the first on normal physiology. To attach frequency, nocturia, and incontinence to the driver of the syndrome had three consequences. The first was that to include and exclude patients in studies one had to find a translation of urgency into a workable definition. For frequency, for instance, this meant more than 8 times per 24 hours. The second was that the applied definition would influence the prevalence OAB. The third and most important consequence was that one had the feeling that a patient fitted into a pathological entity whereas the whole complex could also be a symptom without pathophysiological backing.

The late Norman Zinner addressed this point in an elegant debate with Paul Abrams in Neurourology and Urodynamics. He started by saying : "So OAB is urgency, with or without incontinence, usually with frequency and nocturia. This implies that incontinence, frequency and nocturia alone is not OAB. It also means that urgency without frequency, nocturia or incontinence, is OAB. So urgency alone is OAB, but what is it? We need descriptive terms like urgency to communicate, but not to make them medical terms and a 'syndrome' out of a constellation of unproven ambiguities." [6] Paul Abrams responded to that by saying that perhaps his relationship to the term "OAB" is rather like his relationship to the motor car: I deprecate its effect on the environment, but I am not about to give it up! [7] Zinner stated that the phrase OAB is misleading because it "makes it too easy for clinicians to feel they have made a diagnosis when they have not."[8]

So although there still is a debate about the existence, meaning, and pathophysiological backing of urgency and the OAB syndrome, every clinician dealing with a patient group that fits the definition knows what is meant by it.

The used definition, the translation in various languages, the validation process of questionnaires, and the interpretation of the respondents account for the number of people affected by OAB.

Studies from Milsom and Stewart et al. claimed that about 13–17% of the population suffer from OAB. [9, 10] This equates to about 49 million people in Europe; the prevalence increases with age. OAB is more present in women than in men. Others found other percentages. Wen et al. looked at prevalences in a Chinese population of more than 10 000 people. He found that OAB dry is present in 1.1% of the Chinese population and in 1.0% when one uses the OAB Symptom Score. OAB increases with age and more men than women suffer from it. [11]

OAB is also a chronic disease. Despite all the effort that is put in by caretakers, 88% of women that have OAB will still have it after 10 years. [12]

If the amount of bother is taken into account one must conclude that, as compared to the voiding phase and the post-micturition phase of the micturition cycle, the filling phase problems like OAB cause more bother. [13] OAB bother also compares well in comparison to other chronic diseases like diabetes mellitus or hypertension. [14]

Various reports have been published that look at the costs of the diagnosis and the treatment of overactive bladder complaints. Apart from that, the remnant costs after failed or not-100%-successful treatment of containment are also substantial. If the costs of disability for work are taken into account too, the total costs are very impressive. A study from Onukwugha et al. estimated the disease-specific total costs of OAB from the societal perspective and using an average costing method in the USA. [15]. This was done by analyzing a population-based survey, a claims data analysis, and the published literature. They applied the data in those community dwelling adults reporting the presence of urinary urgency or urgency urinary incontinence as "often" on a Likert scale. Based on the data they estimated the disease related cost at 25 billion dollars. If even the real cost were 25% of this figure one must conclude that OAB has a high impact on society, let alone on the individual patient.

References

1 Abrams P, Blaivas J G, Stanton SL, et al. The standardisation of terminology of lower urinary tract function. *Neurourol Urodyn*. 1988; **7**:403–426.

2 Abrams P, Cardozo L, Fall M, et al. The standardisation of terminology of lower urinary tract function. *Neurourol Urodyn*. 2002;**21**: 167–178.

3 Chapple CR, Artibani W, Cardozo LD, et al. The role of urinary urgency and its measurement in the overactive bladder symptom syndrome: current concepts and future prospects. *BJU Int*. 2005;**95**:335–340.

4 Michel MC, Chapple CR. Basic mechanisms of urgency: preclinical and clinical evidence. *Eur Urol*. 2009;**56**(2):298–307.

5 Blaivas JG, Panagopoulos G, Weiss JP, Somaroo C. Two types of urgency. *Neurol Urodyn*. 2009; **28**:188–190.

6 Zinner NR. OAB: Are we barking up the wrong tree?Neurourol Urodyn. 2011;**30**:1410–1411.

7 Abrams P. Response to OAB: Are we barking up the wrong tree? *Neurourol Urodyn*. 2011;**30**: 1409.

8 Zinner NR. Author's response to Paul Abram's response to OAB. *Neurourol Urodyn*. 2011;**30**: 1412–1414.

9 Milsom I, Abrams P, Cardozo L, et al. How widespread are the symptoms of an overactive bladder and how are they managed? A population-based prevalence study. *BJU Int*. 2001;**87**(9):760–766.

10 Milsom I, Stewart WF, Van Rooyen JB, et al. Prevalence and burden of overactive bladder

in the United States. *World J Urol.* 2003;**20**(6): 327–336.

11   Wen JG, Li JS, Wang ZM, The prevalence and risk factors of OAB in middle-aged and old people in China. *Neurourol Urodyn.* 2014; **33**(4):387–391.

12   Garnett S, Swithinbank L, Ellis-Jones J, Abrams P. The long-term natural history of overactive bladder symptoms due to idiopathic detrusor overactivity in women. *BJU Int.* 2009; **104**(7):948–953.

13   Coyne KS, Wein AJ, Tubaro A, et al: The burden of lower urinary tract symptoms *BJU Int* 2009;**103** (Suppl 3):4–11 (EpiLUTS).

14   Kobelt G, Kirchberger I, Malone-Lee J. Quality-of life aspects of the overactive bladder and the effect of treatment. *BJU Int.* 1999;**83**:583–590.

15   Onukwugha E, Zuckerman IH, McNally D, et al. The total economic burden of overactive bladder in the United States: a disease-specific approach. *Am J Manag Care.* 2009;**15**(4 Suppl): S90–97.

CHAPTER 2

Pathophysiology

Mathieu Boudes and Dirk De Ridder

Laboratory of Experimental Urology, Department of Development and Regeneration, KU Leuven, Leuven, Belgium

---

KEY POINTS

- Urinary incontinence caused by detrusor overactivity (DO) remains a major problem for many people with neurological disorders. According to the Standardization published by the International Continence Society, DO is an urodynamic observation characterized by involuntary detrusor contractions during the filling phase which may be spontaneous or provoked. [1]

- DO may also, whenever possible, be classified as neurogenic detrusor overactivity (NDO) when there is a relevant neurological condition, or idiopathic detrusor overactivity (IDO) when there is no defined cause. A variety of neurological diseases that affect brain structures and spinal pathways involved in the coordination of lower urinary tract function may cause NDO, including multiple sclerosis, spinal cord injury (SCI), meningomyelocele (MMC), stroke, cerebral palsy, and so on.

- Overactive bladder syndrome (OAB) is a symptom complex including urgency, with or without urge incontinence, but usually with frequency and nocturia. This symptom combination is suggestive of detrusor overactivity which can be demonstrated by urodynamics, but it can also be due to other forms of urethrovesical dysfunction.

Introduction

Urinary incontinence caused by detrusor overactivity (DO) remains a major problem for many people with neurological disorders. According to the Standardization published by the International Continence Society, DO is an urodynamic observation characterized by involuntary detrusor contractions during the filling phase which may be spontaneous or provoked. [1] DO may also, whenever possible, be classified as neurogenic detrusor overactivity (NDO) when there is a relevant neurological condition, or idiopathic detrusor overactivity (IDO) when there is no defined cause. A variety of neurological diseases that affect brain structures and spinal pathways involved in the coordination of lower urinary tract function may cause NDO, including multiple sclerosis, spinal cord injury (SCI), meningomyelocele (MMC), stroke, cerebral palsy, and so on. Overactive bladder syndrome (OAB) is a symptom

Overactive Bladder: Practical Management, First Edition. Edited by Jacques Corcos, Scott MacDiarmid and John Heesakkers.
© 2015 John Wiley & Sons, Ltd. Published 2015 by John Wiley & Sons, Ltd.

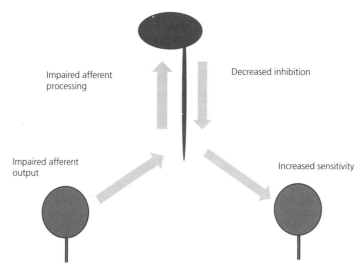

Figure 2.1 Changes in the innervation can lead to impairment of afferent and efferent signaling at different levels. Source: Adapted from Andersson 2004. [2] Reproduced with permission of Nature Publishing Group.

complex including urgency, with or without urge incontinence, but usually with frequency and nocturia. This symptom combination is suggestive of detrusor overactivity which can be demonstrated by urodynamics, but it can also be due to other forms of urethrovesical dysfunction.

Next to DO, sphincteric problems may complicate the clinical picture. Sphincter overactivity and underactivity can both occur. The coordination between bladder and sphincter can be lost, leading to bladder emptying disorders and increased intravesical pressures. Of all these problems DO with sphincter overactivity is probably the most important, since persistent high intravesical pressures may lead to vesico-ureteral reflux and subsequent renal damage.

The underlying mechanisms are complex and involve changes in afferent and efferent processing and also include histological changes in the bladder wall (Figure 2.1).

This chapter will give a short pragmatic overview of the current understanding of the pathophysiology of neurogenic bladder disorders and will give some information about animal models that are being used to study this condition.

The innervation of the bladder

The voluntary control over the bladder function requires complex peripheral and central innervation.

The central innervation
The brain
Different parts of the brain are important for the regulation of the micturition cycle. These centers include the pontine micturition center (also known as Barrington's nucleus), the cerebral cortex, the paraventricular nucleus (PVN), the medial preoptic area (MPOA) and periventricular nucleus

(PeriVN) of the hypothalamus, the periaqueductal gray (PAG), the locus coeruleus (LC) and subcoeruleus, the red nucleus (Red N.), the raphe nuclei, and the A5 noradrenergic cell group. [3]

During the storage phase, afferent input from the spinal cord will travel to the PAG. From there the information is sent to the hypothalamus and thalamus, the anterior cingulate cortex (ACC), the insula and the lateral prefrontal cortex (LPFC). The lateral prefrontal cortex relates to the medial prefrontal cortex (MPFC). At this site the decision to void or not to void is made. During the filling phase, the MPFC will inhibit the PAG and subsequently the PMC. At the initiation of the voiding phase, the MPFC will no longer inhibit the PAG and PMC and voiding will occur through

relaxation of the urethral sphincter and contraction of the detrusor (Figure 2.2) The PMC will send motoric output signals to the sacral nuclei. During voiding afferent input is continuously sent to the PAG until the bladder is empty. [4]

The spinal cord

The regulation of micturition requires connections between the brain and sympathetic, parasympathetic, and somatic systems in the spinal cord. Parasympathetic and sympathetic neurons are located in the intermediate gray matter of the spinal cord sacral and lumbar segments. Parasympathetic neurons send dendrites into the dorsal commissure and into the lateral funiculus and lateral dorsal horn of the spinal cord and exhibit an extensive

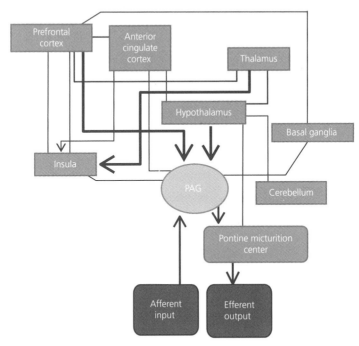

Figure 2.2 The different parts of the brain that play a part in the control of the filling and emptying phase of the bladder cycle. Source: Adapted from Fowler 2008. [4] Reproduced with permission of Nature Publishing Group.

axon collateral system that is distributed bilaterally in the cord. A similar axon collateral system has not been identified in sympathetic preganglionic neurons. The somatic motor neurons that innervate the external urethral sphincter are located in the ventral horn (lamina IX) in Onuf's nucleus, have a similar arrangement of transverse dendrites, and have an extensive system of longitudinal dendrites that travel within Onuf's nucleus.

Interneurons in the lumbosacral spinal cord are located in the dorsal commissure, the superficial dorsal horn, and the parasympathetic nucleus. Some of these interneurons send long projections to the brain, whereas others make local connections in the spinal cord and participate in segmental spinal reflexes.

Afferent nerves from the bladder project to regions of the spinal cord that contain interneurons and parasympathetic dendrites. Pudendal afferent pathways from the urethra and the urethral sphincter exhibit a similar pattern of termination. The overlap between bladder and urethral afferents in the lateral dorsal horn and the dorsal commissure indicates that these regions are probably important sites of viscerosomatic integration that might be involved in coordinating bladder and sphincter activity. [5]

The peripheral innervation

Innervation of the LUT arises from three sets of nerves: (i) pelvic, (ii) hypogastric, and (iii) pudendal. The three nerves convey both motor and sensory input onto the LUT. Whereas the pelvic nerve provides an excitatory input to the bladder, the hypogastric nerve provides inhibitory input to the bladder and excitatory input to the bladder outlet. The pudendal nerve innervates the striated muscle of the sphincter and the pelvic floor.

The **sympathetic** innervation originates in the thoracolumbar of the spinal cord. Sympathetic postganglionic nerves release noradrenaline, which by activating β3-adrenergic receptors on the detrusor muscle is known to relax the bladder and to contract the urethra and the bladder neck with the activation of α-adrenergic receptors. It is worth noting that the last drug developed to relieve patients from OAB specifically targets β3-adrenergic receptors. [6]

The **parasympathetic** and somatic nerves arise from the sacral segments of the spinal cords and convey both efferent and afferent information. Excitation of parasympathetic efferents causes release of acetylcholine and non-adrenergic, noncholinergic (NANC) neurotransmitters. The acetylcholine, which is generally seen as the main neurotransmitter in the voiding cycle, and of ATP at the nerve endings. [7] These transmitters act on muscarinic (mainly mAChR2 and mAChR3) and purinergic (mainly P2X1) receptors, respectively, to cause detrusor smooth muscle contraction. [8, 9] The relative importance of both signaling molecules is highly dependent on the species, which means that data from animal research must be interpreted with care when translated to human pathology. [10] In rats, ATP plays a substantial role in the initiation of the voiding contraction, whereas its role seems to be much less important in humans. [10, 11] Little is known about the effect of the NANC transmitters release in bladder function. They have been reported to modulate urothelium and lamina propria contractility properties in pigs. [12] Moreover, in diabetic and spinal cord injury rats [13, 14], the contraction induced by NANC is modified compared to controls animals. Interestingly, those changes in bladder function may involve additional, P2X-receptor independent mechanisms. [13] However, to date, there is no clear consensus on the molecules hidden behind the NANC.

Somatic cholinergic motor nerves that supply the striated external urethral sphincter arise in S2–S4 motor neurons in Onuf's nucleus and travel through the pudendal nerves. At the same spinal level another (more medial) motor nucleus innervates the pelvic floor muscles.

Sensory information from the bladder travels through the pelvic and hypogastric nerves, whereas sensory input from the bladder neck and the urethra is carried in the pudendal and hypogastric nerves. The afferent nerves consist of myelinated (Aδ) and unmyelinated (C) axons. The thin, myelinated Aδ-fibres convey information about bladder filling. The C-fibers are insensitive to bladder filling under physiological conditions (they are therefore termed "silent" C-fibers) and respond primarily to noxious stimuli such as chemical irritation or cooling. The cell bodies of Aδ-fibers and C-fibers are located in the dorsal root ganglia (DRG) at the level of S2–S4 and T11–L2 spinal segments. A dense nexus of sensory nerves has been identified in the suburothelial layer of the urinary bladder in both humans and animals, with some terminal fibers projecting into the urothelium. This suburothelial plexus is particularly prominent at the bladder neck but is relatively sparse at the dome of the bladder and is thought to be critical in the sensory function of the urothelium.

Alteration at any level of the neuronal control of micturition could theoretically induce NDO. Indeed, a modified afferent activity, decreased capacity of the CNS to process afferent information, decreased suprapontine inhibition, or increased sensitivity to contraction-mediated transmitters in the bladder might be involved in NDO genesis. [2, 15]

The genesis of the NDO: three hypothesis

Three main hypotheses have been proposed to explain the pathophysiological basis of DO: neurogenic, [15] myogenic, [16] and integrative. [17]

The neurogenic hypothesis

The neurogenic hypothesis arises from the observation that plasticity occurs in neuronal control of the bladder after trauma. Various changes in peripheral and central neural pathways could lead to bladder overactivity. These include (i) a reduction in peripheral of central inhibition; (ii) an enhancement of excitatory transmission in the micturition reflex pathway; (iii) increased primary afferent input from the bladder; and (iv) emergence of bladder reflexes that are resistant to central inhibition. Therefore, the damage to central inhibition, or sensitization of peripheral afferent terminals, in the bladder wall can unmask primitive voiding reflexes that trigger bladder overactivity.

The myogenic hypothesis

In NDO animal models and patients, the detrusor ultrastructure is modified, which may facilitate the propagation of electrical coupling between muscle cells, leading to increased excitability. [18] The myogenic hypothesis suggests that the common feature underlying detrusor overactivity in animals and humans is a change in the properties of smooth muscle that allows local activity to spread throughout the bladder wall. The hypothesis stipulates that even though there is a close relationship between end organs and their innervations, and alteration in one is likely to result in alterations in the other, the myogenic basis of bladder overactivity does not preclude the involvement of alterations in the neuronal pathways of the micturition reflex.

The integrative hypothesis

The integrative hypothesis proposes that interstitial cells, urothelium, and peripheral nerves contribute to normal generation of micromotions (localized spontaneous activity) of the bladder wall, leading to low pressure sensing of the filling state. In patients or animal models, the micromotions are enhanced; with a wider propagation of spontaneous activity and sending of exaggerated sensory information, giving rise to urgency. [19–22]

The link to the clinic

Depending on the localization and extension of the neurological lesion of pathology the clinical picture can change. Usually these pathologies are classified as being suprapontine, suprasacral-infrapontine, or infrasacral. This classification relates to the important relay centers that are involved in the neural control of bladder, sphincter, and pelvic floor (brain centers controlling the PMC, the spinal cord with the parasympathetic nuclei and Onuf's nucleus, and the peripheral innervation).

Knowledge about the exact nature and localization of the neurological problem will allow the clinician to predict the urological phenotype to some degree (Figure 2.3).

Suprapontine lesions

The processing of afferent and efferent information may become problematic. Generally speaking the central inhibition of the micturition reflex during the filling phase will become less efficient. Urgency with or without DO can occur. During the

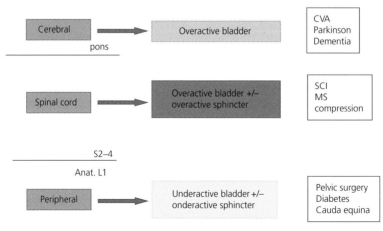

Figure 2.3 Depending on the location of the neurological lesion, several types of bladder and sphincter behavior can be expected.

voiding phase few or no abnormalities are seen, since the spinal mechanisms are still intact, provided that the PMC can be activated. Examples are Parkinson's disease, early multiple sclerosis, traumatic brain injury, brain tumors, cerebrovascular accidents, and so on.

Suprasacral-infrapontine lesions

Afferent information (especially from Aδ fibers) can no longer travel through the spinal tracts and efferent signals traveling down may not reach the sacral centers. C-fiber dependent sacral reflexes will become apparent, leading to inappropriate detrusor contractions and poor coordination between the bladder outlet and the detrusor. High intravesical pressures can arise as a consequence of inappropriate detrusor contractions against a closed sphincter. This phenomenon is called "detrusor-sphincter dyssynergia." These high intravesical pressures can lead to vesico-ureteral reflux with subsequent renal insufficiency. Examples are spinal cord injury, multiple sclerosis, spinal compression, transverse myelitis, and so on.

Peripheral lesions

When the innervation (afferent and efferent) between the end-organs and the spinal cord is disrupted, the bladder and sphincter become more or less denervated. Depending on the extent and nature of the lesions this can lead to an underactive bladder with severely impaired or absent bladder sensations. Clinically this will present with overflow incontinence, retention, and eventually sphincter weakness. This can be seen in a variety of conditions such as cauda equina syndromes, surgical removal of the pelvic plexus during cancer surgery for anorectal or cervical malignancies, and so on.

The neurological pathologies responsible for the development of the neurogenic bladder

Animal models

As human studies and research using human material are inherently limited because of the implications associated with such investigations, our understanding of the lower urinary tract function is incomplete. Much of our knowledge of bladder function has come from *in vitro* but it is difficult to extrapolate the conclusions of these types of studies. Indeed, ideally, animal models should reproduce all the facets of the human condition, but it is inconceivable that any single animal model will replicate all the aspects of a human condition which are by definition different from patient to patient, plus human bladder physiology differs from animals. For instance, the nerve-mediated contractions of rodent bladders are mediated by cholinergic and purinergic neurotransmitters whilst human bladder contraction is almost solely controlled by acetylcholine – although alternative contraction mechanisms (purinergic, non-cholinergic non adrenergic, NANC) appear in pathological states.

Therefore, animal models must be viewed as tools and not as a mirror to understand pathological mechanisms within the limit of the models.

Spinal cord transection/injury

The spinal cord injury model is the most used animal research model to study NDO. The degree of dysfunction is related to the disease process itself, the area of the spinal cord injured, and the severity of the neurological impairment. Immediately after the injury, a spinal shock phase is followed by hyperreflexia of the striated muscle, the sphincter, and the bladder, leading to a huge increase in bladder pressure that might affect bladder tissue cyto-architecture.

Plasticity of the afferent bladder neurons

Following that phase, it is commonly believed that the overactive bladder phenotype is underlined by the appearance of a C-fiber-mediated micturition reflex due to reorganization of synaptic connections in the spinal cord concomitantly with the plasticity of the dorsal root ganglion neurons. Chronic SCI is accompanied by the hypertrophy of bladder afferent neurons [23] and an up-regulation of the calcitonin gene-related peptide (CGRP) [24, 25] and pituitary adenylaceclase-activating polypeptide (PACAP) content that is likely to facilitate bladder reflex contractions and contribute to bladder dysfunction. [26, 27] Moreover, SCI also results in alteration in the electrophysiological properties of bladder-innervating sensory neurons. On the one hand, sodium current expression shifts from high-threshold tetrodotoxin (TTX)-resistant to low-threshold TTX sensitive. On the other hand, A-type potassium currents are suppressed in SCI rats. [28–30] Peptidergic and non-peptidergic sensory neuron connectivity is also altered in chronic SCI as sprouting of the central roots occurs. All together, the afferent neurons innervating the bladder are more likely to trigger action potentials with smaller stimuli. [31]

Plasticity of the spinal cord

SCI induces central reorganization with the formation of new synapses and alteration to preexisting ones. [32] The balance between excitatory and inhibitory transmission in the bladder control pathway might be altered. Indeed, the glutamatergic transmission is modified [33] with a decreased GABA A receptor activation. [34] These neurochemical alterations may be involved in bladder dysfunction.

Parkinson animal models

Parkinson disease is one of the most common neurological causes of NDO and symptoms become more severe as the disease progresses and affect up to 90% of patients. [35] Parkinsonism can be induced in animals by administering a neurotoxin that induces DO. [36] This model has led us to understand the involvement of central dopaminergic pathways that have both excitatory and inhibitory effects on rat bladder function. Activation of the D1-like receptor might tonically inhibit the micturition reflex while D2-like receptors facilitate it. [28]

Experimental auto-immune encephalomyelitis model

The vast majority of patients with multiple sclerosis (MS) develop bladder control and NDO often refractory to antimuscarinics. Moreover, 60% of MS patients show detrusor–sphincter dyssynergia, an abnormality characterized by obstruction of urinary outflow as a result of discoordinated contraction of the urethral sphincter muscle and the bladder detrusor muscle. Myelin basic protein (MBP) can be used as an antigen for inducing experimental allergic encephalomyelitis (EAE) in rodents and has widely been used as a model for MS. It was shown that bladder walls undergo morphological changes. Indeed, a significant increase in the bladder-weight-to-body-weight ratio and marked bladder remodeling with increased luminal area and tissue hypertrophy. Despite increased amounts of all tissue components (urothelium, smooth muscle, and connective tissue), the ratio of connective tissue to muscle increased significantly in EAE mice compared with control mice [37] (Figure 2.4).

Bladder dysfunction in EAE rats is transient, reversible, and leads to more frequent voiding events. Interestingly, the functional alterations occur concomitantly with hind limb paralysis and inflammatory changes in the spinal cord [38] and the

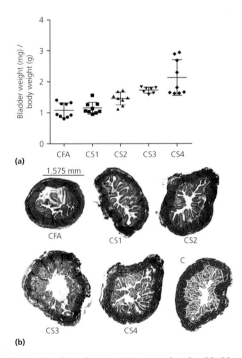

(a)

(b)

Figure 2.4 Clinical score (CS) is correlated to bladder tissue remodeling in EAE mice. (a) The bladder-weight-to-body-weight ratio increase correlates with increasing clinical score (CS) in EAE mice compared to CFA-immunized mice. (b) Histological examination showed bladder hypertrophy and lumen dilation in the EAE mice relative to the CFA control mice, corresponding with increasing CS. (For color detail, please see color plate section).

bladder remodeling corresponds to EAE severity, suggesting that at least part of the urinary symptoms arise from local changes in the bladder. [39]

Multiple system atrophy

Multiple system atrophy (MSA) is a sporadic adult-onset neurodegenerative disorder that features motor impairment and autonomic dysfunction. [40] Non-motor features (i.e., urogenital dysfunction) are often premonitory of MSA onset. [41] Retrospective data analyses indicate that urological symptoms emerge early and may precede the neurological presentation by several years in the majority of MSA patients. [42]

Transgenic mice with targeted overexpression of human αSyn (hαSyn) in oligodendroglia have been developed to reproduce GCIs and to study related mechanisms of neurodegeneration relevant to the human disease. [43] Several recent neuropathological findings in transgenic mice with oligodendroglial overexpression of hαSyn under the proteolipid protein (PLP) promoter, [44, 45] including progressive neurodegeneration of the substantia nigra pars compacta (SNc), locus coeruleus, and Onuf's nucleus suggest possible urinary dysfunction in the MSA model similar to that in human MSA. [46] Indeed, in those mice, urodynamic analysis revealed a less efficient and unstable bladder with increased voiding contraction amplitude, higher frequency of non-voiding contractions, and increased post-void residual volume. MSA mice bladder walls showed early detrusor hypertrophy and age-related urothelium hypertrophy. All together, these results strongly suggest that this mice model could be used in preclinical studies. [47]

Histological changes

Next to the reorganization of the innervation, local changes in the bladder wall can occur as a consequence of neurological diseases. The detrusor, lamina propria, and urothelium will undergo changes that might contribute to altered generation of afferent signals and abnormal responses to efferent output.

The detrusor

At the ultrastructural level, a common feature seen in NDO bladders from patients and animal models is the presence of protrusion junctions and ultraclose abutments between the smooth muscle cells, features occurring only rarely in normal tissue. [48]

The urothelium

The urothelium is the epithelial lining of the urinary tract between the renal pelvis and the urinary bladder. Three cells layers compose the urothelium: a basal cell layer attached to the basement layer, an intermediate layer, and apically a layer composed of large cells named "umbrella cells." Those cells are connected with tight junctions that create a physical barrier towards water, solutes, and urea. Historically, the urothelium has been viewed primarily as a barrier; it is now recognized to be a structure that reacts to chemical and physical stimuli by releasing signaling molecules. Accumulative evidences have shown that urothelium expresses many different receptors involved in noci- and mechanoception, such as neurotrophin receptor (TrkA and p75), norepinephrine (α and β), cytokines, purine receptor (P2Xs and P2Ys), transient receptor channels (i.e., TRPV4).

The urothelium is known to reciprocally communicate with afferent nerves running below and within it and some authors have hypothesized that SCI would impact the urothelial cell barrier function and its morphology unless the exact contribution of the urothelium on the development of NDO is unknown. [49] Indeed, although a lot of studies have focused on alterations in the detrusor muscle and its innervation after SCI, much less is understood about changes in the urothelium morphology and its function. Apodaca et al. described that SCI is accompanied by disruption of the urothelium with a loss of umbrella cells that induced a decrease of the transepithelial resistance and permeability to water and urea. The observed alterations are most likely due to urinary retention and overdistension of the urothelium as when the spinal reflex is recovered, between two and three weeks following the injury, the barrier function was recovered – although the apical cells remained smaller. Prior to SCI, treatment of the animals with hexamethonium (a ganglionic blocker) and capsaicin ameliorated the SCI-induced decreased of the transepithelial resistance, strongly suggesting an intimate relation between the urothelium and the nervous system. [48]

The lamina propria

The lamina propria stands between the urothelium and the detrusor and contains the interstitial cells. Because of their particular organization just underneath the urothelium, the interstitial cells have attracted the interest of many investigators because they could embody a structural and functional link between urothelial cells and sensory nerves and/or between urothelial cells and detrusor smooth muscle cells. The guinea-pig interstitial cells have spontaneous and neurogenic calcium oscillations suggesting their functional innervation and indicating that bladder ICC sub-populations are under direct control of the complex innervation that governs normal bladder function. [50]

Moreover, these cells might be involved in the pathophysiology of functional bladder disorders, where local signaling processes are thought to play important roles. In MS patients, the ultrastructural and immunohistochemical phenotype of interstitial cells show modest changes. In NDO bladders the interstitial cells express fewer actin filaments together with a decreased expression of alpha smooth muscle actin and also fewer caveolae. These changes feature a trend toward a fibroblast phenotype with a different topographical organization of those cells. Furthermore, the interstitial cells area is significantly broadened in NDO bladders with a remarkable less-dense intercellular matrix and a broadened space between cell layers. In NDO bladders, frequent close apposition of lymphocytes and ULP ICLC was found. [51, 52] In SCI rats, the lamina propria and detrusor interstitial cells are ultrastructurally damaged post-SCI with retracted/lost cell processes and were adjacent to areas of cellular debris and neuronal degradation [53] (Figure 2.5).

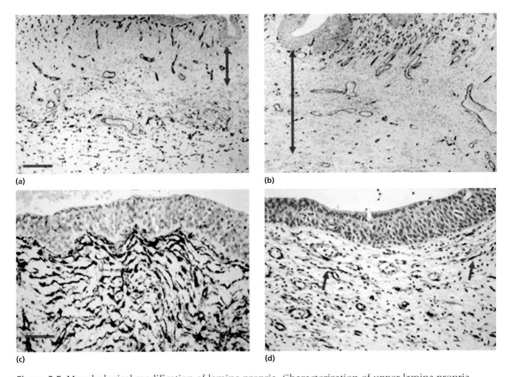

(a)

(b)

(c)

(d)

Figure 2.5 Morphological modification of lamina propria. Characterization of upper lamina propria interstitial cells in bladders from control (a) and (c) and MS patients (b) and (d) with CD34 (a) and (b) and SMA (c) and (d). Scale bar: 50 μm. Source: Adapted from Gevaert 2011 [52]. Reproduced with permission of John Wiley & Sons Ltd. (For color detail, please see color plate section).

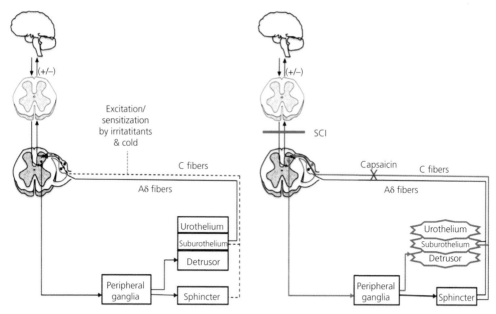

Figure 2.6 The C-fiber reflex. Following spinal cord injury, Aδ-fibers are overruled by C-fibers after a few days or weeks. The activation of these C-fibers can lead to unvoluntary detrusor contractions. Next to these changes in afferent innervation the bladder wall itself also undergoes changes.

The functional implications of these observations remain to be determined, but it is likely that these are some of the many elements contributing to altered bladder function in MS patients. [54]

The neuronal structure

Studies carried out in animal models have demonstrated that procedures such as spinal section of urethral obstruction lead to an increase in size of both the afferent neurons in the dorsal root ganglia [55] and the efferent neurons in the pelvic plexus. [56, 57]

have different impact than progressive diseases such as multiple sclerosis or Parkinson's disease.

Changes can occur in the central mechanisms (brain and spinal cord), but the end organs will also undergo changes. Reorganizing nerves (e.g., the appearance of the C-fiber reflex, Figure 2.6), receptor plasticity, and even changes in the detrusor and urothelium will lead to a complex clinical picture. At this moment few animal models can be used to study these changes in detail. Much more research will be needed to elucidate these complex changes.

Conclusions

Neurological diseases can have a devastating effect on the control of bladder, urethral sphincter, pelvic floor musculature, and bowel. Acute neurological trauma, such as spinal cord or brain injury, will

References

1 Abrams P, Cardozo L, Fall M, et al. The standardisation of terminology of lower urinary tract function: report from the Standardisation Subcommittee of the International Continence Society. *Neurourol Urodyn.* 2002;**21**(2):167–178.

2 Andersson KE. Mechanisms of disease: central nervous system involvement in overactive bladder syndrome. *Nat Clin Pract Urol.* 2004;**1**(2): 103–108.

3 Drake MJ, Fowler CJ, Griffiths D, et al. Neural control of the lower urinary and gastrointestinal tracts: supraspinal CNS mechanisms. *Neurourol Urodyn.* 2010;**29**(1):119–127.

4 Fowler CJ, Griffiths D, de Groat WC. The neural control of micturition. *Nat Rev Neurosci.* 2008;**9**(6):453–466.

5 Birder L, Chai T, Griffiths D, et al. Neural control. In: ICUD-EAU (ed) *Incontinence.* 5th Edition edn: ICUD-EAU; 2013. pp. 179–261.

6 Andersson KE. β3-Receptor agonists for overactive bladder – new frontier or more of the same? *Curr Urol Rep.* 2013;**14**(5):435–441.

7 Kasakov L, Burnstock G. The use of the slowly degradable analog, alpha, beta-methylene ATP, to produce desensitisation of the P2-purinoceptor: effect on non-adrenergic, non-cholinergic responses of the guinea-pig urinary bladder. *Eur J Pharmacol.* 1982;**86**(2):291–294.

8 Lee HY, Bardini M, Burnstock G. Distribution of P2X receptors in the urinary bladder and the ureter of the rat. *J Urol.* 2000;**163**(6):2002–2007.

9 Theobald RJ. Purinergic and cholinergic components of bladder contractility and flow. *Life Sci.* 1995;**56**(6):445–454.

10 Sibley GN. A comparison of spontaneous and nerve-mediated activity in bladder muscle from man, pig and rabbit. *J Physiol.* 1984;**354**:431–443.

11 Andersson KE, Soler R, Füllhase C. Rodent models for urodynamic investigation. *Neurourol Urodyn.* 2011;**30**(5):636–646.

12 Moro C, Chess-Williams R. Non-adrenergic, non-cholinergic, non-purinergic contractions of the urothelium/lamina propria of the pig bladder. *Auton Autacoid Pharmacol.* 2012;**32**(3 Pt 4):53–59.

13 Lai HH, Munoz A, Smith CP, et al. Plasticity of non-adrenergic non-cholinergic bladder contractions in rats after chronic spinal cord injury. *Brain Res Bull.* 2011;**86**(1-2):91–96.

14 Munoz A, Boone TB, Smith CP, Somogyi GT. Diabetic plasticity of non-adrenergic non-cholinergic and P2X-mediated rat bladder contractions. *Brain Res Bull.* 2013;**95**:40–45.

15 de Groat WC. A neurologic basis for the overactive bladder. *Urology.* 1997;**50**(6A Suppl):36–52; discussion 3–6.

16 Brading AF. A myogenic basis for the overactive bladder. *Urology.* 1997;**50**(6A Suppl):57–67; discussion 8–73.

17 Drake MJ, Mills IW, Gillespie JI. Model of peripheral autonomous modules and a myovesical plexus in normal and overactive bladder function. *Lancet.* 2001;**358**(9279): 401–403.

18 Haferkamp A, Dörsam J, Elbadawi A. Ultrastructural diagnosis of neuropathic detrusor overactivity: validation of a common myogenic mechanism. *Adv Exp Med Biol.* 2003; **539**(Pt A):281–291.

19 Drake MJ, Harvey IJ, Gillespie JI. Autonomous activity in the isolated guinea pig bladder. *Exp Physiol.* 2003;**88**(1):19–30.

20 Drake MJ, Hedlund P, Harvey IJ, et al. Partial outlet obstruction enhances modular autonomous activity in the isolated rat bladder. *J Urol.* 2003;**170**(1):276–279.

21 Drake MJ, Harvey IJ, Gillespie JI, Van Duyl WA. Localized contractions in the normal human bladder and in urinary urgency. *BJU Int.* 2005;**95**(7):1002–1005.

22 Coolsaet BL, Van Duyl WA, Van Os-Bossagh P, De Bakker HV. New concepts in relation to urge and detrusor activity. *Neurourol Urodyn.* 1993;**12**(5):463–471.

23 Kruse MN, Bray LA, de Groat WC. Influence of spinal cord injury on the morphology of bladder afferent and efferent neurons. *J Auton Nerv Syst.* 1995;**54**(3):215–224.

24 Zinck ND, Rafuse VF, Downie JW. Sprouting of CGRP primary afferents in lumbosacral spinal cord precedes emergence of bladder activity after spinal injury. *Exp Neurol.* 2007;**204**(2):777–790.

25 Ackery AD, Norenberg MD, Krassioukov A. Calcitonin gene-related peptide immunoreactivity in chronic human spinal cord injury. *Spinal Cord.* 2007;**45**(10):678–686.

26 Zvarova K, Dunleavy JD, Vizzard MA. Changes in pituitary adenylate cyclase activating polypeptide expression in urinary bladder pathways after spinal cord injury. *Exp Neurol.* 2005;**192**(1):46–59.

27 Ishizuka O, Alm P, Larsson B, Mattiasson A, Andersson KE. Facilitatory effect of pituitary adenylate cyclase activating polypeptide on micturition in normal, conscious rats. *Neuroscience.* 1995;**66**(4):1009–1014.

28 Seki S, Igawa Y, Kaidoh K, Ishizuka O, et al. Role of dopamine D1 and D2 receptors in the micturition reflex in conscious rats. *Neurourol Urodyn.* 2001;**20**(1):105–113.

29 Yoshimura N, de Groat WC. Plasticity of Na+channels in afferent neurones innervating rat urinary bladder following spinal cord injury. *J Physiol.* 1997;**503** (Pt 2):269–276.

30 Yoshimura N, White G, Weight FF, de Groat WC. Different types of Na+and A-type K+currents in dorsal root ganglion neurones innervating the rat urinary bladder. *J Physiol.* 1996;**494** (Pt 1):1–16.

31 Cruz CD, Cruz F. Spinal cord injury and bladder dysfunction: new ideas about an old problem. *Scientific World Journal.* 2011;**11**:214–234.

32 de Groat WC, Kawatani M, Hisamitsu T, et al. Mechanisms underlying the recovery of urinary bladder function following spinal cord injury. *J Auton Nerv Syst.* 1990;**30** Suppl:S71–7.

33 Pikov V, Wrathall JR. Altered glutamate receptor function during recovery of bladder detrusor-external urethral sphincter coordination in a rat model of spinal cord injury. *J Pharmacol Exp Ther.* 2002;**300** (2):421–427.

34 Miyazato M, Sasatomi K, Hiragata S, et al. Suppression of detrusor-sphincter dysynergia by GABA-receptor activation in the lumbosacral spinal cord in spinal cord-injured rats. *Am J Physiol Regul Integr Comp Physiol.* 2008;**295**(1):R336–342.

35 Fowler CJ. Urinary disorders in Parkinson's disease and multiple system atrophy. *Funct Neurol.* 2001;**16**(3):277–282.

36 Burns PA, Pranikoff K, Nochajski TH, et al. A comparison of effectiveness of biofeedback and pelvic muscle exercise treatment of stress incontinence in older community-dwelling women. *J Gerontol.* 1993;**48**(4):M167–74.

37 Altuntas CZ, Daneshgari F, Izgi K, et al. Connective tissue and its growth factor CTGF distinguish the morphometric and molecular remodeling of the bladder in a model of neurogenic bladder. *Am J Physiol Renal Physiol.* 2012;**303**(9):F1363–1369.

38 Mizusawa H, Igawa Y, Nishizawa O, et al. A rat model for investigation of bladder dysfunction associated with demyelinating disease resembling multiple sclerosis. *Neurourol Urodyn.* 2000;**19**(6):689–699.

39 Altuntas CZ, Daneshgari F, Liu G, et al. Bladder dysfunction in mice with experimental auto-immune encephalomyelitis. *J Neuroimmunol.* 2008;**203**(1):58–63.

40 Stefanova N, Bücke P, Duerr S, Wenning GK. Multiple system atrophy: an update. *Lancet Neurol.* 2009;**8**(12):1172–1178.

41 Jecmenica-Lukic M, Poewe W, Tolosa E, Wenning GK. Premotor signs and symptoms of multiple system atrophy. *Lancet Neurol.* 2012;**11**(4):361–368.

42 Kirchhof K, Apostolidis AN, Mathias CJ, Fowler CJ. Erectile and urinary dysfunction may be the presenting features in patients with multiple system atrophy: a retrospective study. *Int J Impot Res.* 2003;**15**(4):293–298.

43 Stefanova N, Tison F, Reindl M, et al. Animal models of multiple system atrophy. *Trends Neurosci.* 2005;**28**(9):501–506.

44 Stemberger S, Poewe W, Wenning GK, Stefanova N. Targeted overexpression of human alpha-synuclein in oligodendroglia induces lesions linked to MSA-like progressive autonomic failure. *Exp Neurol.* 2010;**224**(2):459–464.

45 Stefanova N, Reindl M, Neumann M, et al. Oxidative stress in transgenic mice with oligo-dendroglial alpha-synuclein overexpression replicates the characteristic neuropathology of multiple system atrophy. *Am J Pathol.* 2005; **166**(3):869–876.

46 Winge K, Fowler CJ. Bladder dysfunction in Parkinsonism: mechanisms, prevalence, symptoms, and management. *Mov Disord.* 2006; **21**(6):737–745.

47 Boudes M, Uvin P, Pinto S, et al. Bladder dysfunction in a transgenic mouse model of multiple system atrophy. *Mov Disord.* 2013;**28**(3):347–355.

48 Birder L, Andersson KE. Urothelial signaling. *Physiol Rev.* 2013;**93**(2):653–680.

49 Birder LA. Role of the urothelium in urinary bladder dysfunction following spinal cord injury. *Prog Brain Res.* 2006;**152**:135–146.

50 Gray SM, McGeown JG, McMurray G, McCloskey KD. Functional innervation of Guinea-pig bladder interstitial cells of cajal subtypes: neurogenic stimulation evokes in situ calcium transients. *PLoS One.* 2013;**8**(1):e53423.

51 Gevaert T, Owsianik G, Hutchings G, et al. The loss and progressive recovery of voiding after spinal cord interruption in rats is associated with simultaneous changes in autonomous contractile bladder activity. *Eur Urol.* 2009;**56**(1):168–176.

52 Gevaert T, De Vos R, Everaerts W, et al. Characterization of upper lamina propria interstitial cells in bladders from patients with neurogenic detrusor overactivity and bladder pain syndrome. *J Cell Mol Med.* 2011;**15**(12):2586–2593.

53 Johnston L, Cunningham RM, Young JS, et al. Altered distribution of interstitial cells and innervation in the rat urinary bladder following spinal cord injury. *J Cell Mol Med.* 2012;**16**(7):1533–1543.

54 Ciancio SJ, Mutchnik SE, Rivera VM, Boone TB. Urodynamic pattern changes in multiple sclerosis. *Urology.* 2001;**57**(2):239–245.

55 Steers WD, Ciambotti J, Etzel B, et al. Alterations in afferent pathways from the urinary bladder of the rat in response to partial urethral obstruction. *J Comp Neurol.* 1991;**310**(3):401–410.

56 Steers WD, Ciambotti J, Erdman S, de Groat WC. Morphological plasticity in efferent pathways to the urinary bladder of the rat following urethral obstruction. *J Neurosci.* 1990;**10**(6):1943–1951.

57 Gabella G, Berggren T, Uvelius B. Hypertrophy and reversal of hypertrophy in rat pelvic ganglion neurons. *J Neurocytol.* 1992;**21**(9):649–662.

SECTION 2
Evaluation

CHAPTER 3

Timing for evaluation

Jack C. Hou and Philippe E. Zimmern

UT Southwestern Medical Center, Dallas, TX, USA

KEY POINTS

- Many OAB patients remain untreated despite the fact that OAB symptoms can significantly improve in the hands of qualified physicians.
- Successful treatment of OAB depends on a detailed evaluation to confirm the diagnosis and on vigilant follow-up.
- Recognizing patients who could benefit from a specialist evaluation is key to avoid delay in management.
- Patients and their physicians need to set defined goals with realistic expectations leaning more towards improvement in quality of life than complete OAB symptom resolution.

Overactive bladder (OAB) is a common problem with a detrimental effect on quality of life. The overall prevalence of overactive bladder symptoms in individuals aged over 40 years has been estimated at 10.7–17.4%. [1–3] Despite this prevalence rate and the significant impact on quality of life, OAB is widely underdiagnosed, with fewer than 50% of those affected receiving medical attention. [4] The perception that the problem is a natural consequence of aging, embarrassment, and fear of surgery are all common reasons reported by older adults for not seeking professional help. Although geriatricians are familiar with the condition, not all primary care physicians have received the same formal training to provide basic evaluation and management. The focus of this chapter is to describe the timing of evaluation and indications for specialist referral.

As the prevalence of overactive bladder symptoms increases with advancing age, physicians can expect to be faced with patients with OAB symptoms more frequently than in the past. Family practice physicians and geriatricians are often the first to encounter patients with OAB symptomatology. Recent data indicates a dynamic progression for OAB and urinary incontinence, with remission in some but mostly persistence and gradual increase in symptom severity over time. [5] Therefore, the physician should be attentive to the patient's OAB complaint as it will not only remain but likely worsen over time. There is a body of literature suggesting that an effective basic evaluation of OAB patients can be provided by primary care physicians. [6, 7] Primary care physicians, geriatricians, and family doctors can recognize, evaluate, and treat OAB symptoms and provide individualized therapy to patients. These patients can be living on their own or in assisted-care, residential, or long-term care facilities. Prompt evaluation for OAB symptoms should be available with treatment goals to improve quality of life. Furthermore, OAB patients undergoing treatment should have realistic expectations set at the start of therapy to maximize adherence to therapy. An algorithm for primary care physicians and geriatricians has been developed to facilitate appropriate and effective work-up of patients with urinary symptoms. [7, 8] It is imperative that primary care providers be trained to assess and evaluate OAB patients and to safely exclude other causes of lower urinary tract symptoms. For example, it is imperative that reversible causes of OAB be addressed, including urinary tract infections, stool impaction, and even delirium. [9] Furthermore, chronic retention leading to frequency, urgency, and sometimes overflow incontinence can be masked and attributed to OAB if a cursory abdominal examination misses a distended bladder or post-void residual is not checked. More concerning even would be the lack of recognition of carcinoma *in situ* of the bladder which may present with irritative symptoms and can go unrecognized for a while until a urine cytology is requested.

Once OAB diagnosis is confirmed, conservative treatment options such as lifestyle changes and pelvic floor exercises should be considered, especially in elderly patients if they are motivated and have the ability to learn and remember. [10] It is the opinion of the authors that timely referral to a physiotherapist with interest in pelvic floor rehabilitation will optimize treatment outcomes for patients motivated to undergo pelvic floor exercises as their treatment of choice. Regular follow-up to monitor progress is essential in ensuring patients are experiencing durable symptomatic improvement. [11] If patients are unresponsive to conservative non-pharmacologic treatments then physicians will need to consider other treatment alternatives, such as pharmacologic therapy.

Anticholinergic therapy is a commonly used approach in the treatment of OAB. Geriatricians are often concerned about side-effects of OAB therapy in their older population, despite increasing data on OAB drugs and their relative safety in that age group. Dubeau et al. assessed the efficacy and tolerability of anticholinergic therapies in subjects with overactive bladder (OAB) stratified by age. They noted significant improvement with adverse event rates similar among age groups. [12]

Treatment with anticholinergic agents often requires dose adjustment to achieve optimal benefit, while balancing efficacy and tolerability. Such a regimen is often first prescribed by the primary care provider. However, adherence to treatment is a major challenge in the successful management of OAB with anticholinergic drugs. Some studies evaluating compliance with anticholinergic medications have found that the proportion of patients still on their original treatment at three months was as low as 40%, and down to 17% by 12 months. [13, 14] Among patients discontinuing OAB medications, 45% reported unmet treatment expectations as the reason for discontinuation. Many patients expect significant improvement or complete dryness with treatment, which is not a realistic expectation for the most part. [15] The high discontinuation rate of OAB medications has implications for patients' quality of life and might be even associated with loss of faith in the clinician with subsequent refusal for follow-up. [16] Also, inability to recognize poor compliance with OAB medications that have potential serious side-effects can lead to inappropriate dose escalation, changes in OAB medications, invasive diagnostic tests, and an increased overall cost to manage OAB symptoms. Unfortunately, the optimal timing and duration of anticholinergic therapy for OAB is still under investigation. The lack of understanding of the natural history and pathophysiology of OAB makes it difficult to give a firm recommendation as to the optimum duration of therapy required before considering alternative therapies, leading to further confusion for patients. [16, 17]

What is certain is that the management of OAB symptoms needs to be individualized, taking into account dosing, side-effects, and patient satisfaction. Behavioral therapy has been added to OAB drug therapy to enhance the outcomes of those suffering with urge incontinence. In the BE-DRI (Behavior Enhances Drug Reduction of Incontinence) study, following 10 weeks of OAB medication and intensive supervised behavioral training, a higher proportion of patients on combined therapy had at least a 70% reduction in incontinence episodes. [18]

After a basic evaluation followed by a brief trial period of anticholinergic therapy alone or associated with behavioral therapy, a patient showing no sign of symptomatic improvement should be further evaluated. Indications for specialist referral are mostly based on expert opinion and consensus without much literature evidence. Timing of referral to a specialist is vaguely defined

Table 3.1 Indications for specialist referral in patients with OAB symptoms not responding to first-line management

- Persistent OAB symptoms after trials with behavioral treatment, drug treatment, or both
- Persistent OAB symptoms with history of prior lower urinary tract surgeries (e.g., sling, prolapse repair, bladder injury
- OAB symptoms with new onset neurologic symptoms or muscle weakness
- OAB symptoms in the presence of pelvic organ prolapse
- OAB symptoms associated with recurrent urinary tract infections
- OAB symptoms with post void residual volumes greater than 150 ml

and usually results from uncertainties in OAB diagnosis or a lack of response to chosen therapy. However, certain clinical situations warrant timely referral to a specialist. Table 3.1 summarizes generally agreed upon criteria for specialist referral.

Conclusion

OAB symptoms are highly prevalent as people age. Unfortunately, many OAB patients remain undiagnosed and untreated despite the fact that OAB symptoms can significantly improve in the hands of well-informed and well-trained physicians. Successful treatment of OAB depends on a detailed evaluation and treatment in a timely fashion with vigilant follow-up. Recognizing patients who could benefit from specialist evaluation is the key to avoid delays in management. It is also important that the patients and their physicians set defined goals with realistic expectations leaning more towards improvement in quality of life than complete OAB symptom resolution.

References

1 Milsom I, Abrams P, Cardozo L, et al. How widespread are the symptoms of an overactive bladder and how are they managed? A population-based prevalence study. *BJU Int.* 2001;**87**(9):760–766. PubMed PMID: 11412210. Epub 2001/06/20. eng.

2 Irwin DE, Kopp ZS, Agatep B, et al. Worldwide prevalence estimates of lower urinary tract symptoms, overactive bladder, urinary incontinence and bladder outlet obstruction. *BJU Int.* 2011;**108**(7):1132–1138. PubMed PMID: 21231991. Epub 2011/01/15. eng.

3 Lee UJ, Scott VC, Rashid R, et al. Defining and managing overactive bladder: disagreement among the experts. *Urology.* 2013;**81**(2):257–262. PubMed PMID: 23374774. Epub 2013/02/05. eng.

4 Burgio KL, Ives DG, Locher JL, et al. Treatment seeking for urinary incontinence in older adults. *J Am Geriatr Soc.* 1994;**42**(2):208–212. PubMed PMID: 8126338. Epub 1994/02/01. eng.

5 Irwin DE, Milsom I, Chancellor MB, Kopp Z, Guan Z. Dynamic progression of overactive bladder and urinary incontinence symptoms: a systematic review. *Eur Urol.* 2010;**58**(4):532–543. PubMed PMID: 20573443. Epub 2010/06/25. eng.

6 Cheung WW, Khan NH, Choi KK, et al. Prevalence, evaluation and management of overactive bladder in primary care. *BMC Fam Prac.* 2009;**10**:8. PubMed PMID: 19166611. Pubmed Central PMCID: PMC2642771. Epub 2009/01/27. eng.

7 Voytas J. The role of geriatricians and family practitioners in the treatment of overactive bladder and incontinence. *Rev Urol.* 2002;**4** Suppl 4:S44–49. PubMed PMID: 16986021. Pubmed Central PMCID: PMC1476021. Epub 2006/09/21. eng.

8 Lavelle JP, Karram M, Chu FM, et al. Management of incontinence for family practice physicians. *Am J Med.* 2006;**119**(3 Suppl 1):37–40. PubMed PMID: 16483867. Epub 2006/02/18. eng.

9 Urinary incontinence. In: Abrams WB, Berkow R, Beers MH, (eds). *The Merck Manual of Geriatrics.* 2nd edn. Whitehouse Stations, NJ: Merck Research Laboratories, 1995.

10 Hay-Smith EJ, Bo Berghmans LC, Hendriks HJ, et al. Pelvic floor muscle training for urinary incontinence in women. Cochrane Database Syst Rev (Online). 2001;(1):CD001407. PubMed PMID: 11279716. Epub 2001/05/02. eng.

11 Burgio KL, Goode PS, Locher JL, et al. Behavioral training with and without biofeedback in the treatment of urge incontinence in older women: a randomized controlled trial. *JAMA.* 2002;**288**(18):2293–2299. PubMed PMID: 12425706. Epub 2002/11/13. eng.

12 DuBeau CE, Morrow JD, Kraus SR, et al. Efficacy and tolerability of fesoterodine versus tolterodine in older and younger subjects with overactive bladder: a post hoc, pooled analysis from two placebo-controlled trials. *Neurourol Urodynam.* 2012;**31**(8):1258–1265. PubMed PMID: 22907761. Epub 2012/08/22. eng.

13 Wagg A, Compion G, Fahey A, Siddiqui E. Persistence with prescribed antimuscarinic therapy for overactive bladder: a UK experience. *BJU Int.* 2012;**110**(11):1767–1774. PubMed PMID: 22409769. Epub 2012/03/14. eng.

14 Haab F, Castro-Diaz D. Persistence with antimuscarinic therapy in patients with overactive bladder. *Int J Clin Pract.* 2005;**59**(8):931–937. PubMed PMID: 16033615. Epub 2005/07/22. eng.

15 Schabert VF, Bavendam T, Goldberg EL, et al. Challenges for managing overactive bladder and guidance for patient support. *American J Manag Care.* 2009;**15**(4 Suppl):S118–122. PubMed PMID: 19355801. Epub 2009/04/16. eng.

16 Abrams P, Larsson G, Chapple C, Wein AJ. Factors involved in the success of antimuscarinic treatment. *BJU Int.* 1999;**83** Suppl 2:42–47. PubMed PMID: 10210604. Epub 1999/04/22. eng.

17 Basra RK, Wagg A, Chapple C, et al. A review of adherence to drug therapy in patients with overactive bladder. *BJU Int.* 2008;**102**(7):774–779. PubMed PMID: 18616691. Epub 2008/07/12. eng.

18 Burgio KL, Kraus SR, Menefee S, et al. Behavioral therapy to enable women with urge incontinence to discontinue drug treatment: a randomized trial. *Ann Intern Med.* 2008;**149**(3):161–169. PubMed PMID: 18678843. Epub 2008/08/06. eng.

CHAPTER 4

Clinical evaluation

Anand Singh and Vik Khullar

St. Mary's Hospital, NHS Trust, Imperial College London, London, UK

KEY POINTS

- An accurate symptom history is a useful guide for the correct physical examination and appropriate further investigations.

- A systematic approach to defining a patient's lower urinary tract symptoms as well as highlighting the most bothersome symptoms is fundamental to achieving a successful clinical outcome.

- Urinary symptoms can be subdivided into storage, voiding, and incontinence symptoms.

- Nocturnal enuresis, dysuria, and defecatory symptoms as well as a comprehensive past medical, gynaecological, and surgical history are also key to a complete evaluation.

- Physical examination should include a relevant neurological and abdominal assessment, in addition to the gynecological exam.

- It must be noted that the reliability of provocative stress tests to demonstrate stress urinary incontinence maybe questionable if such Manoeuvres also provoke a detrusor contraction.

- Whilst the Q-tip test is a good measure of bladder neck mobility, it has not been shown to add any addition useful information which would affect definitive management.

- The POP-Q has been used extensively in research settings to objectively assess the short and long term outcomes of pelvic floor surgery. This method of quantification has been shown to have good inter and intra-observer reliability.

- Questionnaires, such as the OABq, SAGA, and KHQ, allow the measurement of qualitative, relatively subjective concepts of wellbeing in a quantitative, objective manner.

Introduction

Most clinicians will spend the majority of their professional lives taking clinical histories and examining patients. Fundamental to eliciting a good clinical history and performing a detailed examination is good communication which, in turn, is influenced by the patient's anxieties, interpretations of normality, and expectations of management as well as cultural preconceptions. Eliciting the history provides additional challenges in that it often uncovers sensitive, distressing, and potentially embarrassing symptoms

Overactive Bladder: Practical Management, First Edition. Edited by Jacques Corcos, Scott MacDiarmid and John Heesakkers.
© 2015 John Wiley & Sons, Ltd. Published 2015 by John Wiley & Sons, Ltd.

that may carry social stigmas and lower self-esteem, which precludes openness to volunteer information. Furthermore, the physical symptoms of lower urinary tract pathology are subjective; the severity is influenced by a woman's coping strategies and in turn influence her quality of life. Good communication between the clinician and patient is essential to facilitating a focused yet comprehensive history.

History

The symptom history is both an important summary of a patient's problems as well as a useful guide to help direct physical examination. The symptoms can help improve the clinician's diagnostic accuracy. However, history is not useful as the sole method of diagnosis; diagnosis based on history and examination is correct in only 65% of patients. [1] This not only enables the clinician to develop an idea of what symptoms are most bothersome to the patient, but also allows a contemporaneous account of the patient's symptoms and coping mechanisms as well as aids an autonomous platform on which they can volunteer potentially embarrassing symptoms. Often the patient will not describe all their bladder symptoms independently and validated questionnaires serve as useful adjuncts to complete the symptom enquiry. Questionnaires have also been shown, if self-completed, to be more accurate an assessment of the patient's disease state than direct questioning by an interviewer. [2, 3] A thorough understanding of the underlying mechanisms and pathophysiology of the overactive bladder is pertinent to undertaking a focused clinical history. A logical, systematic approach is always important to illustrate a comprehensive clinical history and avoid missing important symptoms.

Urinary symptoms can be subdivided into storage, voiding, and incontinence symptoms. [4]

Storage symptoms

Frequency – *The number of times a woman voids in her waking hours.* Normal daytime frequency ranges between four and seven voids per day. Despite women with detrusor overactivity (DO) voiding more frequently, frequency is not diagnostic of DO [5] or of urodynamic stress incontinence (USI). [6] From the reverse perspective, women who void infrequently are at risk of developing voiding difficulty. [7]

Causes of abnormal urinary frequency can be divided into four main groups:

1 Increased fluid intake and urine output (normal bladder capacity) (e.g., osmotic diuresis, abnormal antidiuretic hormone secretion, polydipsia).
2 Reduced functional bladder capacity (e.g., inflamed bladder, DO, habitual, increased bladder sensation).
3 Reduced structural bladder capacity (e.g., fibrosis after infection or irradiation, interstitial cystitis, post-surgical, detrusor hypertrophy).
4 Decreased urinary frequency (e.g., detrusor hypotonia, impaired bladder sensation, reduced fluid intake).

Clustering voids during a particular time of day may suggest diuretic use, habitual, dependent oedema, or excessive drinking.

Nocturia – *the number of times a woman is woken from sleep to pass urine.* The clinician should be careful not to confuse this with nocturnal enuresis or voiding whilst the woman is awake at night. Normal number of voids varies with age, with anything more than once at night for a woman less than 70 years being abnormal and one additional void per decade thereafter being normal (e.g., two or less for an 80 year old, three or less for a 90 year old). Subclinical cardiac failure in the elderly may cause increased pooling of fluid in the extracellular compartment during the day, which in turn shifts from the intravascular compartment particularly in dependent areas such as the legs during the night when the patient becomes supine, thereby stimulating diuresis. [8] Reducing fluid intake in the evening does not reduce nocturia. [9]

Urgency – *the sudden compelling desire to pass urine which is difficult to defer.* Often this symptom can lead to urgency urinary incontinence if not relieved immediately and should be considered an abnormal symptom if it occurs more than once per week. The term overactive bladder often encompasses the symptom of urgency and is defined as *urgency with or without urgency incontinence usually with frequency and nocturia in the absence of an underlying metabolic or pathological condition.* The impact of this symptom on the patient can often be quantified by a bladder diary recording episodes of urgency or using a visual analog scale (see later).

Bladder pain – severity may correlate with bladder filling, however it can persist post micturition as the bladder walls touch. In patients with DO, the pain may coincide with detrusor contractions. The pain can vary in nature and is typically located either supra- or retropubically. Aetiology may include inflammation, endometriosis, bladder calculi, or tumors, all of which require further investigation with a

cystoscopy and/or bladder wall biopsy. Pelvic inflammatory disease may be considered in patients with urethral pain as this is described as a burning sensation when passing urine or during sexual intercourse. This diagnosis should be considered in the context of concomitant symptoms (e.g., suprapubic pain, pyrexia, or vaginal discharge).

Voiding symptoms

Hesitancy – *difficulty in initiation of micturition resulting in a delay in the onset of voiding after the patient is ready to pass urine.* It is important to note the volumes voided if this symptom is suggested in the history, as this a rare symptom in women and is more common in men. [10] Furthermore, women with DO may report symptoms of hesitancy secondary to small volumes being passed due to urgency and frequency. Hesitancy with a full bladder is suggestive of detrusor sphincter dysynergia (a contracting urethral sphincter during detrusor contraction), urethra strictures, detrusor acontractility, or psychological inhibition of the voiding reflex. The symptom is neither discriminatory nor diagnostic in any of these pathologies.

Straining – *the increased and sustained muscular effort used to increase the intra-abdominal pressure to maintain or improve the urinary stream.* Bladder emptying may be improved through a Valsalva manoeuvre thereby increasing the intravesical pressure. The urinary stream may be intermittent with each transient increase in flow correlating with a temporary increase in intra-abdominal pressure. Chronic straining may lead to pelvic floor prolapse, which in turn can compound the symptom of straining by creating a functional urethral obstruction.

Poor and intermittent flow – *the urinary flow stops and starts on one or more occasion during micturition.* This symptom may precede straining and may be also associated with a poor stream. The urinary flow is dependent on the volume of urine passed, so that volumes increasing up until 150 ml lead to increased urinary flow rates, but volumes over 700 ml lead to a decreased flow rate due to bladder over distension. The maximum flow rate increases as the volume in the bladder decreases in cases of detrusor hypotonia. In this situation the detrusor pressure generated by the bladder increases as the bladder volume declines.

A frequency volume chart aids proper assessment of this symptom by documenting the volumes voided and should be used if the volume of urine passed is less than 150 ml at free flow rate. Aetiology may include reduced volumes voided, bladder outflow obstruction (2% women) or decreased contractility (which may be neuropathic or myopathic).

Incomplete emptying – *the feeling of incomplete bladder emptying experienced by the patient after micturition is complete.* The symptom maybe secondary to urine remaining in the bladder, a sensory abnormality (increased or nonspecific sensory abnormalities often seen in neurological patients), or in patients with DO in whom after-contractions are present. It is important to bear in mind that the symptom does not necessarily correlate with an actual raised post-micturition residual volume.

Post-micturition dribble – *the involuntary loss of urine immediately after the patient has completed micturition usually as they arise from the toilet.* The symptom should be distinguished from terminal dribbling, which is continuous with the main flow of urine. Aetiology includes a urethral diverticulum, a cystourethrocele, or after-contractions in detrusor overactivity (where the urgency is often reported).

Incontinence symptoms

Urinary incontinence describes any involuntary loss of urine. Symptoms should be carefully delineated to determine the cause of leakage. It is important to recognize that urinary incontinence is not a diagnosis but a symptom or a sign, often with a complex integration of one or more pathological processes, coping strategies, health seeking behavior, and effects on quality of life. Severe urinary incontinence produces many symptoms common to different diagnostic categories.

The type, frequency, pattern, precipitating factors, and severity of incontinence should be elicited in the history as well as the social impact and effects on hygiene. Continuous urinary loss is rare and is usually seen when there is an ectopic ureter or a fistula (e.g., as a complication of pelvic surgery, obstetric injury, or radiotherapy). Intermittent urinary incontinence may be seen in women who have had multiple previous operations and have a fixed, fibrosed "drain pipe" (Blaivas type 3) urethra. [11] Women who report urinary loss "all the time" may have severe detrusor overactivity. Precipitating factors should be linked to the pattern of urinary loss, for example leakage may be associated with strenuous physical activity or sexual intercourse. The severity can be more objectively quantified via frequency volume charts, the number of pads or underwear changed in 24 hours, or the magnitude of the provoking stimulus.

There is often little correlation between urodynamic diagnosis and symptoms described by the patient. This often reflects the lifestyle modifications and coping strategies the woman undertakes to help relieve her incontinence symptoms in her daily life; this highlights the importance of a clear and comprehensive clinical history in addition to urodynamic investigation.

Urgency urinary incontinence – *the involuntary leakage of urine accompanied by or preceded by urgency.* The characteristics of incontinence should be delineated here, that is a small, episodic loss of urine between micturition or a large leakage precipitated by certain events (e.g., running water, keys in the front door, during orgasm or external temperature variations). It is important to bear in mind that women often cope by increasing their frequency of micturition to avoid embarrassing incontinent events. The symptom of UUI has limited sensitivity (78%) and specificity (39%) in the diagnosis of detrusor overactivity. [12]

Stress urinary incontinence – *the involuntary loss of urine on effort or exertion, or on coughing or sneezing.* There is no associated urgency and the symptom must be carefully differentiated from urgency urinary incontinence which may coexist, with up to 9% of patients reporting symptoms of pure SUI having a diagnosis of detrusor overactivity on urodynamic testing. [13] Only 39% of women reporting stress urinary incontinence actually have urodynamic stress incontinence. [14]

Mixed incontinence – it is very common for women to report symptoms of both SUI and UUI; therefore it is important to determine the balance of symptoms, chronological order of presentation, [15] and respective burden of these symptoms on the patient's quality of life.

Coital incontinence – *the leakage of urine during sexual arousal, penetration, during intercourse or at orgasm.* Careful and sensitive questioning may help elude the aetiology of coital incontinence; often urinary leakage on penetration is more likely to be a symptom of urethral sphincter incompetence, [16] whilst leakage at orgasm may be more likely associated with DO. [17, 18]

Other

Nocturnal enuresis – *the loss of urine during sleep.* Nocturnal enuresis can be primary (starts in childhood and persists through to adulthood) or secondary (when the incontinence starts in adulthood following a period of night time continence). Careful enquiry should include questions about diurnal symptoms, family history of symptoms, symptoms of overactive bladder, and sleep patterns. Delayed bladder control in adulthood is associated with DO in adulthood.

Dysuria – *pain on passing urine often experienced in the urethra.* The importance of a clear history of associated symptoms is underlined with this symptom of multiple aetiologies. Often described as "a burning sensation" whilst passing urine and immediately after micturition is complete, dysuria may be associated with hematuria (trauma, calculi, tumor, infection), bladder pain, loin pain (renal pathology), fever, vaginal discharge (pelvic inflammatory disease), superficial dyspareunia (endometriosis). The character of the sensation may help elude a cause (e.g., stinging and infection, discomfort and obstruction, or pressure and prolapse). Pain must also be characterized by its frequency (including possible cyclical nature), duration, precipitating and relieving factors, and exact location. Dysuria associated with bladder pain or hematuria should always warrant further cystoscopic investigation.

Constipation – although constipation is not a lower urinary tract symptom per se, careful questioning in the clinical history remains an essential part of managing urinary symptoms. Despite there being no absolute definition of constipation, it is typically described as infrequent bowel movements (three or less per week) which are hard to pass (straining more than 25% of the time). [19] The physiological process of normal defecation of the bowel is similar to the process of micturition from the bladder. The relationship between constipation and lower urinary tract symptoms has been extensively reviewed. [20] Overlapping neural pathways in the peripheral nervous system explain a complex and intimate relationship between bowel and bladder function. Whereas it may often be assumed that chronic constipation may be a cause of LUTS, the clinician must be careful not to ignore the possibility of a common underlying pathology. Finally, whilst treatment for chronic constipation may indeed decrease OAB symptoms, OAB treatment may paradoxically create constipation. [21]

Prolapse symptoms

Pelvic organ prolapse symptoms may be volunteered by a woman without direct questioning or indeed require specific enquiry if she considers these less bothersome and potentially less relevant than her urinary symptoms. The feeling of a lump, bulge, heaviness or dragging sensation ("something coming down from the vagina") either continuously or on straining is often described. This may often cause only mild discomfort or pressure symptoms with certain postures rather than pain.

Further detailed enquiry including associated back ache, vaginal bleeding, and the duration of symptoms should be documented. Women may describe the need to reduce the prolapse via self-digitation in order to defecate or pass urine. Prolapse may be associated with urinary storage or voiding symptoms, and therefore concomitant management may be influenced by the degree of prolapse and severity of symptoms. Over 40% of women with urodynamic stress incontinence will also have significant cystoceles. [22] The anterior vaginal wall prolapse can often kink the mid urethral point creating a "pseudo-sphincter" thereby masking urodynamic stress incontinence in women who may report mild stress urinary incontinence, therefore it is important to reduce vaginal prolapse during urodynamics and when checking for urodynamic stress incontinence during urodynamic investigation. [23]

Neurological history

The micturition reflex is regulated via the transmitted sequence of complex neuronal messages in the spinal cord, brainstem, and brain. The neurogenic origin of LUTS presents when these signals become perturbed, leading to deregulation of normal lower urinary tract function or even loss of voluntary bladder control. [24] The incidence and prevalence of LUT dysfunctions rise with increasing progression of the underlying neurological disease, [25] and whilst LUTS are rarely the presenting symptoms, they are often early in onset, highly complicated, and have significant impact on the patient's quality of life. [24]

A logical approach should be followed if neurogenic urinary dysfunction is suspected. The clinician should ask about altered sensation and power in the lower limbs and perineum. There may be a reduced sensation during sexual intercourse, absent sensation of bladder filling or a desire to void, difficulty with erectile/ejaculatory function in men, fecal incontinence or fecal urgency leading to soiling of clothing. Back pain or recent spinal injury or surgery may precipitate voiding dysfunction, which should be worked up expeditiously as this may signify serious underlying pathology. Multisystem atrophy and multiple sclerosis are the most common neurological conditions complicated with LUTS. [26, 27]

Impaired bladder sensation may be the result of iatrogenic denervation (e.g., during neurosurgery or abdominoperineal resection of the rectum) or chronic diabetes mellitus (resulting in frequency as a result of overflow incontinence secondary to a hypotonic bladder).

Lower urinary tract symptoms as a manifestation of neurogenic sequelae should also be considered in advanced cerebrovascular accidents, Parkinson's disease, cerebral and spinal cord lesions. Neurological aetiology should also be considered if the LUTS are complex and do not correlate well with urodynamic diagnoses. Close liaison with a neurologist or uro-neurologist will help direct investigation and treatment appropriately.

General gynecological history

Many women with LUTS have coexisting gynecological pathology. [28] Prolapse symptoms have already been discussed earlier, although at this stage it is important to enquire about previous operations for both prolapse and incontinence symptoms, since this may result in scarring, denervation, distortion, or narrowing of the urethral sphincter as well as influence the success of future surgery. The woman's menopausal state should be documented as both estrogen and progesterone have a variety of effects along the lower urinary tract. Although the subject remains contentious, the general consensus remains that stress urinary incontinence appears to be more related to estrogen deficiency, whilst urgency urinary incontinence appears to be more age related. [28] The number of proven urinary tract infections in the past two years should be documented and any history of childhood urinary symptoms (e.g., nocturnal enuresis) should be recorded in adults.

Operations on the uterus may affect bladder function (e.g., the effect of a radical hysterectomy for endometrial carcinoma on the innervation of the bladder), and vault brachytherapy can result in fibrosis of the bladder wall resulting in OAB symptoms. [29] A history of leiomyoma should be sought since the mechanical pressure of large, anterior uterine wall, subserosal fibroids may reduce normal bladder capacity or cause symptoms of bladder outlet obstruction.

Obstetric history

A general obstetric history to include parity, duration of labor, mode of delivery, birth weights of children, year of delivery, intrapartum complications (e.g., obstetric anal sphincter injury, periurethral lacerations or wound breakdowns), as well as *de novo* post-partum urinary symptoms (e.g., urinary retention requiring prolonged catheterization or stress urinary incontinence) which may be precipitated by cesarean section, epidural block or prolonged labor. [30, 31]

Other relevant past medical and surgical history

Subtle associations between past and current medical history and concomitant LUTS should be carefully interpreted in the context of onset of symptoms and medical management (see next section). Chronic diabetes mellitus has already been discussed, but diabetes insipidus can result in polyuria through polydipsia. Any condition that may increase intrabdominal pressure, such as a chronic cough or straining to defecate or micturate, will only increase the risk of pelvic floor prolapse (discussed earlier), but may also augment the symptoms of SUI. Any condition resulting in extravasation of fluid into the third space may create diurnal variations in voiding patterns (e.g., congestive cardiac failure or chronic renal impairment and hypertension). Finally, a past psychiatric history may reveal possible clues to abnormal voiding patterns in women with dementia [32] or rarer causes of detrusor overactivity in women with schizophrenia. [33]

All major pelvic or abdominal surgery should be recorded in the medical notes, including intra-operative complications if any (e.g., bladder injury or denervation during difficult pelvic side wall resection). Prolonged catheterization due to post-operative urinary retention should be noted as over distension of the bladder may lead to detrusor hypotonia. [34]

Drug history

The clinician should be able to decide whether certain drug therapy with a known urinary symptom side-effect profile is directly causal, contributory, or merely coincidental to the LUTS described by the patient. Often the only way of knowing is to discontinue the medication for a specified period of time and monitor the impact this action has on the LUTS. Obviously the risks of discontinuing medical treatment must be weighed up against the potential diagnostic benefit.

Diuretics, alcohol, and caffeine can cause urgency, frequency, and urgency urinary incontinence. [35] Alcohol can also alter the sensation of bladder filling. Sympathomimetics can produce voiding difficulty via increase bladder outlet resistance. Drugs which have an anticholinergic effect will impair detrusor contractility leading to urinary retention and possible overflow incontinence (e.g., antipsychotics, antiparkinson agents, antidepressants, antispasmodics, and opiates).

Examination

The physical examination forms an essential part of the complete evaluation of women with LUTS. The woman must first be reassured that despite the possibility of demonstrable urinary leakage during the examination, she should not be embarrassed by this. The woman's height and weight must be recorded in order to calculate her BMI, which has been shown to be a significant risk factor for incontinence. [36]

Neurological examination should be performed, with attention to the sacral neuronal pathways from S1 to S4. Assessment of gait, abduction, dorsiflexion, tone, and strength of the toes (S3) and sensory innervation to sole and lateral aspect of the foot (S1), posterior aspects of the thigh (S2), and perineum (S3) and cutaneous sacral reflexes (bulbo-cavernosus and anal reflexes) may be assessed. A rectal examination will provide a subjective assessment of resting and voluntary anal tone (S2–S4) whilst during cough will allow an assessment of reflex anal sphincter contraction. A contraction of the external anal sphincter may be elicited by stroking the skin lateral to the anus and is indicative of an intact sacral reflex. It must also be noted that in the elderly or neurologically impaired, restricted mobility may lead to functional incontinence and lack of manual dexterity may preclude self-catheterization.

Abdominal inspection and examination may provide cues for further multidisciplinary investigation of LUTS, for example abdominal striae may signify disorders of collagen metabolism pertaining to prolapse symptoms [37] or a large fibroid uterus palpable per abdomen may cause bladder outlet obstruction. A distended bladder maybe visible or palpable suprapubically via percussion.

The gynecological examination is the mainstay of physical assessment for women with LUTS and should always be performed during initial consultation. The clinician should begin with inspection of the vulval skin for signs of irritation secondary to urine exposure such as excoriations or erythema. The clinical sign of urinary incontinence maybe demonstrable at his point, without digital examination, whereby the patient is asked to cough vigorously and urine is seen leaking from the urethra. One must be careful not to forget that leakage of urine can also be extra-urethral in the case of ectopic ureters, other congenital urogenital abnormalities, or urogenital fistulas. Optimal examination for this test should be done with a comfortably full bladder, in the absence of the urinary urgency, and initially in supine position. The patient should be asked to stand if no leakage is demonstrable, yet the clinical history points towards stress urinary incontinence. The reliability of provocative stress tests to demonstrate stress urinary incontinence maybe questionable if such maneuvres also provoke a detrusor contraction.

Vaginal mucosal atrophy should be noted on inspection, particularly in women more than ten years after the menopause. The role of topical hormone replacement therapy in the treatment of women with LUTS remains controversial; topical estrogen is superior to placebo when considering symptoms of urgency incontinence, frequency, and nocturia although only vaginal estrogen administration has been found to be superior for the symptom of urgency. There remains conflicting evidence for the use of combination treatment of antimuscarinic and topical estrogen. [38] Finally, whilst the role of topical estrogen therapy in the reduction of urinary tract infections is strong, there still remains a paucity of robust evidence in the literature supporting its role in the management of pelvic organ prolapse.

The mobility of the urethra vesicle junction could give important clues into the strength and support the urethra has and its involvement in the mechanism of incontinence. With the woman lying supine and during a Valsalva manoeuvre, the anterior vaginal wall can be seen deflecting posteriorly and the urethral meatus anteriorly, toward the ceiling. Both signs are evidence of loss of urethral support. A Q-tip cotton bud placed into the urethra to the level of the bladder neck is a good test of bladder neck mobility. [39] The rotational movement of the bladder neck around the symphysis pubis whilst the patient is asked to strain deflects the Q-tip in a cranial direction. The resting and straining angles are measured. Urethrovesical junction hypermobility is defined by a maximum strain axis exceeding 30 degrees from the horizontal. The Q-tip has not been shown to be predictive of Valsalva leak point pressures in women with urethral hypermobility and stress urinary incontinence and does not add any extra information to the history and examination. [40–42] The test may have a role in predicting failure of incontinence surgery and efficacy of surgical treatments of women diagnosed with USI. [43, 44]

When proceeding to the examination of the pelvic organs, it is important to perform a bimanual exam to help identify any concomitant pelvic organ pathology such as large uterine fibroids, endometriotic nodules, vaginal or ovarian cysts. Pelvic masses can cause pressure symptoms which result in increased frequency. Inspection of the urethra may reveal a suburethral mass or diverticula.

Pelvic organ prolapse and urinary incontinence can often coexist, although remain separate clinical diagnoses. Pelvic organ prolapse is best assessed using a Sims' speculum in left lateral position and during Valsalva effort. If the prolapse is not demonstrable to the degree which the patient eludes to in her history, then digital examination of vaginal prolapse whilst standing

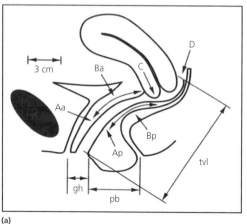

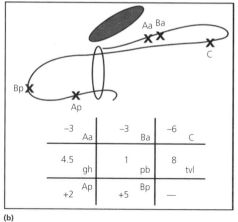

(a)   (b)

Figure 4.1 (a and b) Diagram of the Pelvic Organ Prolapse Questionnaire with Grid example.(a) Points and landmarks for POP–Q system examination. Aa, point A anterior, Ap, point A posterior, Ba, point B anterior, C, cervix or vaginal cuff (these three points form the anterior reference points); Bp, point B posterior; D, posterior fornix (the latter three points form the posterior reference points) gh, genital hiatus; pb, perineal body; tvl, total vaginal length. (b) Grid and line diagrams for the POP to demonstrate a predominantly posterior support defect. Leading point of prolapse is upper posterior vaginal wall, point Bp (+5). Point Ap is 2 cm distal to hymen (+2) and vaginal cuff scar is 6 cm above hymen (−6). Cuff has undergone only 2 cm of descent because it would be at −8 (total vaginal length) if it were properly supported. This represents stage III Bp prolapse. (Bump RC, Mattiasson A, Bø K et al. The standardization of terminology of female pelvic organ prolapse and pelvic floor dysfunction. Am J Obstet Gynecol 1996; 175: 10–17) and asking her to recreate her provocative maneuvres will aid assessment. To demonstrate stress urinary incontinence, the woman should be examined with a comfortably full bladder. Methods of objectively measuring the degree of pelvic organ prolapse have evolved through simple classification of mild, moderate, or severe to first, second, third degree descent, to the Baden-Walker halfway classification. [45, 46] These methods have been superseded by the International Continence Society Pelvic Organ Prolapse Quantification (ICS POP-Q). [47] This method of quantification has been shown to have good inter- and intra-observer reliability. [48] The POP-Q has been used extensively in research settings to objectively assess the short and long term outcomes of pelvic floor surgery.

There are six defined points for measurement in the POPQ system – Aa, Ba, C, D, Ap, Bp and three others landmarks: GH, TVL, PB. Each is measured in centimeters above or proximal to the hymen (negative number) or centimeters below or distal to the hymen (positive number) with the plane of the hymen being defined as zero (0), which acts as the fixed reference point throughout the examination.

The gynecological examination is completed with a digital rectal examination to assess sphincter tone and pelvic floor muscle strength and exclude provocative causes of urinary incontinence such as fecal impaction and rectal masses.

Questionnaires and quality of life

Patient self-completed questionnaires are the most suitable method for assessing the patient's perspective of their lower urinary tract, vaginal, and bowel symptoms. There are many questionnaires available for use, each fulfilling a different purpose. They may be used directly to assess a patient's bladder condition, as screening tools for certain LUTS, as methods of monitoring progress on or after treatment, in epidemiological studies or with economic and health service evaluation. Finally, and perhaps most relevant to this section, questionnaires can be used to assess the impact of a condition on a patient's quality of life.

Quality of life (QoL) is a term derived from the World Health Organisation [49] as a *"state of physical, social and emotional wellbeing and not merely the absence of disease."* Measurement of a person's quality of life can be enormously subjective and individualized, with multiple complex influences of a person's experiences and perceptions. A specific symptom that one person finds irrelevant, another may find integral to their day to day physical, psychological, and social wellbeing. Questionnaires allow the measurement of these qualitative, relatively subjective concepts in a quantitative, objective manner and in so doing underpin the notion that often the goal of treatment is not necessarily cure of symptoms, but improving a patient's QoL. Health related quality of life (HRQoL) assessment allows the clinician to focus on components relevant to health status rather than those which may encompass QoL in the broader sense. [50]

Questionnaires related to LUTS must not only be validated (measure what they are intended to measure) and reliable (are the measures reproducible?) but also short, easy to use, sensitive to change, and relevant to clinical practice. These specific criteria are evaluated by the International

Consultation on Incontinence in order to achieve a grading system of recommendation for the questionnaire. Whilst many questionnaires assess symptoms beyond the scope of this book, currently 14 questionnaires of Grade A recommendation (Highly recommended) are in use for women with LUTS. [51] The symptoms of overactive bladder and impact on QoL are represented in most of these questionnaires; however one questionnaire, the OABq, achieves the highest levels of recommendation specific for OAB symptoms. [52] The negative impact a LUTS has on HRQoL can be assessed via a sub question or "bother" item. This item enables the patient to indicate areas that cause the greatest burden on HRQoL as perceived by them. This can be a more sensitive indicator of treatment goals than frequency of symptoms alone.

Successful management of LUTS often requires individual treatment plans which are tailored to meet individual patient goals. Identifying autonomous and realistic treatment goals for women with OAB symptoms is pertinent to achieving successful treatment outcome. Furthermore, mutual agreement between the clinician and patient of perceptions of impact of symptoms and treatment outcomes is best achieved in this way. The Self-Assessment Goal Achievement (SAGA) questionnaire was developed for use in both clinical practice and in clinical trials to facilitate the establishment of patients' goals concerning their treatment for LUTS, including symptoms of OAB. It has been validated as a measure of patients' goals and goal achievement and may improve healthcare provider–patient interactions and treatment outcomes in a number of languages. [53]

Summary

Urinary symptoms need to be collected in a methodical and organized manner to facilitate the accurate evaluation of symptoms that will help diagnosis and management. The impact of symptoms on patient's lives can only be adequately assessed by using health related quality of life questionnaires and these are sensitive techniques of assessing the outcomes of treatments such as drug therapy. It is vital that whatever method is used it should be validated and self-completed by the patient to produce the greatest benefit.

References

1. Digesu GA, Khullar V, Cardozo L, Salvatore S. Overactive bladder symptoms: do we need urodynamics? Neurourol Urodyn. 2003;22(2):105–108. *Erratum in: Neurourol Urodyn.* 2003;**22**(4):356.

2. Khan MS, Chaliha C, Leskova L, Khullar V. The relationship between urinary symptom questionnaires and urodynamic diagnoses: an analysis of two methods of questionnaire administration. *BJOG.* 2004;**111**(5):468–474.

3. Khan MS, Chaliha C, Leskova L, Khullar V. A randomized crossover trial to examine administration techniques related to the Bristol female lower urinary tract symptom (BFLUTS) questionnaire. *Neurourol Urodyn.* 2005;**24**(3): 211–214.

4. Haylen BT1, de Ridder D, Freeman RM, et al. An International Urogynecological Association (IUGA)/International Continence Society (ICS) joint report on the terminology for female pelvic floor dysfunction. *Int Urogynecol J.* 2010; **21**(1):5–26.

5. Larsson G, Abrams P, Victor A. The frequency/volume chart in detrusor instability. *Neurourol Urodyn.* 1991;**10**: 533–543.

6. Larsson G, Victor A. The frequency/volume chart in genuine stress incontinence. *Neurourol Urodyn.* 1992;**11**:23–31.

7 Swinn MJ, Lowe E, Fowler CJ. The clinical features of non-psychogenic urinary retention. *Neurourol Urodyn.* 1998; **17**: 383–384.

8 Carter PG, McConnell AA, Abrams P. the significance of atrial natriuretic peptide in nocturnal urinary symptoms in the elderly. *Neurourol Urodyn* 1992;**11**:420–421.

9 Hill S, Cardozo LD, Khullar V. Does eveing fluid restriction improve nocturia? *Int Urogynaecol J* 1995;**6**:242.

10 Groutz A, Gordon D, Lessing JB, Wolman I, Jaffa A, David MP.Prevalence and characteristics of voiding difficulties in women: are subjective symptoms substantiated by objective urodynamic data?*Urology.* 1999;**54**(2):268-72.

11 Blaivas JG, Appell RA, Fantl JA et al. Definition and classification of urinary incontinence: recommendations of the Urodynamic Society. *Neurourol Urodyn* 1997;**16**:149–151.

12 Sand PK, Ostergard DR. Incontinence history as a predictor of detrusor stability. *Obstet Gynecol* 1988;**71**:257–259.

13 James M, Jackson S, Shepherd A, Abrams P. Pure stress leakage symptomatology: is it safe to discount detrusor instability? *Br J Obstet Gynaecol.* 1999;**106**(12):1255–1258.

14 Abrams P. The clinical contribution of urodynamics. In: Abrams P, Feneley R, Torrens M (eds) *Urodynamics.* Berlin: Springer-Verlag, 1983: pp. 118–174.

15 Scotti RJ, Angell G, Flora R, Greston WM. Antecedent history as a predictor of surgical cure of urgency symptoms in mixed incontinence. *Obstet Gynecol* 1998;**91**:51–54.

16 Kelleher CJ, Cardozo LD, Wise BG, Cutner A. The impact of urinary incontinence on sexual function. *Neurourol Urodyn.* 1992;**11**:359–360.

17 Field SM, Hilton P. The prevalence of sexual problems in women attending for urodynamic investigation. *Int Urogynecol J* 1993;**4**:212–215.

18 Sutherst JR. Sexual dysfunction and urinary incontinence. *Br J Obstet Gynaecol* 1979;**86**: 387–388.

19 Digesu GA, Panayi D, Kundi N, et al. Validity of the Rome III Criteria in assessing constipation in women. *Int Urogynecol J.* 2010;**21**(10): 1185–1193.

20 Coyne KS, Sexton CC, Kopp ZS, et al. The impact of overactive bladder on mental health, work productivity and health-related quality of life in the UK and Sweden: results from EpiLUTS. *BJU Int.* 2011;**108**(9):1459–1471.

21 Chapple CR, Khullar V, Gabriel Z, et al. The effects of antimuscarinic treatments in overactive bladder: an update of a systematic review and meta-analysis. *Eur Urol.* 2008;**54**(3): 543–562.

22 Rosenzweig BA, Pushkin S, Blumenfeld D, Bhatia NN. Prevalence of abnormal urodynamic test results in continent women with severe genitourinary prolapse. *Obstet Gynecol.* 1992;**79**(4):539–542.

23 Hextall A, Boos K, Cardozo L, et al. Videocystourethrography with a ring pessary in situ. A clinically useful preoperative investigation for continent women with urogenital prolapse? *Int Urogynecol J Pelvic Floor Dysfunct.* 1998;**9**(4):205–209.

24 Magari T1, Fukabori Y, Ogura H, Suzuki K. Lower urinary tract symptoms of neurological origin in urological practice. *Clin Auton Res.* 2013;**23**(2):67–72.

25 Mehnert U1, Nehiba M. Neuro-urological dysfunction of the lower urinary tract in CNS diseases: pathophysiology, epidemiology, and treatment options. *Urologe A.* 2012;**51**(2):189–197.

26 Sakakibara R, Uchiyama T, Yoshiyama M, Hattori T. Urinary dysfunction. *J Clin Neurosci.* 2001; **19**:1285–1288.

27 Carr LK. Lower urinary tract dysfunction due to multiple sclerosis. *Can J Urol.* 2006;**13**:2–4

28 Benson JT. Gynecologic and urodynamic evaluation of women with urinary incontinence. *Obstet Gynecol.* 1985;**66**: 691–694.

29 Wiebe E1, Covens A, Thomas G. Vaginal vault dehiscence and increased use of vaginal vault brachytherapy: what are the implications? *Int J Gynecol Cancer.* 2012;**22**(9):1611–1616.

30 Kerr-Wilson RHJ, Thompson SW, Orr JW et al. Effect of labor on the postpartum bladder. *Obstet Gynecol.* 1984;**64**:115–118.

31 Kerr-Wilson RHJ, McNally S. Bladder drainage for caesarean section under epidural analgesia. *Br J Obstet Gynaecol.* 1986;**93**: 28–30.

32 Takahashi O, Sakakibara R, Panicker J, et al. White matter lesions or Alzheimer's disease: which contributes more to overactive bladder and incontinence in elderly adults with dementia? *J Am Geriatr Soc.* 2012;**60**(12): 2370–2371.

33 Bonney W, Gupta S, Arndt S et al. Neurobiological correlates of bladder dysfunction in schizophrenia. *Neurourol Urodyn.* 1993;**12**: 347–349.

34 Hinman F. Postoperative overdistension of the bladder. *Surg Gynecol Obstet.* 1976;**142**: 901–902.

35 Fantl JA, Wyman JF, Wilson M et al. Diuretics and urinary incontinence in community-dwelling women. *Neurourol Urodyn.* 1990;**9**:25–34.

36 The Norwegian EPINCONT Study. *Brit J Obstet Gynaecol.* 2003;**110**(3):247–254.

37 Norton PA. Pelvic floor disorders: the role of fascia and ligaments. *Clin Obstet Gynecol.* 1993; **36**(4):926–938.

38 Robinson D1, Cardozo L. Estrogens and the lower urinary tract. *Neurourol Urodyn.* 2011;**30**(5):754–757.

39 Crystle CD, Charme LS, Copeland WE. Q-tip test in stress urinary incontinence. *Obstet Gynecol.* 1971;**38**(2):313–315.

40 Fantl JA, Hurt WG, Bump RC et al. Urethral axis and sphincteric function. *Am J Obstet Gynecol.* 1986;**155**: 554–558.

41 Walters MD, Diaz K. Q-tip test: a study of continent and incontinent women. *Obstet Gynecol.* 1987;**70**:208–211.

42 Walters MD, Shields LE. The diagnostic value of history, physical examination and the Q-tip cotton swab test in women with urinary incontinence. *Am J Obstet Gynecol.* 1988;**159**: 145–149.

43 Bergman A, Koonings PP, Ballard CA. Negative Q-tip test as a risk factor for failed incontinence surgery in women. *J Reprod Med.* 1993; **34**: 193–197.

44 Walsh LP1, Zimmern PE, Pope N, Shariat SF; Urinary Incontinence Treatment Network. Comparison of the Q-tip test and voiding cystourethrogram to assess urethral hypermobility among women enrolled in a randomized clinical trial of surgery for stress urinary incontinence. *J Urol.* 2006;**176**(2):646–649; discussion 650.

45 Baden WF, Walker TA. Physical diagnosis in the evaluation of vaginal relaxation. *Surg Gynecol Obstet.* 1963;**117**:761–773.

46 Baden WF, Walker TA. Physical diagnosis in the evaluation of vaginal relaxation. *Clin Obstet Gynecol.* 1972;**15**(4):1055–1069.

47 Bump RC, Mattiasson A, Bø K et al. The standardization of terminology of female pelvic organ prolapse and pelvic floor dysfunction. *Am J Obstet Gynecol.* 1996;**175**:10–17.

48 Hall AF, Theofrastous JP, Cundiff GW et al. Interobserver and intraobserver reliability of the proposed International Continence Society, Society of Gynecologic Surgeons, and American Urogynecologic Society pelvic organ prolapse classification system. *Am J Obstet Gynecol.* 1996;**175**:1467–1470.

49 WHO. Definition of Quality of Life. 1978.

50 Shumaker SA, Wyman JF, Uebersax JS, et al. Health-related quality of life measures for women with urinary incontinence: the Incontinence Impact Questionnaire and the Urogenital Distress Inventory. Continence Program in Women (CPW) Research Group. *Qual Life Res.* 1994;**3**(5):291–306.

51 Avery KN, Bosch JL, Gotoh M, et al. Questionnaires to assess urinary and anal incontinence: review and recommendations. *J Urol.* 2007;**177**(1):39–49.

52 Coyne K, Revicki D, Hunt T, et al. Psychometric validation of an overactive bladder symptom and health-related quality of life questionnaire: the OAB-q. *Qual Life Res.* 2002;**11**(6): 563–574.

53 Khullar V, Marschall-Kehrel D, Espuna-Pons M, et al. European content validation of the Self-Assessment Goal Achievement (SAGA) questionnaire in patients with overactive bladder. *Int Urogynecol J.* 2013;**24**(9): 1529–1536.

CHAPTER 5

Urodynamic evaluation of the overactive bladder

Barry G. Hallner,[1] Ryan M. Krlin[2] and J. Christian Winters[2]

[1] *Department of Obstetrics & Gynecology, Louisiana State University Health Sciences Center, New Orleans, LA, USA*
[2] *Department of Urology, Louisiana State University Health Sciences Center, New Orleans, LA, USA*

Introduction

The term Urodynamics was first described by Davis in 1953. [1, 2] In its simplest form urodynamics is monitoring the changing function of the lower urinary tract over time. A clear understanding of the physiology of urine storage and voiding and the disease process of voiding dysfunction is critical to formulate questions to be answered by urodynamic testing. [3] The urinary system can be divided into either the storage of urine or the emptying of urine, each with its own set of diagnostic tests. To evaluate the bladder storage, one can do simple urodynamics (aka eye ball urodynamics) or single or multichannel cystometry. The urodynamic tests used to evaluate bladder emptying are post-void residual (PVR) assessment, uroflowmetry, and pressure–flow studies (PFS). It is important that the urodynamic test reproduce the patients' symptoms. [4] A study that does not is not diagnostic. [5] For instance if a patient states he/she only leaks urine in an upright position, doing this test in a supine position may offer little information. [6] However, not being able to reproduce an abnormality on urodynamics assessment does not rule out its existence. [5]

The American Urological Association Guidelines Panel [7] concluded that UDS may have a role when conservative and drug therapies fail in a patient who desires more invasive treatment options for OAB. Patients with OAB may have concomitant findings on UDS that affect the ultimate treatment decision. A patient with refractory urgency incontinence may have concomitant urodynamic diagnoses of stress urinary incontinence (SUI) or bladder outlet obstruction (BOO), and correction of these associated conditions may greatly improve the symptoms related to urinary urgency. In the setting of mixed urinary incontinence (MUI), UDS may contribute by aiding in symptom correlation. However, it should be noted that these tests may not precisely predict outcomes of treatment. [7]

Overactive Bladder: Practical Management, First Edition. Edited by Jacques Corcos, Scott MacDiarmid and John Heesakkers.

OAB and urodynamics

Overactive bladder is a syndrome, which represents a constellation of symptoms, thus OAB cannot be precisely measured by urodynamics. OAB consists of the symptoms of frequency, urgency, nocturia, and urgency with incontinence. [8] These symptoms cannot be directly measured during urodynamic testing; however, various urodynamic events correlate to or may explain the etiology of these OAB symptoms. Patient management is often initially guided by office evaluation alone in most straightforward cases, and this strategy is supported by several guidelines. [7] The initial management of uncomplicated OAB usually consists of behavioral modification and or antimuscarinic therapy. [7] It is recommended in situations where the diagnosis is unclear or when patients have not responded to therapy that urodynamics be considered. Even though urodynamics cannot diagnose OAB, information gained during bladder filling (i.e., presence of detrusor overactivity (DO), early sensation and concomitant SUI), and bladder emptying (bladder outlet obstruction or impaired contractility) can aid in the management of patients with OAB symptoms. [16] To comprehend the role of UDS in OAB it is essential to understand the components of urodynamic testing during bladder filling and storage. In 2002 The International Continence Society (ICS) defined terms that are used in reporting cystometric results.

Filling cystometry and OAB

Cystometry is classified broadly as either a single channel or a multichannel study. In single channel cystometry bladder pressure (P_{ves}) is measured and recorded during the filling or storage phase. In multichannel cystometry abdominal pressure (P_{abd}) is measured along with bladder pressure, which is then subtracted from P_{ves} to give detrusor pressure (P_{det}). The most commonly used filling media are sterile water, physiologic saline, and radiographic contrast. Ideally, the position of the patient should represent the stress that is involved in the patients' symptoms. Sitting in an inclined chair or semi-erect are the preferred positions but standing and supine may also be used. Most studies are preferred with fluids at room temperature. Bladder filling may be accomplished by either retrograde filling using a transurethral catheter by a water pump or by simple gravity. At our facility filling rates via a water pump on average are between 30 to 50 ml/min. The ICS no longer divides filling rates into slow, medium, and fast. Provocation Maneuvers may include all or individual maneuvers of straining, coughing, hearing running water, heel bouncing, walking, and washing hands.

KEY POINTS

- Cystometry may be single or multichannel.
- P_{ves} = intravesical pressure recording.
- P_{abd} = intraabdominal pressure via rectal, vaginal, or extraperitoneal pressure recording.
- $P_{det} = P_{ves} - P_{abd}$. Ideally P_{det} at rest should be 0 cm H$_2$O

Cystometrogram

Cystometry is the mainstay of investigation for bladder storage function and is the only method of objectively diagnosing detrusor overactivity (DO). Values are subjective, and the absolute volumes at which these symptoms occur are clinically less relevant. The more important issues are whether bladder sensation is increased, decreased, or absent and whether a particular sensation such as urgency correlates or not with urodynamic findings during cystometrography. [4] Parameters that are measured by cystometrography include the following:

Bladder sensation during filling cystometry [8]

A **Normal bladder sensation** can be judged by three defined points noted during filling cystometry and evaluated in relation to the bladder volume at that moment and in relation to the patient's symptomatic complaints.

1 **First sensation** of bladder filling is the feeling the patient has, during filling cystometry, when he/she first becomes aware of the bladder filling.

2 **First desire to void** is defined as the feeling, during filling cystometry, that would lead the patient to pass urine at the next convenient

moment, but voiding can be delayed if necessary.

3 **Strong desire to void** is defined, during filling cystometry, as a persistent desire to void without the fear of leakage.

B **Increased bladder sensation** is defined, during filling cystometry, as an early first sensation of bladder filling (or an early desire to void) and/or an early strong desire to void, which occurs at low bladder volume and which persists.

C **Reduced bladder sensation** is defined, during filling cystometry, as diminished sensation throughout bladder filling.

D **Absent bladder sensation** means that, during filling cystometry, the individual has no bladder sensation.

E **Bladder pain**, during filling cystometry, is a self-explanatory term and is an abnormal finding.

F **Urgency**, during filling cystometry, is a sudden compelling desire to void.

G **Maximum capacity**, in patients with normal sensation, is the volume at which the patient feels he/she can no longer delay micturition.

H **Compliance.** Bladder compliance describes the relationship between changes in bladder volume and changes in detrusor pressure. It is calculated by dividing the volume change (ΔV) by the change in detrusor pressure (ΔP_{det}) during that change in bladder volume ($C = \Delta V / \Delta P_{det}$). It is expressed in ml/cm H_2O.

1 It is a measure of bladder vesicoelasticity and reflects the sum of two factors:

i The passive mechanoelastic property of the bladder.

ii The active neuromuscular force.

a) The normal bladder has high compliance and is able to expand to capacity with minimal changes in intravesical pressure usually < 15 to 20 cm H_2O. [3]

iii Decreased compliance is defined as less than 20 ml/cm H_2O. [9]

a) Decreased compliance may be caused by infection, inflammation, obstruction, chronic indwelling catheter, neurologic disease, or surgical denervation, or it may be an artifact of too-rapid bladder filling.

2 Compliance is the most reliable and reproducible urodynamic parameter, largely because it is not patient dependent.

i Additionally, it is a passive measurement and provides valuable information with respect to potential upper tract damage.

ii A sustained increase in bladder pressure can cause upper tract damage. [10] This is measured by evaluating the detrusor leak point pressure on the urodynamics tracing.

a) These urodynamic events do not diagnose OAB, but can be correlated to OAB symptoms.

I **Detrusor Leak Point Pressure** (DLPP) is defined as the lowest Pdet at which leakage occurs in the absence of detrusor contraction or increased abdominal pressure. [8]

1 When outlet resistance is high, high bladder pressure is needed to overcome this resistance and cause leakage. Bladder pressure higher than 40 cm H_2O impedes ureteral

peristalsis, causes hydroureters, and damages the upper tracts. [10]

2 Patients with low bladder compliance and a low DLPP may be floridly incontinent, but their upper tracts are safe because the low-resistance urethra functions as a pop-off mechanism to relieve the high detrusor pressure. [4]

3 Patients with low bladder compliance and a DLPP higher than 40 cm H_2O risk upper tract damage unless the outlet resistance is reduced or compliance is improved with medication or surgery. [4]

4 In the neurogenic population, the use of the DLPP has been identified to predict a risk for upper tract complications. [10]

Detrusor function during filling cystometry [8]

A **Normal detrusor function:** allows bladder filling with little or no change in pressure. No involuntary phasic contractions occur despite provocation.

B **Detrusor overactivity** is an urodynamic observation characterized by involuntary detrusor contractions during the filling phase which may be spontaneous or provoked.

1 A ΔP_{det} of more than 15 cm H_2O was previously the minimum pressure required to diagnose detrusor overactivity, but any involuntary pressure increase that is associated with urgency now qualifies as overactivity. [4]

There are certain patterns of detrusor overactivity [8]

A **Phasic detrusor overactivity** is defined by a characteristic waveform and may or may not lead to urinary incontinence.

B **Terminal detrusor overactivity** is defined as a single, involuntary detrusor contraction, occurring at cystometric capacity, which cannot be suppressed and results in incontinence usually resulting in bladder emptying.

C **Detrusor overactivity incontinence** is incontinence due to an involuntary detrusor contraction.

D **Neurogenic detrusor overactivity** when there is a relevant neurological condition. This term replaces the term "detrusor hyperreflexia."

E **Idiopathic detrusor overactivity** when there is no defined cause. This term replaces "detrusor instability."

OAB during filling cystometry

OAB symptoms such as frequency, urgency, nocturia, and urgency incontinence are not urodynamic measurements. In fact, these symptoms in our opinion are probably best measured by a voiding diary. However, urodynamic events during filling cystometry may be correlated to this syndrome. Urinary frequency may be associated with early sensation to void, decreased cystometric capacity, and motor detrusor overactivity with or without incontinence.

Involuntary bladder contractions (detrusor overactivity) on filling cystometry may also explain symptoms such as frequency and urgency (Figure 5.1). In addition, these involuntary contractions are the probable cause of urgency urinary incontinence. It is important to note, however, that involuntary detrusor contractions may occur in the absence of symptoms, and thus these contractions may occur in the absence of the OAB syndrome. DO may be characterized by involuntary rises in detrusor pressure of a short duration followed by a return to baseline pressures. These more common familiar waveforms are known as phasic detrusor overactivity and are the most common type of DO. In patients with sustained involuntary elevations of detrusor storage pressure above baseline, this tonic detrusor overactivity may represent a disorder of bladder compliance. Whether a loss of compliance is due to prolonged, tonic, and sustained elevations in detrusor pressure or morphologic changes in the bladder wall resulting in loss of accommodation is unclear. However, it is important for the clinician to understand the concepts of low urinary storage pressures, particularly in patients with neurogenic bladder.

KEY POINTS

- OAB symptoms such as frequency, urgency, nocturia, and urgency incontinence are not urodynamic measurements.

- Urinary frequency may be associated with early sensation to void, decreased cystometric capacity, and motor detrusor overactivity with or without incontinence.

- Involuntary detrusor contractions may occur in the absence of symptoms, and thus these contractions may occur in the absence of the OAB syndrome.

- In patients with sustained involuntary elevations of detrusor storage pressure above baseline may represent a disorder of bladder compliance.

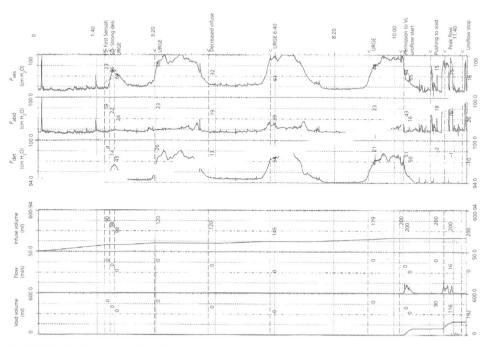

Figure 5.1 Detrusor overactivity without urinary incontinence. Note the rise in detrusor pressure (P_{det}) and vesical pressure (P_{ves}) without a rise in intra-abdominal pressure (P_{abd}). Increased sensation and urgency are noted at low fill volumes. This tracing also illustrates terminal DO. (For color detail, please see color plate section).

Does OAB equal urodynamic DO? A clinical correlation

OAB may either be a pure sensory or pure motor dysfunction, but also a combination of the two. A significant percentage of patients with OAB may have DO on UDS, but many do not. In fact, the most consistent symptom of OAB is urinary urgency with or without urgency incontinence. [11] In these cases, increased bladder sensation is a common finding with patients experiencing first sensation, normal desire, strong desire, and urgency at lower than anticipated filling volumes.

A large number of studies have tried to answer whether OAB symptoms equal urodynamic DO with varying results especially when evaluating DO in females versus males. A symptomatic diagnosis of OAB does not always correlate with urodynamic DO. [12] Digesu found that 18.7% (843) of 4500 women with lower urinary tract symptoms (LUTS) could be classified as having OAB; 54.2 % (457 of 843) of these women had urodynamic proven DO. Of the 4500 women undergoing urodynamic testing with LUTS, 36.5 % (1641) had urodynamic DO, but only 27.5% (457 of 1641) of these women had OAB symptoms. [13] The sensitivity and specificity of DO for OAB symptoms were 54 and 68% respectively. [13] On the other hand, symptoms of urge incontinence are strongly correlated with DO in men. A retrospective study of 139 adults noted a correlation between DO and OAB symptoms; 75% of males with OAB symptoms had DO on cytometrogram and only 36.8% of female patients. [14]

A study of 1457 adult male and female patients was retrospectively conducted based on OAB symptoms to determine how well the symptoms of OAB correlated with urodynamic DO using ISC definitions. Again, a better correlation in results between OAB symptoms and urodynamic DO was observed in men than in women. The authors concluded that the bladder is a better and more reliable witness in men than in women. [15]

KEY POINTS

- Patients with OAB tend to experience increased bladder sensations, experiencing first sensation, normal desire, strong desire, and urgency at lower than anticipated filling volumes.

- The symptomatic diagnosis of OAB does not always correlate with urodynamic DO.

- A better correlation in results between OAB symptoms and urodynamic DO is observed in men more than in women.

Pressure–flow studies and OAB

OAB and PFS: clinical correlation

The use of pressure–flow studies (PFS) to evaluate bladder emptying does not lead to a diagnosis of complex OAB symptoms. PFS are useful in identifying the mechanism of voiding, as to whether or not it is a function of normal bladder contractility. PFS allow bladder outlet obstruction to be differentiated from detrusor underactivity. High-pressure associated with low flow rates is diagnostic of functional or anatomic outlet obstruction. These disorders of bladder emptying may lead to OAB symptoms. Symptoms of urgency and frequency may improve following correction of bladder outlet obstruction (BOO) secondary to benign prostatic hypertrophy (BPH), post-sling obstruction, and prolapse. Thus, in these patients, should outlet obstruction be diagnosed by PFS, subsequent treatment may result in complete or near complete resolution of symptoms. [16] The AUA urodynamic guidelines also recommend pressure–flow studies in women with persistent symptoms following outlet procedures to evaluate for iatrogenic BOO. [7] Surgical intervention is recommended in this scenario due to the potential association of prolonged BOO and irreversible voiding dysfunction. [17] In appropriate patients with refractory OAB, PFS should be considered to evaluate for obstruction as treatment may be associated with symptom resolution.

KEY POINTS

- Pressure–flow studies allow bladder outlet obstruction to be differentiated from detrusor under activity.
- Disorders of bladder emptying may lead to OAB symptoms.
- In patients with refractory OAB, should PFS reveal obstruction, its subsequent treatment may result in complete or near complete resolution of symptoms

---

Video urodynamics

First described in the late 1960s, the use of fluoroscopy adds real-time, high-resolution anatomic details to a cystometrogram and pressure–flow study. [4] It allows structural-functional correlations to be investigated because transducer pressures, patients' symptoms, and live fluoroscopic images are studied simultaneously. The disadvantages are cost, radiation use, training, and personnel required to operate the equipment. [9] It provides for more detailed anatomic diagnosis of vesicoureteral reflux, detrusor–external sphincter dyssynergia (DESD), bladder diverticula, urinary fistula, and urethral leakage. These findings may then be correlated to OAB symptoms.

KEY POINT

- It allows structural-functional correlations to be investigated because transducer pressures, patients' symptoms, and live fluoroscopic images are studied simultaneously.

Ambulatory urodynamics

The technique was described by Abrams in 1997 and involves the recording of three micturition cycles; a resting cycle, an ambulant cycle, and an exercising cycle. [3] Ambulatory urodynamic monitoring is performed in an effort to observe more realistic or more physiological observations and should be considered when conventional cystometry is unable to reproduce the patient's symptoms and fails to provide a pathophysiologic explanation of the patients' symptoms.

Ambulatory urodynamic monitoring (AUM) is suggested to be more sensitive for detecting and quantifying uninhibited detrusor contractions than standard cystometry in various patient groups based on conventional cystometric criteria. [18] However, it remains a highly technical and labor-intensive study that clinically remains of little use in most centers. Heslington examined 22 asymptomatic healthy females and performed both conventional cystometry and ambulatory cystometry. DO was noted in 18% of patients by conventional cystometry and 68% on ambulatory monitoring. [19] AUM studies have shown a 30% incidence of DO in neurologically intact asymptomatic women. [3] These findings may also then be correlated to OAB symptoms.

KEY POINTS

- AUM is suggested to be more sensitive for detecting and quantifying uninhibited detrusor contractions than standard cystometry in various patient groups based on conventional cystometric criteria.
- AUM is a highly technical and labor-intensive study that clinically remains of little use in most centers.

Summary

Urodynamics may not be necessary in the evaluation of simple OAB symptoms, but it may provide critical information in the diagnosis and management of OAB and associated voiding dysfunction. In complicated urologic presentations, urodynamic evaluation is imperative and should be tailored to answer specific clinical questions. The clinician should then assess whether the study has answered the specific clinical questions. If the study has not adequately answered those questions, it may need to be repeated or adjusted. It is equally important to recall that not being able to reproduce a patient's symptoms does not rule out its existence. Urodynamic studies should be individualized and their application tailored to meet the unique needs of the patient. Multichannel UDS or an individual test component alone can provide invaluable information in clinical diagnosis, patient counseling, as well as medical and or surgical management.

References

1 Davis DM. *The Mechanism of Urology Disease.* Philadelphia: WB Saunders, 1953.
2 Kraklau DM, Bloom DA. The cystometrogram at 70 years. *J Urol.* 1998;**160**:316–319.

3 Karram MM, Walters MD. *Urogynecology and Reconstructive Pelvic Surgery*. 3rd edn. Philadelphia: Mosby, 2007: pp. 78–113.

4 Raz S, Robriquez L. *Urodynamics, Female Urology*. 3rd edn. Philadelphia: WB Saunders, 2008: pp. 140–153.

5 Nitt VW, Combs AJ. Urodynamics: When, why, and how. In N.H VW (ed.) *Practical Urodynamics*. Philadelphia: WB Saunders, 1998: pp: 15–26.

6 Winters JC, Appell RA. Urinary Incontinence and frequency and urgency syndromes in women. In Nitti VW (ed.) *Practical Urodynamics*. Philadelphia: WB Saunders, 1998: pp 184–196.

7 Winters JC, Dmochowski R, Goldman H, et al: Urodynamics studies in adults: AUA/SUFU Guideline. *J Urol.* 2012;**188**:2464–2472.

8 Abrams P, Cardozo L, Fall M, et al. The standardisation of terminology of lower urinary tract function: Report from the Standardisation Sub-Committee of the International Continence Society. *Neurourol Urodyn.* 2003;**21**:167–178.

9 Siddighi S, Hardesty J, *Urogynecology & Female Pelvis Reconstructive Surgery: Just the Facts*, 1st edn. McGraw Hill, 2006: pp: 49–68.

10 Mcguire EJ, Woodside JR, Borden TA, et al. Prognostic value of urodynamic testing in myelodysplastic patients. *J Urol.* 1981;**126**:205–209.

11 Abrams P, Wein AJ, et al. The overactive bladder: from basic science to clinical management. Consensus Conference. *Urology* 1997;**50**:Suppl: 1–114.

12 Hann-Chorng K. The role of urodynamic study in the evaluation and management of overactive bladder. *Incont Pelvic Floor Dysfunct.* 2008;**2**(3):95–97.

13 Digesu GA, Khullan V, Cardozo L et al. Overactive bladder symptoms: do we need urodynamics? *Neurourol Urodyn.* 2003;**22**:105–108.

14 Sekido N, Hinotsu S, Kawai K et al. How many uncomplicated male and female overactive bladder patients reveal detrusor overactivity during urodynamic study? *Int J Urol.* 2006;**13**(10):1276–1279.

15 Hashim H, Abrams P. Is the bladder a reliable witness for prediciting detrusor overactivty? *J Urol.* 2006:**175**(1):191–194; discussion 194–195.

16 de Boer TA, Salvatore S, Cardozo L, et al. Pelvic organ prolapse and overactive bladder. *Neurourol Urodyn.* 2010;**29**:30–39.

17 Leng WW, Davies BJ, Tarin T. Delayed treatment of bladder outlet obstruction after sling surgery: association with irreversible bladder dysfunction. *J Urol.* 2004;**172**: 1379–1381.

18 Oh SJ, Son H, Jeong JY, Ku JH. Patients experience with ambulatory urodynamics. *A prospective study. Scand J Urol Nephrol.* 2006; **40**(5):391–396.

19 Heslington K, Hilton P. Ambulatory monitoring and conventional cystoscopy in asymptomatic female volunteers. *Br J Obstet Gynaecol.* 1996;**103**(5):434–441.

CHAPTER 6

Other testing

Hessel Wijkstra and Lara C. Gerbrandy-Schreuders

Department of Urology, AMC University Hospital, Amsterdam, The Netherlands

---

KEY POINTS

- Most probably, myogenic and neurogenic functions play a role in lower urinary (dys-)function.
- Non-invasive tests to diagnose overactive bladder and detrusor overactive bladder are under development and clinical validation.
- The most promising non-invasive tests for clinical diagnosis are detrusor/bladder wall thickness and biomarkers.
- Functional MRI and other functional brain imaging techniques reveal the involvement of the central nervous system in lower urinary (dys-)function.
- Near infrared spectroscopy and bladder strain imaging are new techniques that need further clinical validation.

This chapter discusses non-invasive techniques for diagnosis of overactive bladder (OAB) and detrusor overactivity (DO). In clinical practice the diagnosis of OAB is mostly based on subjective information. DO is assessed by a urodynamic investigation which is invasive and not very reliable. A poor correlation was demonstrated between symptoms and urodynamic findings. [1]

Bladder/detrusor wall thickness

It is assumed that DO is associated with bladder wall hypertrophy. [2] Ultrasound is a non-invasive imaging technique that can visualize the bladder or detrusor wall with high accuracy. Detrusor wall thickness (DWT) includes the detrusor muscle only, while bladder wall thickness (BWT) includes all three layers of the bladder wall. The measurement is poorly standardized with regard to the measurement position, bladder filling, if BWT or DWT should be used, and threshold. [3] Experts do agree that high frequency ultrasound is essential for an accurate measurement. Because the bladder/detrusor wall becomes thinner when bladder volume increases, measurements should be performed at a well-defined bladder volume. Three different anatomical approaches have been

---

Overactive Bladder: Practical Management, First Edition. Edited by Jacques Corcos, Scott MacDiarmid and John Heesakkers.

described: transvaginal, translabial/transperineal, and suprapubic.

In women, the transvaginal approach is considered the most reliable method because of the small distance between the ultrasound probe and the bladder wall. [4] In most studies, bladder wall thickness measurements are performed with an empty bladder (<50 ml) at three locations: trigone, anterior wall, and dome. [5] The mean value of the three measurements is used as the BWT value which proved a sensitive method for diagnosing DO. [4, 6] In a recent study, a BWT value of 6.5 mm had a 100% positive predictive value for DO. [7] BWT values do differ between studies and methods are not standardized. Only a few studies did not find a relation between DWT or BWT and DO. [8, 9] The first study used DWT and the second measured the thickness at the trigone only. BWT also correlates with OAB symptoms. [10]

Data regarding the translabial/transperineal approached are scarce. DWT measured as the mean value of the trigone, anterior wall, and dome thickness, was 4.7 mm in the DO group versus 4.1 mm in non-DO subjects resulting in a poor sensitivity. [11] The larger distance between the ultrasound probe and bladder as compared to the transvaginal approach can influence measurement accuracy.

The suprapubic approach has been described for measuring bladder outlet obstruction in men. [12] Few data regarding DO diagnosis have been published. DWT was measured in a study comparing the values between OAB and without OAB [13] and no statistical differences were found. The authors conclude that the technique should not be recommended for diagnosing DO.

A few studies compared the three different anatomical approaches. Kuhn et al. found significant differences between the different measurement locations, [14] demonstrating that the three approaches cannot be compared.

In conclusion, the most promising and reliable technique to measure BWT in women is the transvaginal approach and studies have shown reproducible results for diagnosing OAB and DO in women. Data regarding the other approaches are scarce. Standardization of the technique is lacking. [3] Prospective well-standardized studies are needed to determine the value of DWT/BWT in routine clinical practice.

Biomarkers

The definition of a biomarker is a "characteristic that is objectively measured and evaluated as an indicator of normal biological processes, pathogenic processes, or pharmacologic responses to a therapeutic intervention." [15] There are multiple potential targets of opportunity to use a biomarker: as a clinical tool for diagnosis and staging of disease, as an indicator of prognosis, or as an application for prediction and monitoring clinical response to an intervention. [15] Ideally, a biomarker is easily accessible, reliable, and reproducible with a high level of specificity and sensitivity, adding extra information to the clinical assessment and improving outcome. [16, 17]

The classic overactive bladder (OAB) biomarker is detrusor overactivity (DO), assessed by urodynamic investigation. A poor correlation was demonstrated between symptoms and urodynamic findings. [1] In clinical practice the diagnosis of OAB is mostly made on subjective information. Urinary biomarkers for OAB could therefore improve diagnostic accuracy and assist in monitoring treatment response. At this moment, neurotrophic factors NGF (nerve growth factor) and to a lesser extent BDNF (brain-derived neurothrophic factor) seem to be emerging as key players in bladder pathophysiology and are potential OAB biomarker candidates. NGF is a tissue-derived trophic factor involved in the development of bladder innervation and an important regulator of neuronal function along micturition pathways. [18] The role of brain-derived neurotrophic factor (BDNF) is less clear, but seems important in inflammation and nociception. [19] Both NGF and BDNF are expressed in urothelium and detrusor, and bind to tyrosine kinase (Trk) receptors, cell-surface transmembrane glycoproteins fully expressed in bladder urothelial cells, and sensory neurons innervating the bladder wall. [18, 20]

Biomarkers for OAB
NGF
Multiple studies demonstrated an increased NGF production in the lower urinary tract in pathologic conditions, that is OAB-wet (urgency urinary incontinence), urodynamic DO, mixed urinary incontinence, and bladder outlet obstruction. [21] In a rat model with neurogenic DO after spinal cord injury or with cyclophosphamide-induced cystitis and overactivity, NGF was elevated in the dorsal root ganglia, spinal cord, and bladder. [22] Chronic administration of NGF into the bladder or spinal cord of rats induced bladder hyperactivity and increased firing frequency of bladder efferent neurons. [23–25] When administering a NGF

sequestering molecule, the bladder over-activity in an experimental cystitis model reduced. [26]

Urinary NGF levels in patients with OAB are significantly higher compared to controls. [21, 27, 28] Intensity of urgency seems to be correlated with the urinary NGF concentration [21, 29]. However, not all OAB patients had elevated urinary NGF levels, which was up to 30% in some cohorts. [30] Reduction in urinary NGF levels was found in OAB patients after initiating antimuscarinic drug therapy, which was reversed after cessation of therapy. [30, 31] In patients with DO who underwent onabotulinum toxin A detrusor injections, the urinary NGF levels dropped significantly. [32]

BDNF
Most evidence for the role of BDNF in bladder dysfunction is in studies about pain and cystitis. Experimental models showed an increase in TrKB receptor expression and urinary BDNF after bladder inflammation or spinal cord injury. [33–35] Another animal study assessed the relevance of BDNF to bladder overactivity and pain in cystitis, with sequestration of BDNF leading to bladder function improvement. [36]

In a recent observational study, the BDNF/creatinine ratio (pg/mg) was significantly lower in 40 healthy volunteers compared to 17 patients with OAB. [26] A higher area under the curve (AUC) in a receiver–operator characteristic (ROC) analysis was found for BDNF (0.78) compared to NGF (0.68). [37].

Prostaglandins
Prostaglandins play a role in regulating lower urinary tract function. [38] Detrusor

muscle stretch, bladder nerve stimulation, urothelial damage, or inflammation triggers prostaglandin synthesis in the bladder muscle and mucosa. [28] Intravesical instillation of prostaglandin E2 (PGE2) induced detrusor contraction in rats. [39] There is conflicting evidence of urinary PGE2 levels in OAB patients. [28, 40] More studies are necessary to define the role of prostaglandins in bladder (patho) physiology.

Cytokines, chemokines, and growth factors

Cytokines and chemokines could affect neurotransmitter metabolism in micturition. Levels of seven urinary cytokines, chemokines, and growth factors were found to be significantly increased in OAB patients compared to controls. [41] These urinary markers are involved in tissue repair and inflammation and their elevation in OAB patients points toward an inflammatory etiology in OAB. Further studies are necessary to define their role in bladder (patho)physiology.

C-reactive protein

C-reactive protein (CRP) is a general serum marker for inflammation and infection. An association between CRP and OAB was demonstrated in a large population-based epidemiologic survey. [42] Serum CRP levels were found to be significantly raised in a study with patients with OAB and IC/BPS compared to controls. [43] Another study also demonstrated this finding in OAB patients, but urinary CRP levels and mRNA expression of CRP in bladder biopsies were not raised. [44] The specificity as a OAB biomarker is quite low as

serum CRP is raised in many medical conditions.

Genetic biomarkers

OAB susceptibility genes are possible biomarkers, as twin studies have suggested. [45, 46] Investigating the possibility of using peripheral blood mononuclear cells using microarray analysis, 16 genes were identified as being differentially regulated in OAB patients compared to healthy controls. [47] Further studies should be done to elucidate the possibility of genetics as OAB biomarkers.

Conclusion

Accumulating evidence has shown the involvement of NGF and BDNF in sensory neural bladder function, and their role in bladder diseases like OAB, idiopathic and neurogenic DO, IC/BPS, and bladder outflow obstruction. However, to confirm the potential role of NGF and BDNF as OAB biomarkers, several issues should be resolved. Large multicenter trials must increase the generalizability of the results. There should be standardization in interpretation, laboratory preparation, as well as urine collection, as bladder volume can possibly influence outcome. [16, 48] Furthermore, there should be validation of the test. The finding of increased urinary NGF levels in bladder diseases other than OAB lowers its specificity as an OAB biomarker. Sensitivity is also questioned, as up to 30% of OAB patients did not show a urinary NGF level increase. Finally, cost-effectiveness data are lacking. [16] All these issues have to be resolved, and until then it is unclear whether urinary NGF and BDNF will find clinical application as a biomarker in the future.

Near infrared spectroscopy

Near infrared spectroscopy (NIRS) is an optical technique that detects hemodynamic changes during bladder filling and voiding. Near-infrared light can penetrate the skin and underlying tissue layers and it is possible to monitor hemodynamic changes in the bladder wall. [49, 50] Near-infrared light is absorbed by oxyhemoglobin (O_2Hb) and de-oxyhemoglobin (HHb). Total hemoglobin (Hb_{sum}) is an indicator of total blood perfusion and can be derived from the sum of O_2Hb and HHb. Involuntary bladder contractions are believed to cause variations in, for example, oxygen supply and may cause changes that can be detected by NIRS. Farag et al. demonstrated that transcutaneous near infrared spectroscopy can detect DO episodes with a high sensitivity. [51] They included 34 men and 7 women with OAB symptoms in a study comparing NIRS with cystometry. Three observers rated the NIRS curves as predictors for DO as measured with cystometry. NIRS had a "substantial" intraobserver agreement and was highly sensitive in detecting DO episodes; 92% for HB_{sum}.

The main problems of the technique are motion artifacts, including movements of the bladder wall, and difficulty in detecting changes in patients with a thick abdominal wall. In fact, Farag et al. excluded approximately one quarter of all measurement parts because of motion artifacts. [51] They also found approximately 18% false positives in controls without detrusor overactivity. In conclusion, near infrared spectroscopy correlates well with urodynamic findings and therefore it is a potential non-invasive new diagnostic tool for detecting detrusor overactivity in OAB patients. However, before it

can be introduced in the clinical environment, especially the problem of motion artifacts should be solved. Last but not least, the technique should be validated in larger, preferably multicenter studies.

Bladder wall strain imaging

A recently introduced technique measures the activity of the bladder wall activity with radiofrequency ultrasound strain imaging. [52, 53] Radiofrequency (RF) ultrasound is used to estimate the deformation (strain) in the bladder wall. Idzenga et al. examined the value of this technique in volunteers and in a BOO patient undergoing a urodynamic investigation. [53] Contraction of the detrusor and flow-rate influenced the measured strain. Also during an increase in detrusor pressure without flow (isovolumetric contraction) a correlation was found. Movement artifacts are still a problem; however this could be solved by using 3D ultrasound in combination with movement correction techniques. Future studies should provide evidence of whether this technique is sensitive enough to detect DO in OAB patients.

Autonomic nervous system

The pathophysiology of idiopathic OAB remains unclear and next to myogenic also neurogenic dysfunction is a possible cause. It is stated that in OAB persons the parasympathetic fibers remain stimulated after bladder emptying and this causes the bladder to contract during the filling phase. These fibers are part of the autonomic nervous system (ANS). [54] In practice, it is difficult to quantify the activity of the ANS. However, a direct relationship between heart rate variability and parasympathetic effects has been reported. [54] Hubeaux et al. found that heart rate variability did not change during bladder filling in stress urinary incontinence; however, the sympathetic tone in women with OAB did change significantly at the end of the bladder filling. [55] Comparable results were found by Liao et al. [54] They concluded that by quantifying heart rate variability, their analysis technique could provide a simple, non-invasive test to assess disturbances in ANS activity.

Functional brain imaging

Functional brain imaging techniques are used to investigate the activity changes of brain regions that are involved in bladder control. [56] The presence or absence of certain activations and deactivations can reflect the ability or inability of the central nervous system (CNS) to suppress, for example, DO and to prevent incontinence. [57] Griffiths et al. and Tadic et al. investigated functional magnetic resonance imaging (fMRI) in normal and overactive bladders. [57, 58] Differences in activation and deactivations were demonstrated when comparing normal and OAB subjects, suggesting that abnormalities in CNS activation patterns may play a role in OAB and other bladder control problems.

Conclusions

Control of lower urinary tract function is a complex system in which most probably myogenic and neurogenic functions both play an important role. Dysfunction, for example OAB and DO, can be caused by several parts of this complex system. Most invasive and non-invasive tests measure changes of the bladder wall. Over the last decade more and more information has become available that neurological systems do play an important role.

The testing methods described in this chapter are mainly focused on replacing the invasive urodynamic investigation with more non-invasive tests. At this moment, detrusor/bladder wall thickness and bio-markers are the most promising techniques that could play a role in clinical diagnosis in the future. fMRI and other functional brain imaging techniques will bring us more important information regarding the involvement of the CNS in lower urinary function. NIRS and strain imaging are techniques under development. More studies are needed to provide us with information about the usefulness of these new techniques.

References

1 Hashim H, Abrams P. Is the bladder a reliable witness for predicting detrusor overactivity? *J Urol.* 2006;**175**(1):191–194, discussion194–195.

2 Cartwright R, Afshan I, Derpapas A, et al. Novel biomarkers for overactive bladder. *Nat Rev Urol.* 2011;**8**(3):139–145.

3 Oelke M. International Consultation on Incontinence-Research Society (ICI-RS) report on non-invasive urodynamics: the need of standardization of ultrasound bladder and detrusor wall thickness measurements to quantify bladder wall hypertrophy. *Neurourol Urodyn.* 2010;**29**(4): 634–639.

4 Oelke M, Khullar V, Wijkstra H. Review on ultrasound measurement of bladder or detrusor wall thickness in women: techniques, diagnostic utility, and use in clinical trials. *World J Urol.* 2013;**31**(4):823–827.

5 Khullar V, Salvatore S, Cardozo L, et al. A novel technique for measuring bladder wall thickness in women using transvaginal ultrasound. *Ultrasound Obstet Gynecol.* 1994;**4**(3): 220–223.

6 Khullar V, Cardozo LD, Salvatore S, Hill S. Ultrasound: a noninvasive screening test for detrusor instability. *Br J Obstet Gynaecol.* 1996;**103**(9):904–908.

7 Serati M, Salvatore S, Cattoni E, et al. Ultrasound measurement of bladder wall thickness in different forms of detrusor overactivity. *Int Urogynecol J Pelvic Floor Dysfunct.* 2010;**21**(11):1405–1411.

8 Yang J-M, Huang W-C. Bladder wall thickness on ultrasonographic cystourethrography: affecting factors and their implications. *J Ultrasound Med.* 2003;**22**(8):777–782.

9 Kuo H-C. Measurement of detrusor wall thickness in women with overactive bladder by transvaginal and transabdominal sonography. *Int Urogynecol J Pelvic Floor Dysfunct.* 2009;**20**(11):1293–1299.

10 Panayi DC, Khullar V, Fernando R, Tekkis P. Transvaginal ultrasound measurement of bladder wall thickness: a more reliable approach than transperineal and transabdominal approaches. *BJU Int.* 2010;**106**(10):1519–1522.

11 Lekskulchai O, Dietz HP. Detrusor wall thickness as a test for detrusor overactivity in women. *Ultrasound Obstet Gynecol.* 2008;**32**(4): 535–539.

12 Oelke M, Höfner K, Jonas U, et al. Diagnostic accuracy of noninvasive tests to evaluate bladder outlet obstruction in men: detrusor wall thickness, uroflowmetry, postvoid residual urine, and prostate volume. *Eur Urol.* 2007;**52**(3):827–834.

13 Chung S-D, Chiu B, Kuo H-C, et al. Transabdominal ultrasonography of detrusor wall thickness in women with overactive bladder. *BJU Int.* 2010;**105**(5):668–672.

14 Kuhn A, Bank S, Robinson D, Klimek M et al. How should bladder wall thickness be measured? A comparison of vaginal, perineal and abdominal ultrasound. *Neurourol Urodyn.* 2010;**29**(8):1393–1396.

15 Biomarkers Definitions Working Group. Biomarkers and surrogate endpoints: preferred definitions and conceptual framework. *Clin Pharmacol Ther.* 2001;**69**(3):89–95.

16 Seth JH, Sahai A, Khan MS, et al. Nerve growth factor (NGF): a potential urinary biomarker for overactive bladder syndrome (OAB)? *BJU Int.* 2013;**111**(3):372–380.

17 Mayeux R. Biomarkers: potential uses and limitations. *NeuroRx.* 2004;**1**(2):182–188.

18 Ochodnický P, Cruz CD, Yoshimura N, Michel MC. Nerve growth factor in bladder dysfunction: contributing factor, biomarker, and therapeutic target. *Neurourol Urodyn.* 2011;**30**(7):1227–1241.

19 Zhao J, Seereeram A, Nassar MA, et al. Nociceptor-derived brain-derived neurotrophic factor regulates acute and inflammatory but not neuropathic pain. *Molecular and Cellular Neuroscience.* 2006 Mar;**31**(3):539–548.

20 Allen SJ, Dawbarn D. Clinical relevance of the neurotrophins and their receptors. *Clin Sci.* 2006;**110**(2):175–191.

21 Liu H-T, Chen C-Y, Kuo H-C. Urinary nerve growth factor in women with overactive bladder syndrome. *BJU Int.* 2011;**107**(5):799–803.

22 Vizzard MA. Changes in urinary bladder neurotrophic factor mRNA and NGF protein following urinary bladder dysfunction. *Exp Neurol.* 2000;**161**(1):273–284.

23 Yoshimura N, Bennett NE, Hayashi Y, et al. Bladder overactivity and hyperexcitability of bladder afferent neurons after intrathecal delivery of nerve growth factor in rats. *J Neurosci.* 2006;**26**(42):10847–10855.

24 Lamb K, Gebhart GF, Bielefeldt K. Increased nerve growth factor expression triggers bladder overactivity. *J Pain.* 2004;**5**(3):150–156.

25 Zvara P, Vizzard MA. Exogenous overexpression of nerve growth factor in the urinary bladder produces bladder overactivity and altered micturition circuitry in the lumbosacral spinal cord. *BMC Physiol.* 2007;**7**:9.

26 Hu VY, Zvara P, Dattilio A, et al. Decrease in bladder overactivity with REN1820 in rats with cyclophosphamide induced cystitis. *J Urol.* 2005;**173**(3):1016–1021.

27 Yokoyama T, Kumon H, Nagai A. Correlation of urinary nerve growth factor level with pathogenesis of overactive bladder. *Neurourol Urodyn.* 2008;**27**(5):417–420.

28 Kim JC, Park EY, Seo SI, et al. Nerve growth factor and prostaglandins in the urine of female patients with overactive bladder. *J Urol.* 2006;**175**(5):1773–1776, discussion 1776.

29 Kuo H-C, Liu H-T, Chancellor MB. Can urinary nerve growth factor be a biomarker for overactive bladder? *Rev Urol.* 2010;**12**(2–3):e69–77.

30 Liu H-T, Chancellor MB, Kuo H-C. Decrease of urinary nerve growth factor levels after antimuscarinic therapy in patients with overactive bladder. *BJU Int.* 2009; **103**(12):1668–1672.

31 Liu H-T, Kuo H-C. Urinary nerve growth factor levels are increased in patients with bladder outlet obstruction with overactive bladder symptoms and reduced after successful medical treatment. *Urology* 2008;**72**(1):104–108, discussion108.

32 Liu H-T, Chancellor MB, Kuo H-C. Urinary nerve growth factor levels are elevated in patients with detrusor overactivity and decreased in responders to detrusor botulinum toxin-A injection. *Eur Urol.* 2009;**56**(4):700–706.

33 Qiao L-Y, Vizzard MA. Cystitis-induced upregulation of tyrosine kinase (TrkA, TrkB) receptor expression and phosphorylation in rat micturition pathways. *J Comp Neurol.* 2002;**454**(2):200–211.

34 Qiao L, Vizzard MA. Up-regulation of tyrosine kinase (Trka, Trkb) receptor expression and phosphorylation in lumbosacral dorsal root ganglia after chronic spinal cord (T8-T10) injury. *J Comp Neurol.* 2002;**449**(3):217–230.

35 Qiao L-Y, Vizzard MA. Spinal cord injury-induced expression of TrkA, TrkB, phosphorylated CREB, and c-Jun in rat lumbosacral dorsal root ganglia. *J Comp Neurol.* 2005;**482**(2):142–154.

36 Pinto R, Frias B, Allen S, et al. Sequestration of brain derived nerve factor by intravenous delivery of TrkB-Ig2 reduces bladder overactivity and noxious input in animals with chronic cystitis. *Neuroscience* 2010;**166**(3):907–916.

37 Antunes-Lopes T, Carvalho-Barros S, Cruz C-D, et al. Biomarkers in overactive bladder: a new objective and noninvasive tool? *Adv Urol.* 2011;**2011**:382431.

38 Mikhailidis DP, Jeremy JY, Dandona P. Urinary bladder prostanoids – their synthesis, function and possible role in the pathogenesis and treatment of disease. *J Urol.* 1987;**37**(3):577–582.

39 Yokoyama O, Miwa Y, Oyama N, et al. Antimuscarinic drug inhibits detrusor overactivity induced by topical application of prostaglandin E2 to the urethra with a decrease in urethral pressure. *J Urol.* 2007;**178**(5):2208–2212.

40 Liu H-T, Tyagi P, Chancellor MB, Kuo H-C. Urinary nerve growth factor but not prostaglandin E2 increases in patients with interstitial cystitis/bladder pain syndrome and detrusor overactivity. *BJU Int.* 2010;**106**(11):1681–1685.

41 Tyagi P, Barclay D, Zamora R, et al. Urine cytokines suggest an inflammatory response in the overactive bladder: a pilot study. *Int Urol Nephrol.* 2010;**42**(3):629–635.

42 Kupelian V, McVary KT, Barry MJ, et al. Association of C-reactive protein and lower urinary tract symptoms in men and women: results from Boston Area Community Health survey. *Urology.* 2009;**73**(5):950–957.

43 Chung S-D, Liu H-T, Lin H, Kuo H-C. Elevation of serum c-reactive protein in patients with OAB and IC/BPS implies chronic inflammation in the urinary bladder. *Neurourol Urodyn.* 2011;**30**(3):417–420.

44 Chuang Y-C, Tyagi V, Liu R-T, Chancellor MB, Tyagi P. Urine and serum c-reactive protein levels as potential biomarkers of lower urinary tract symptoms. *Urolog Sci.* 2010;**21**(3): 132–136.

45 Wennberg A-L, Altman D, Lundholm C, et al. Genetic influences are important for most but not all lower urinary tract symptoms: a population-based survey in a cohort of adult swedish twins. *Eur Urol.* 2011;**59**(6): 1032–1038.

46 Rohr G, Kragstrup J, Gaist D, Christensen K. Genetic and environmental influences on urinary incontinence: a Danish population-based twin study of middle-aged and elderly women. *Acta Obstet Gynecol Scand.* 2004;**83**(10):978–982.

47 Cheung W, Bluth MJ, Johns C, Khan S, Lin YY, Bluth MH. Peripheral blood mononuclear cell gene array profiles in patients with overactive bladder. *Urology.* 2010;**75**(4):896–901.

48 Kuo H-C, Liu H-T, Chancellor MB. Urinary nerve growth factor is a better biomarker than detrusor wall thickness for the assessment of overactive bladder with incontinence. *Neurourol Urodyn.* 2010;**29**(3):482–487 .

49 Macnab AJ, Stothers L. Development of a near-infrared spectroscopy instrument for applications in urology. *Can J Urol.* 2008;**15**(5):4233–4240.

50 Macnab AJ, Stothers L. Near-infrared spectroscopy: validation of bladder-outlet obstruction assessment using non-invasive parameters. *Can J Urol.* 2008;**15**(5):4241–4248.

51 Farag FF, Martens FM, D'Hauwers KW, et al. Near-infrared spectroscopy: a novel, noninvasive, diagnostic method for detrusor overactivity in patients with overactive bladder symptoms--a preliminary and experimental study. *Eur Urol.* 2011;**59**(5):757–762.

52 Idzenga T, Farag F, Heesakkers J, et al. Noninvasive measurement of bladder muscle activity using radiofrequency ultrasound strain imaging. Ultrasonics Symposium (IUS), 2011 IEEE International. 2011:2229–2232.

53 Idzenga T, Farag F, Heesakkers J, et al. Noninvasive 2-dimensional monitoring of strain in the detrusor muscle in patients with lower urinary tract symptoms using ultrasound strain imaging. *J Urol.* 2013;**189**(4): 1402–1408.

54 Liao W-C, Jaw F-S. A noninvasive evaluation of autonomic nervous system dysfunction in women with an overactive bladder. *Int J Gynaecol Obstet.* 2010;**110**(1):12–17.

55 Hubeaux K, Deffieux X, Ismael SS, et al. Autonomic nervous system activity during bladder filling assessed by heart rate variability analysis in women with idiopathic overactive bladder syndrome or stress urinary incontinence. *J Urol.* 2007;**178**(6):2483–2487.

56 Blok BF, Willemsen AT, Holstege G. A PET study on brain control of micturition in humans. *Brain.* 1997;**120** (Pt 1):111–121.

57 Tadic SD, Griffiths D, Schaefer W, et al. Brain activity underlying impaired continence control in older women with overactive bladder. *Neurourol Urodyn.* 2012;**31**(5):652–658.

58 Griffiths D, Derbyshire S, Stenger A, Resnick N. Brain control of normal and overactive bladder. *J Urol.* 2005;**174**(5):1862–1867.

SECTION 3
First Line Management

CHAPTER 7

Changes in lifestyle

Diane K. Newman

Division of Urology, University of Pennsylvania Medical Center, Philadelphia, PA, USA

KEY POINTS

- Evidence-based research indicates that modification of certain lifestyle practices can improve lower urinary tract symptoms.
- Lifestyle changes involve elimination of dietary irritants, managing fluid intake, weight control, bowel regularity, and smoking cessation.
- Weight loss improves lower urinary tract symptoms in overweight women.
- Controlling extreme amounts of daily fluid intake and eliminating bladder irritants from the diet can improve bladder urgency and frequency.

Introduction

Epidemiological studies have shown that lower urinary tract symptoms (LUTS), including urinary incontinence (UI) and overactive bladder (OAB), are commonly seen in adult men and women. According to evidence-based research and guidelines, lifestyle changes are effective and recommended as first-line treatment for LUTS. Lifestyle changes are aimed at improving symptoms through modifications, including the establishment of elimination of bladder irritants from the diet, fluid intake management, weight control, management of bowel regularity, and smoking cessation. The ultimate goal is for the patient to adopt specific strategies that will eliminate symptoms. These interventions are one component of conservative management as they improve symptoms through identification of lifestyle habits and changing a person's behavior, environment, or activity that are contributing factors or triggers of LUTS. [1–3] They can be initiated after simple assessment in many patients and should be considered the mainstay of care of men and women with voiding and pelvic floor disorders. They have a large body of evidence-based research [4] and have been recommended as treatment for UI and non-neurogenic OAB by multiple organizations [5, 6] and international guidelines. [4]

Overactive Bladder: Practical Management, First Edition. Edited by Jacques Corcos, Scott MacDiarmid and John Heesakkers.

© 2015 John Wiley & Sons, Ltd. Published 2015 by John Wiley & Sons, Ltd.

Lifestyle modifications

The lifestyle practices that contribute to LUTS and are modifiable include:
- Smoking cessation.
- Weight reduction.
- Extremes of daily fluid intake.
- Dietary bladder irritants.
- Constipation and straining during defecation.

Obesity

Obesity, defined as a body mass index $\geq 30 \text{kg/m}^2$ in adults by the National Institutes of Health, is an independent and modifiable risk factor for LUTS in women and men. There is a growing amount of research, including several systematic reviews, demonstrating positive association between body mass index (BMI) > 25 and stress UI (SUI) and a high risk factor for urinary tract symptoms including urgency, frequency, OAB, and urgency UI (UUI). [7–9] There is evidence that obesity increases intra-abdominal pressure, places strain and stress on the pelvic floor structures, leading to weakening of the pelvic floor muscle, nerves, and blood vessels, while coexisting metabolic syndrome predisposes to urgency UI. The resultant impact on vascular perfusion and neural innervation may be the cause of OAB symptoms and incontinence. Also, increases in waist circumference are associated with new incidence or progression of current UI.

In a secondary analysis of a population-representative, cross-sectional Internet survey of 30 000 men and women in the US, UK, and Sweden, conducted to assess the prevalence, resulting bother, and health-related quality of life impact of LUTS, found that those men and women who were overweight (BMI 25.0–29.9) or obese (BMI > 30) were significantly more likely to report incontinence symptoms than those with a BMI in the normal range (BMI 14.0–24.9). [10] Women were more likely to report any UI, and, in particular, SUI, and men were more likely to report other forms of incontinence, such as post-micturition leakage.

So what is the impact of weight loss? Weight loss through lifestyle modification and bariatric surgery improves stress UI. [11, 12] Subak et al. [13] conducted a six-month lifestyle behavioral weight loss treatment and outcomes included reduced frequency of self-reported UI episodes (mean weekly reduction of 47%) among overweight and obese women as compared with a control group (28%) and reduced UUI episodes by 42% (compared with 26% in control group). Even moderate weight loss of 5–10% of body weight can decrease UI episodes as much as 50–60% and is sustainable over a 12-month period. [14, 15] Wasserberg et al. [16] demonstrated that morbidly obese women who undergo bariatric surgery and achieve significant weight loss experience a decrease in LUTS, and Burgio and colleagues [17] noted that 71% of women who lost 18 or more BMI points regained continence.

So the message for clinicians is that men and women who maintain a healthy weight in the normal BMI range may be able to reduce their risk for developing UI, and those who undergo moderate to extreme weight loss may be able to decrease their episodes of UI. As there is ample evidence-based research to support recommendations of weight loss, as part of lifestyle interventions in obese patients, clinicians should encourage overweight men and women with LUTS to lose weight.[18]

Smoking

Previous and current cigarette smoking increase the risk of both SUI and UUI with heavy smokers having the highest risk. [7, 19] Smoking over time eventually leads to chronic coughing which causes increased intra-abdominal pressure, directly increasing the pressure in the bladder. Usually, the sphincter muscle is able to contract tightly to avoid leakage of urine. However, it is felt that persons who cough repetitively cause downward pressure on the pelvic floor causing repeated stretch injury to the pudendal and pelvic nerves and weakening the ligaments of the pelvic floor muscles that support the external sphincter, and incontinence, specifically stress UI, can occur. Nicotine may contribute to detrusor contractions and tobacco products have anti-estrogenic hormonal effects that may impact the production of collagen synthesis.

No data has been reported examining whether smoking cessation in women resolves incontinence. But stopping smoking is a health benefit for many reasons so clinicians should educate women who smoke on the relationship between smoking and UI and strategies designed to discourage women from smoking are often suggested.

Extremes of daily fluid intake

Individuals may subscribe to either restrictive or excessive fluid intake behavior. Working women report fluid intake limitations and avoidance of caffeinated beverages as strategies to avoid urinary symptoms. [20] On the other end of the spectrum, women who diet and exercise go through the day carrying a water bottle. So over or under-hydration can contribute to LUTS. Adequate fluid intake is needed to eliminate irritants from the bladder. Under-hydration may play a role in the development of urinary tract infections and decrease the functional capacity of the bladder. Surveys of community residing elders with LUTS report self-care practices to include the self-imposed restrictions of fluids, as they fear UI, urinary urgency, and frequency. [21, 22] Excessive fluid intake can also be a problem as large volume intake can trigger incontinence and OAB symptoms of urgency and frequency. [23] Fluid intake averaging >3700 ml/day has been associated with a higher voiding frequency and incidence of UI compared with an intake of approximately 2400 ml/day. [4] Hashim and Abrams [24] recommend decreasing fluid intake by 25% to reduce frequency, urgency, and nocturia, provided baseline consumption is not less than one liter a day, and that increasing fluid intake by 25 and 50% can result in a worsening of daytime frequency.

What is not known is the ideal daily fluid intake. The general health recommendation is an intake of eight servings of 8-ounce glasses of water per day, yet no scientific or medical basis for this recommendation can be found in the literature. The Institute of Medicine issued a report in 2004 with guidelines for total water intake for healthy people. [25] That recommendation for women was 2.7 liters per day, but was intended to include water consumed both through beverages and food. This food vs. fluid component has been a source of confusion for the public and professionals alike, with a misperception of fluid source as only deriving from beverage intake.

Fluid intake should be regulated to 30 cc/kg body weight per day with a 1500 ml/day minimum at designated times unless contraindicated by a medical condition.

In older adults, there appears to be a strong relationship between evening fluid intake, nocturia, and nocturnal voided volume. Aging causes an increase in nocturia, defined as the number of voids recorded from the time the individual goes to bed with the intention of going to sleep, to the time the individual wakes with the intention of rising. To decrease nocturia precipitated by drinking fluids primarily in the evening or with dinner, the patient is instructed to reduce fluid intake after 6 pm and shift intake towards the morning and afternoon. [26, 27] Wagg [28] recommends that late afternoon administration of a diuretic may reduce nocturia in persons with lower extremity venous insufficiency or congestive heart failure unresponsive to other interventions.

Dietary bladder irritants

Common dietary staples can cause diuresis or bladder irritability contributing to LUTS. Caffeine intake has been associated with LUTS in both men [29] and women [30]. Caffeine is an ingredient found in certain beverages, foods, and medications and is felt to impact urinary symptoms by causing a significant rise in detrusor pressure and an excitatory effect on detrusor contraction. Daily oral caffeine (150 mg/kg) results in detrusor overactivity and increased bladder sensory signaling

in the mouse. [31] The consumption of caffeinated beverages, foods, and medications should not be underestimated. In the USA, over 80% of the adult population consumes caffeine in the form of coffee, tea, soft drinks, and energy drinks on a daily basis. The Boston Area Community Health (BACH) [32] reported on beverage intake and LUTS in a large cohort ($n = 4144$). Women who increased coffee intake by at least two servings/day had 64% higher odds of progression of urgency ($p = 0.003$). Women who had recently increased soda intake, particularly caffeinated diet soda, had higher symptom scores of urgency and LUTS progression. Greater coffee or total caffeine intake at baseline increased the odds of LUTS (storage symptoms) progression in men (coffee: >two cups/day vs. none, odds ratio = 2.09, 95% confidence interval: 1.29, 3.40, p-trend = 0.01; caffeine: p-trend < 0.001). Citrus juice intake was associated with 50% lower odds of LUTS progression in men ($p = 0.02$). Lohsiriwat [33] (2011) found that caffeine at a dose of 4.5 mg/kg caused diuresis and decreased the threshold of bladder sensation at filling phase, with an increase in flow rate and voided volume. Nocturia was also found to be associated with caffeine consumption, especially if caffeine was consumed in the evening hours.

Other findings suggest that high but not lower caffeine intake is associated with a modest increase in the incidence of frequent UUI. [34] It has been postulated that a fourth of the cases with the highest caffeine consumption would be eliminated if high caffeine intake were eliminated. [35] Confirmation of these findings in other studies is needed before recommendations can be made.

Assessment of daily caffeine intake on all patients with UI and OAB and instructions on the correlation between symptoms and caffeine intake is integral to clinical practice. It is recommended that patients with incontinence and OAB avoid excessive caffeine intake (e.g., no more than 200 mg/day, two cups).

In addition to caffeine, alcohol is also felt to have a diuretic effect that can lead to increased frequency. Anecdotal evidence suggests that eliminating dietary factors such as artificial sweeteners (aspartame) and certain foods (e.g., highly spiced foods, citrus juices, and tomato-based products) may play a role in continence. Current questionnaire-based data suggests that citrus fruits, tomatoes, vitamin C, artificial sweeteners, coffee, tea, carbonated and alcoholic beverages, and spicy foods tend to exacerbate LUTS, while calcium glycerophosphate and sodium bicarbonate tend to improve IC/BPS symptoms. [36] The patient is instructed on an elimination diet by identifying possible irritating products on a "one by one" basis to see if symptoms decrease or resolve.

Constipation and straining at stool

Chronic constipation (defined as having less than three stools per week) and straining during defecation can contribute to LUTS, specifically UI and OAB. Constipation is associated with impaired bladder emptying and worsening of irritative bladder symptoms. The close proximity of the bladder and urethra to the rectum and their similar nerve innervations make it likely that there are reciprocal effects between them. According to Kaplan and colleagues,

[37] animal studies and clinical data support bladder-bowel cross-sensitization, or crosstalk between the bowel and bladder. The Epidemiology of Lower Urinary Tract Symptoms (EpiLUTS) II [38] survey of men and women ($n = 2160$), aged 40 years old indicated that OAB is more likely to be reported if either gender had chronic constipation or fecal incontinence compared with those without OAB. In a case-control study of women with LUTS ($n = 820$) and matched controls ($n = 148$), constipation and straining during defecation were significantly more common among the women with LUTS including detrusor overactivity and urgency than among the controls. [39] Jelovsek [40] reported a 36% overall rate of constipation in women with UI and advanced pelvic organ prolapse.

Many experts believe that if excessive straining on defecation is a lifetime habit, it may have a cumulative effect on pelvic floor and bladder function causing denervation of the external anal sphincter and pelvic floor muscles. Patients with LUTS often report self-care practices to cope with LUTS by limiting fluid intake, a strategy that only worsens constipation. The use of antimuscarinic medications in patients with constipation can compound the problem as constipation is a side-effect of these medications. So determining the patient's bowel habits is an important first step in identifying changes that if reported should be managed, and a regimen that normalizes defecation should be recommended. Self-care practices that promote bowel regularity are an integral part of any treatment care plan. Suggestions to reduce constipation include the addition of fiber to the diet, increased fluid intake, regular exercise, external stimulation, and establishment of a routine defecation schedule.

High fiber intake must be accompanied by sufficient fluid intake. Improved bowel function can also achieved by determining a timetable for bowel evacuation so that the patient can take advantage of the urge to defecate. [27]

Summary

Lifestyle modifications are evidence-based interventions that can be effective in improving lower urinary treatment symptoms. Clinicians should proactively assess patients for LUTS and recommend lifestyle practices and changes that may be contributing or even causing a specific symptom. An important part of this assessment is determining the patient's readiness to change as adherence to certain lifestyle changes may be difficult for an individual to follow long term. Sharing with the patient the evidence base for these changes may give them the motivation to try to change.

References

1 Newman, DK, Wein, A.J. Office-based behavioral therapy for management of incontinence and other pelvic disorders. *Urol Clin North Am.* 2013;**40**(4):613–635.

2 Burgio KL, Newman DK, Rosenberg MT, Sampselle C. Impact of behaviour and lifestyle on bladder health. *Int J Clin Pract.* 2013;**67**(6): 495–504. doi: 10.1111/ijcp.1214.

3 Wyman, JF, Burgio, KL, Newman, DK. Practical aspects of lifestyle modifications and behavioural interventions in the treatme nt of overactive bladder and urgency urinary incontinence. [Review] *Int J Clin Pract.* 2009;**63**(8), 1177–1191.

4 Moore, K, Bradley, C, Burgio, B, et al. Adult conservative treatment. In Abrams P, Cardozo L, Khoury S, Wein A (Eds.): *Incontinence: Proceedings from the 5th International Consultation on*

Incontinence. Plymouth UK: Health Publications, 2013: pp. 1101–1228.

5 Gormley EA, Lightner DJ, Burgio KL, et al. Diagnosis and treatment of overactive bladder (non-neurogenic) in adults: AUA/SUFU guideline. *J Urol.* 2012 ;**188**(6 Suppl):2455–63. doi: 10.1016/j.juro.2012.09.079. Epub 2012 Oct 24.

6 Shamliyan T, Wyman JF, Ramakrishnan R, et al. Systematic review: randomized, controlled trials of nonsurgical treatments for urinary incontinence in women. *Ann Intern Med.* 2008; Mar 18;**148**(6):459–473.

7 Milson, I, Altman, D, Cartwright, R, et al. Epidemiology of urinary incontinence (UI) and other lower urinary tract symptoms (LUTS), pelvic organ prolapse (POP) and anal incontinence (AI). In Abrams P, Cardozo L, Khoury S, Wein A (Eds.): *Incontinence: Proceedings from the 5th International Consultation on Incontinence.* Plymouth: Health Publications, 2013: pp. 15–107.

8 Vaughan CP AA, Cartwright R, Johnson TM 2nd, et al. *Impact of obesity on urinary storage symptoms: results from the FINNO study.* 2012;**189** (4):1377–1382. doi: 10.1016/j.juro.2012.10.058. Epub 2012 Oct 24. 2013.

9 Subak LL, Richter HE, Hunskaar S. Obesity and urinary incontinence: epidemiology and clinical research update. *J Urol.* 2009;**182**: S2–7.

10 Khullar V, Sexton CC, Thompson CL, et al. The relationship between BMI and urinary incontinence subgroups: Results from EpiLUTS. *Neurourol Urodyn.* 2013;**18**.

11 Knoepp LR, Semins MJ, Wright EJ, Steele K, Shore AD, Clark JM, Makary MA, Matlaga BR, Chen CC. Does bariatric surgery affect urinary incontinence? *Urology* 2013;**82**(3):547–551.

12 Osborn DJ, Strain M, Gomelsky A, et al. (2013). Obesity and female stress urinary incontinence. *Urology 201*;**82**(4):759–763.

13 Subak LL, Wing R, West DS, et al. Weight loss to treat urinary incontinence in overweight and obese women. *N Engl J Med.* 2009;**360**: 481–490.

14 Wing RR, Creasman JM, West DS, et al. Improving urinary incontinence in overweight and obese women through modest weight loss. *Obstet Gynecol.* 2010;**116**:284–292.

15 Wing RR, West DS, Grady D, et al. Effect of weight loss on urinary incontinence in

overweight and obese women: results at 12 and 18 months. *J Urol.* 2010; **184**:1005–1010.

16 Wasserberg N, Petrone P, Haney M, et al. Effect of surgically induced weight loss on pelvic floor disorders in morbidly obese women. *Ann Surg.* 2009;**2249**:72–76.

17 Burgio KL, Richter HE, Clements RH, et al. (2007). Changes in urinary and fecal incontinence symptoms with weight loss surgery in morbidly obese women. *Obstet Gynecol.* 2007; **110**:1034–1040.

18 Vissers D, Neels H, Vermandel A, et al. The effect of non-surgical weight loss interventions on urinary incontinence in overweight women: a systematic review and meta-analysis. *Obes Rev.* 2014;**15**(7):610–617.

19 Hannestad YS, Rortveit G, Daltveit AK et al. Are smoking and other lifestyle factors associated with female urinary incontinence? *The Norwegian EPINCONT study. BJOG.* 2003;**110**: 247–254.

20 Fitzgerald, S, Palmer, MH, Berry, SJ, Hart, K. Urinary incontinence: Impact on working women. *AAOHN Journal* 2000;**48**(3):112–118.

21 Diokno AC, Burgio K, Fultz NH, et al. Medical and self-care practices reported by women with urinary incontinence. *Am J Manag Care* 2004;**10**:69–78.

22 Johnson TM, 2nd, Kincade JE, Bernard SL, et al. Self-care practices used by older men and women to manage urinary incontinence: results from the national follow-up survey on self-care and aging. *J Am Geriatr Soc.* 2000;**48**: 894–902

23 Segal S, Saks EK, Arya LA. Self-assessment of fluid intake behavior in women with urinary incontinence. *J Womens Health (Larchmt).* 2011; **20**(12):1917–1921. doi: 10.1089/jwh.2010.2642. Epub 2011 Oct 4. PMID: 21970566

24 Hashim H, Abrams, P. How should patients with an overactive bladder manipulate their fluid intake? *BJU Int.* 2008;**102**:62–66.

25 Institute of Medicine and Food and Nutrition Board. *Dietary reference intakes for water, potassium, sodium, chloride, and sulfate.* Washington, DC: National Academies Press; 2004.

26 Newman, DK, Burgio, KL, Markland, AD, Goode, PS. Urinary incontinence: Nonsurgical treatments. In T L Griebling (Ed.) *Geriatric Urology.* London: Springer-Verlag Ltd, 2014: pp. 141–168.

27 Newman DK, Wein AJ. *Managing and Treating Urinary Incontinence,* 2nd Edn. Baltimore, MD: Health Professions Press, 2009: pp. 245–306.

28 Wagg, AS, Chen, LK, Kirschner-Hermanns, R, et al. Incontinence in the frail elder. In Abrams P, Cardozo L, Khoury S, Wein A (Eds.) *Incontinence: Proceedings from the 5th International Consultation on Incontinence.* Plymouth UK: Health Publications, 2013:1001–1228.

29 Davis NJ, Vaughan CP, Johnson TM 2nd, et al. Caffeine intake and its association with urinary incontinence in United States men: results from National Health and Nutrition Examination Surveys 2005–2006 and 2007– 2008. *J Urol.* 2013;**189**(6):2170–2174. doi: 10.1016/j.juro.2012.12.061. Epub 2012 Dec 28. PMID: 23276513.

30 Gleason JL RH, Redden DT, Goode PS, et al. Caffeine and urinary incontinence in US women. *Int Urogynecol J.* 2013;**24**(2):295–302. doi: 10.1007/s00192-012-1829-5. Epub 2012 Jun 15.

31 Kershen R, Mann-Gow T, Yared J, et al. Caffeine ingestion causes detrusor overactivity and afferent nerve excitation in mice. *J Urol.* 2012;**188**(5):1986–1992. doi: 10.1016/j. juro.2012.07.010. Epub 2012 Sep 20.

32 Maserejian NN, Wager CG, Giovannucci EL, et al. Intake of caffeinated, carbonated, or citrus beverage types and development of lower urinary tract symptoms in men and women. *Am J Epidemiol.* 2013;**177**(12): 1399–1410. doi: 10.1093/aje/kws411. Epub 2013 May 30. PMID: 23722012.

33 Lohsiriwat SHM, Chaiyaprasithi B. Effect of caffeine on bladder function in patients with overactive bladder symptoms. *Urol Ann.* 2011;**3**(1):14–18. doi:10.4103/0974-7796. 75862.

34 Townsend MK RN, Grodstein F. Caffeine intake and risk of urinary incontinence progression among women. *Obstet Gynecol.* 2012;**119**(5): 950–7. doi: 10.1097/AOG.0b013e31824fc604.

35 Jura YH TM, Curhan GC, Resnick NM, Grodstein F. Caffeine intake, and the risk of stress, urgency and mixed urinary incontinence. *J Urol.* 2011;**185**(5):1775–1780. doi: 10. 1016/j.juro.2011.01.003. Epub 2011 Mar 21.

36 Shorter B, Lesser M, Moldwin R, Kushner L. Effect of comestibles on symptoms of interstitial cystitis. *J Urol.* 2007;**178**:145–152.

37 Kaplan R, Dmochowski BD, Cash ZS et al. *Systematic review of the relationship between bladder and bowel function: implications for patient management Int J Clin Pract.*2013;**67**(3): 205–216, doi: 10.1111/ijcp.12028.

38 Coyne KS, Cash B, Kopp Z et al. The prevalence of chronic constipation and faecal incontinence among men and women with symptoms of overactive bladder. *BJU Int* 2011;**107**:254–61.

39 Manning J, Korda A, Benness C, Solomon M. The association of obstructive defecation, lower urinary tract dysfunction and the benign joint hypermobility syndrome: a case-control study. *Int Urogynecol J Pelvic Floor Dysfunct.* 2003;**14**: 128–132.

40 Jelovsek JE, Barber MD, Paraiso MF, et al. Functional bowel and anorectal disorders in patients with pelvic organ prolapse and incontinence. *Am J Obstet and Gynecol.* 2005; **193**:2105–2111.

Lifestyle changes that can improve bladder symptoms

Maintain a healthy weight

Being overweight can put pressure on your bladder, which may cause leakage of urine when you laugh or cough. If you are overweight, weight loss can reduce this increased pressure on your bladder (Table A2).

Stop smoking

Cigarette smoking is irritating to the bladder muscle. It can also lead to coughing spasms which can cause urinary leakage (Table A2).

Table A1 Caffeine content of some foods and drugs

	Size	Caffeine content (mg)
Coffee	8 oz	133 (range, 102–200)
Tea	8 oz	53 (range, 40–120)
Soft drinks	12 oz	35–72
Energy drinks	8–20 oz	48–300
Chocolate candies	varies	9–33
Excedrin (extra-strength)	2 tablets	130
Anacin (maximum strength)	2 tablets	64
Vivarin, NoDoz	1 tablet	200

Source: Adapted from: Moore, K et al. In Abrams P, Cardozo L, Khoury S, Wein A (Eds.): Incontinence: Proceedings from the 5th International Consultation on Incontinence. Plymouth UK: Health Publications, 2013;1101–1228.

Moderate liquid and beverage intake

Many people who have bladder problems will drink less, hoping they will need to urinate less often. While drinking less liquid does result in less urine in your bladder, a much smaller amount of urine may be more highly concentrated and irritate the lining of your bladder. Concentrated urine (dark yellow, strong smelling) may cause you to go to the bathroom more frequently. Also, drinking too little fluids can cause dehydration. Do not limit your fluids to control your bladder symptoms unless your doctor or nurse tells you to.

Other people may increase the amount they drink because they think more urine in the bladder will cause less bladder pain and discomfort. But drinking too much fluid will cause you to go to the bathroom more often. You should avoid extremes in the amount you drink (neither too much nor too little).

Normal fluid intake is 50–70 ounces (1 oz = 30 ml) of liquid each day. This means that each day, you should consume the equivalent of six to eight 8-ounce glasses of liquids (any beverages and soups). This should produce a healthy 40–50 ounces of urine in 24 hours. People who work in hot climates or exercise heavily need more

Table A2 Levels of evidence and recommendations lifestyle modifications

Lifestyle practice	Levels of evidence	Recommendations
Fluid	Fluid intake may play a minor role in the pathogenesis of UI.	Minor decrease of fluid intake by 25% may be recommended provided baseline consumption is not less than 30 ml/kg a day **Grade of Recommendation: B**
Caffeine	Caffeine consumption may play a role in exacerbating UI. Small clinical trials do suggest that decreasing caffeine intake improves continence. **Level of Evidence: 2**	Caffeine reduction may help in improving incontinence symptoms **Grade of Recommendation: B**
Bowel function	There is some evidence to suggest that chronic straining may be a risk factor for the development of UI. **Level of Evidence: 3**	Further research is needed to define the role of straining during defecation in the pathogenesis of UI.
Obesity	Massive weight loss (15 to 20 BMI points) significantly decreases UI in morbidly obese women. **Level of Evidence: 2** Moderate weight loss may be effective in decreasing UI especially if combined with exercise **Level of Evidence: 1**	Weight loss in obese and morbidly should be considered a first line treatment to reduce UI prevalence **Grade of Recommendation: A.**
Smoking		Further prospective studies are needed to determine whether smoking cessation prevents the onset, or promotes the resolution, of UI.

fluids because of loss through perspiration, but their urine output should still be approximately 40–50 ounces. Do not drink large amounts at one time; instead, sip 2 to 3 ounces every 20 to 30 minutes between meals. It is very unlikely that you will need to drink more than 2 quarts (or 8 cups) of total fluids each day (Table A2).

Monitor your diet

Certain food and beverages can irritate the bladder and make symptoms worse. These include alcoholic beverages, caffeinated foods (soft drinks, coffee or tea, chocolate, energy drinks), and/or carbonated beverages, tomato-based products, citrus fruits and juices, spicy foods, and artificial sweeteners (e.g., Equal). Also some over-the-counter drugs and prescription medications can worsen bladder problems such as Excedrin, Midol, Anacin. Do not stop taking prescription drugs without first talking to your healthcare provider. Here is the caffeine content of some foods and drugs (Table A1) (Table A2).

your diet such as beans, pasta, oatmeal, bran cereal, whole wheat bread, fresh fruits and vegetables; (ii) exercise to maintain regular bowel movements; (iii) drink plenty of non-irritating fluids (water); (iv) see your doctor if you have bowel problems (Table A2).

© 2011 Diane K Newman

Maintain bowel regularity

Keeping regular and healthy bowel habits may lessen bladder symptoms. Some suggestions include: (i) increase fiber-rich foods in

CHAPTER 8

Physical therapy

Kari Bø

Norwegian School of Sport Sciences, Department of Sports Medicine, Oslo, Norway

---

KEY POINTS

- A voluntary pelvic floor muscle contraction can inhibit urgency to void and detrusor contraction.

- Patients can be taught the correct pelvic floor muscle contraction by vaginal palpation of a trained physical therapist.

- Training of a voluntary contraction in situations where urgency is likely to occur may help the person to inhibit bladder contraction and enable them to reach the toilet without leaking.

- There are several training regimens presented, but there is no evidence regarding the most effect training program.

- There is an immediate need for high quality randomized controlled trials in selected groups of patients with overactive bladder symptoms only.

Physical therapy

Physical therapy for the pelvic floor implies management by a trained physical therapist and includes history taking; assessment of pelvic floor muscle function using observation, palpation, and measurement with manometer, dynamometer, and/or ultrasound; and the set-up of an individual treatment plan targeting the goals of the patient.

Conservative treatment of overactive bladder (OAB) symptoms includes bladder training, pelvic floor muscle training (PFMT) with and without biofeedback, electrical stimulation, and often many of the interventions are combined. Unfortunately, to date most systematic reviews on conservative treatments of OAB symptoms do not separate studies on patients with symptoms or urodynamic diagnosis of stress urinary incontinence (SUI), urgency urinary incontinence (UUI), or mixed urinary incontinence (MUI). The combination of heterogeneous patient groups in systematic reviews and meta-analyses may obscure the real cure rate for each of the diagnoses.

The mechanisms of OAB symptoms are not yet thoroughly understood, and pathophysiological factors may vary among

---

Overactive Bladder: Practical Management, First Edition. Edited by Jacques Corcos, Scott MacDiarmid and John Heesakkers.
© 2015 John Wiley & Sons, Ltd. Published 2015 by John Wiley & Sons, Ltd.

patients. Optimally, the physical therapy intervention should relate to the underlying pathophysiological condition to be effective.

Methods

This review is based on four former systematic reviews on conservative treatments for UI and OAB symptoms [1–4], Cochrane reviews [5–8]), Guidelines of the European Association of Urology (EAU) [9] and the International Consensus on Incontinence (ICI). [10]

Scheduled voiding/bladder training

Scheduled voiding is "a treatment program designed to gradually increase a person's control over voiding function and urgency and to reduce episodes of incontinence." [9] It has also been named bladder training, bladder drill, bladder discipline, and bladder re-education. Bladder training will be used in this chapter as this is the commonly used term in published studies up till now. Different strategies have been used in different protocols and the patients are often also instructed on bladder function and fluid intake, for example caffeine restriction and bowel habits. One method is to ask the patient to void according to a fixed voiding schedule; another is to motivate patients to follow their own bladder diary/voiding chart (habit training). Timed voiding is voiding initiated by the patient, while prompted voiding is voiding initiated by the caregiver. [9] Bladder training is simple, relatively inexpensive, and free from unpleasant side-effects. [4]

Rationale

According to Wyman [4] it is unclear how bladder training achieves its effect. The following explanations have been proposed:

- Improved cortical inhibition over involuntary detrusor contractions.
- Improved cortical facilitation over urethral closure during bladder filling.
- Improved central modulation of afferent sensory impulses.
- The individual becoming more knowledgeable and aware of circumstances that cause incontinence and so changes behavior in ways that increase the reserve capacity of the lower urinary tract system.

Evidence

Bladder training has traditionally been advocated for OAB and contradictory results have been shown for stress urinary incontinence (SUI). Wyman et al. [11] found effect both in SUI and urgency urinary incontinent women and no difference in effect of PFMT and bladder training in the SUI group. However, Sherburn et al. [12] showed significantly better effect of PFMT than bladder training in a group of elderly women with SUI. Most studies on bladder training are on females, and Moore et al. [10] concluded that there is insufficient evidence available to comment on the effectiveness of bladder training/timed voiding in men (limited level 3 evidence). The evidence summary from the European Association of Urology (EAU) on bladder training is as follows: [9]

- There is limited evidence that supervised bladder training is better than no treatment in women with UUI and mixed urinary incontinence: 1b.
- The effectiveness of bladder training diminishes after the treatment has ceased: 2.

- There is inconsistent evidence to show whether bladder training is better than drug therapy: 2.
- A combination of bladder training with antimuscarinic drugs does not result in greater improvement of UI but may have other benefits: 2.
- Bladder training is better than pessary alone: 1b.
- Timed voiding reduces leakage episodes in cognitively impaired men and women: 1b.

Clinical recommendations

The EAU recommendations on bladder training are: [9]

- Bladder training should be offered as a first line therapy to adults with urgency urinary incontinence or mixed urinary incontinence: A.
- Timed voiding should be offered to adults with urinary incontinence who are cognitively impaired: A.

Wyman [4] recommended that bladder training programs should be initiated by assigning an initial voiding interval based on baseline voiding frequency and that this is often set at 1 h intervals during waking hours (shorter intervals, e.g., 30 min, may be necessary). The schedule can then be increased by 15–30 min per week depending on the patients' tolerance to the schedule. Self-monitoring of voiding behavior using voiding diaries should be used. Moore et al. [10] gave a grade D recommendation that health professionals should provide the most intensive bladder training supervision that is possible within service constraints. If there is no improvement after three weeks of bladder training, the patient should be offered other treatment options.

Pelvic floor muscle training

Systematic reviews of RCTs in the general female population conclude that PFMT has Level 1, Grade A evidence for effectiveness, and there is consensus that PFMT should be first line treatment for SUI and MUI. [5, 10] The effect of PFMT on OAB symptoms, is however, still under debate.

Rationale

Shafik and Shafik [13] investigated the effect of a voluntary PFM contraction on detrusor and urethral pressures in 28 patients with OAB (mean age 48. 8 years ± 10.2 years, 18 men and 10 women) and 17 healthy volunteers (mean age 42.6 years ± 9.8 years, 12 men and 5 women). They found that during PFM contraction the urethral pressure significantly increased and vesical pressure significantly decreased in both patients and healthy subjects. The change during PFM contraction was significantly larger in the healthy volunteers. The authors concluded that PFM contractions led to a decline of detrusor pressure, an increase of urethral pressures, and suppression of the micturition reflex, and that the results encourage PFM contractions in treatment of OAB.

It is known from clinical experience that patients can successfully inhibit urgency, detrusor contraction, and urinary leakage by walking, bending forwards, crossing their legs, using hip adductor muscles with or without conscious co-contraction of the PFM, or by conscious contraction of the PFM alone. After inhibition of the urgency to void and detrusor contraction, the patients may gain time to reach the toilet and thereby prevent leakage. The reciprocal inhibition reflex runs via cerebral control, recruiting ventral horn motor neurons for voluntary PFM contraction and inhibiting the parasympathetic excitatory pathway for the micturition reflex via Onuf's ganglion. This mechanism has been exploited as part of bladder training regimens. [14] There may therefore be two main hypotheses for the mechanism of PFMT to treat urgency incontinence:

- intentional contraction of the PFM during urgency, and holding of the contraction till the urge to void disappears;
- strength training of the PFM with long-lasting changes in muscle morphology, which may stabilize neurogenic activity.

None of the studies in this field (neither uncontrolled studies nor RCTs) have evaluated whether changes in the inhibitory mechanisms really occur after PFMT. In addition, research in this area is relatively new, and there does not seem to be any consensus on the optimal exercise protocol to prevent or treat OAB. [2] The theoretical basis of how PFMT may work in the treatment of OAB therefore remains unclear. [1, 15]

Evidence

Four RCTs using PFMT alone to treat symptoms of OAB were found. [15–18]

Nygaard et al. found [16] significant improvement in many variables in the subgroup of women with detrusor instability. There was no difference in outcome between the two randomized groups, and no comparison with non-treated controls. Berghmans et al. [15] did not demonstrate any significant effect of their exercise protocol compared to an untreated control group. Wang et al. [18] found that the significant subjective improvement/cure rate of OAB was the same between the electrical stimulation group and in the biofeedback-assisted PFMT group, but lower

in the PFMT home training group. Millard [17] did not show any additional benefit for a simple PFMT protocol (two-page written instruction, no assessment of ability to contract, and no follow-up or supervised training). To date the effect of PFMT on OAB is therefore questionable.

The quality of the interventions and dose–response issues are difficult to judge because there are no direct recommendations on how PFMT should be conducted to inhibit urgency and detrusor contraction. The published studies have all used different exercise protocols. Berghmans et al. [15] and Millard [17] included intentional contraction of the PFM to inhibit detrusor contractions in addition to a strength training program. However, Millard [17] did not report adherence, and Berghmans et al. [15] also included bladder training in their protocol. The protocol from Berghmans et al. did not show any effect when compared with untreated controls. In Millard's study [17] a very weak exercise protocol was conducted. There was no control of ability to contract the PFM, patients were left alone to exercise, and there was no report on adherence to the exercise protocol. The exercise period varied between 9 and 12 weeks in duration in the four RCTs. This may be too short to treat a complex condition such as OAB.

In conclusion, there are few RCTs in this area and the results are difficult to interpret. The exercise protocols may not have been optimal. Because the pathophysiological background for OAB is not clear, it is difficult to plan an optimal training protocol. Based on the theoretical knowledge and symptoms of OAB it seems reasonable to put more emphasis on the inhibition mechanisms of the PFM contraction, and teaching and follow-up of patients trying to contract the PFM when there is an urge to void. There is a need for more basic research to understand the role of a voluntary PFM contraction in inhibition of the micturition reflex. Future RCTs with high interventional and methodological quality are recommended.

Clinical recommendations

Clinical experience and basic research show that it may be possible to learn to inhibit detrusor contraction by intentionally contracting the PFM and holding the contraction to stop the urge to void. A protocol based on patients' experiences needs to be tested in a high-quality RCT.

Electrical stimulation

Electrical stimulation has a long tradition in physical therapy, although there is an ongoing debate on the rationale and evidence for its effectiveness. [19] For symptoms of OAB, urologists and gynecologists have used different modalities of electrical stimulation since the late 1970s.

Rationale

Godec et al. [20] studied 40 patients with cystometrograms, taken during and after 3 min of 20 Hz functional electrical stimulation (FES). The results showed that, during FES, hyperactivity of the bladder was diminished or completely abolished in 31 of 40 patients. One minute after stimulation cessation, the inhibition was still present. Mean bladder capacity also increased significantly, from 151 ± 126 ml to 206 ± 131 ml ($p < 0.05$).

De Groat [21] noted that during the storage of urine, distension of the bladder produces low-level vesical afferent firing.

This stimulates the sympathetic outflow to the bladder outlet (base and urethra), and the pudendal outflow to the external urethral sphincter. He stated that these responses occur by spinal reflex pathways, representing "guarding reflexes" that promote continence. Sympathetic firing also inhibits the detrusor muscle and bladder ganglia. Morrison [22] claimed that the excitatory loop through Barrington's micturition center is switched on at bladder pressures between 5 and 25 mmHg, whereas the inhibitory loop through the raphe nucleus is active predominantly above 25 mmHg. The inhibition is at the automatic level, with the person not being conscious of the increasing tone in the PFM and urethral wall striated muscles.

Evidence

There are no Cochrane reviews on the effect of electrical stimulation for OAB symptoms. In a systematic review of Berghmans, [23] nine RCTs were found. Methodological quality was rated with PEDro score (0–10 with 10 as the highest possible score) and ranged from 3 to 8. Electrical stimulation studies offered an infinite combination of current types, waveforms, frequencies, intensities, electrode placements, and electrical stimulation probes and so on. Without a clear biological rationale for the cause of OAB symptoms, Berghmans [23] stated that it is difficult to make choices of effective electrical stimulation parameters. Berghmans [23] concluded that there was:

• some evidence that intensive office bound and home electrical stimulation is better than no or placebo treatment for women with OAB and/or UUI symptoms (some of the studies included both men and women);

- insufficient evidence to determine whether electrical stimulation is better than PFMT with and without biofeedback or medication;
- no studies evaluating if there is extra benefit of adding electrical stimulation to other treatments.

Lucas et al. [9] in the EAU Guidelines concluded that evidence for electrical stimulation is inconsistent for whether electrical stimulation alone can improve UI, and that there were no consistent evidence of efficacy of magnetic stimulation (the chair) for the cure or improvement of UI. For posterior percutaneous tibial nerve stimulation (PTNS) it was concluded that there are not enough data to make a conclusion about the effectiveness in men, that it is effective in women with UUI who cannot tolerate anticholinergic medication (2a), and that it does not give benefit for women with UUI who have not responded to anticholinergic medication (1b). No serious adverse effects have been reported for PTNS in UUI. [9] Moore et al. [10] concluded that the included studies on electrical stimulation were generally assessed as having a high risk of bias and that heterogeneity between studies meant it was not appropriate to pool the data.

Clinical recommendations for electrical stimulation for OAB: [23]

- intensive treatments with both office and home use;
- stochastic frequency: 4–10 Hz; frequency modulation 0.1 s;
- intensity: $I_{max;}$
- pulse duration: 200–500 µs;
- biphasic, duty circle: 13 s 5/8;
- shape of current: rectangular;
- number and time schedule of sessions: daily at home 2 X 20 min 7 day; office 1 x 30 min/week;
- duration of treatment period: 3–6 months.

In conclusion, so far the evidence for physical therapy in treatment of OAB – bladder training, PFMT, and electrical stimulation – are not convincing. There are, however, few RCTs of high interventional and methodological quality in this area. There is a theoretical rationale and support from basic science for a possible effect through inhibition of the detrusor contraction, and there is an immediate need for further high quality studies.

References

1 1.Berghmans L, Hendriks H, de Bie RA et al. Conservative treatment of urge urinary incontinence in women: a systematic review of randomized clinical trials. *BJU Int.* 2000;**85**(3): 254–263.

2 Bø K, Berghmans L. Overactive bladder and its treatments. *Non-pharmacological treatments for overactive bladder: pelvic floor exercises. Urology* 2000;**55**(suppl 5A):7–11.

3 Greer JA, Smith AL, Arya LA. Pelvic floor muscle training for urgency urinary incontinence in women: a systematic review. *Int Urogynecol J.* 2012;**23**:687–697.

4 Wyman J. Bladder training for overactive bladder. In: Bø K, Berghmans B, Mørkved S van Kampen M (Eds): *Evidence-Based Physical Therapy For The Pelvic Floor – Bridging Science And Clinical Practice.* Butterworth Heinemann, Elsevier, 2007: pp. 208–218.

5 Dumoulin C, Hay-Smith J. Pelvic floor muscle training versus no treatment, or inactive control treatments, for urinary incontinence in women. Cochrane Database of Systematic Reviews: CD005654, 2010.

6 Hay-Smith EJC, Herderschee R, Dumoulin C, Herbison PG. Comparisons of approaches to pelvic floor muscle training for urinary incontinence in women. Cochrane Database of Systematic Reviews: CD009508, 2011.

7 Herderschee R, Hay-Smith EJC, Herbison GP, et al. Feedback or biofeedback to augment pelvic floor muscle training for urinary incontinence in women. Cochrane Database of Systematic reviews: CD009252, 2011.

8   Rai BP, Cody JD, Alhasso A, Stewart L. Anticholinergic drugs versus non-drug active therapies for non-neurogenic overactive bladder syndrome in adults. Cochrane Database of Systematic reviews. The Cochrane Library, Issue 12. Art no: CD003193, 2012.

9   Lucas MG, Bosch JLHR, Cruz FR, et al. Guidelines on Urinary incontinence. European Association of Urology (EAU) Guidelines 2012 Edition. *Drukkerij Gelderland bv Arnhem: the Netherlands*, **2012**.

10 Moore K, Dumoulin C, Bradley C, et al. Adult conservative management. In: Abrams P, Cardozo L. Khouy S, Wein A (Eds) *Incontinence*. 5th Edn. Committee 12, 2013: pp.1101–1227

11 Wyman JF, Fantl JA, McClish DK et al. Comparative efficacy of behavioral interventions in the management of female urinary incontinence. *Am J Obstet Gynecol* 1998;**179**:999–1007.

12 Sherburn M, Bird M, Carey M, et al. Incontinence improves in older women after intensive pelvic floor muscle training: an assessor blinded randomized controlled trial. *Neurourol Urodyn.* 2011;**30**:317–324.

13 Shafik A, Shafik IA. Overative bladder inhibition in response to pelvic floor muscle exercises. *World J Urol.* 2003;**20**:374–377.

14 Burgio K, Locher J, Goode P et al .Behavioral vs drug treatment for urge urinary incontinence in older women. *JAMA* 1998;**280**, 23:1995–2000.

15 Berghmans B, van Waalwijk van Doorn E, Nieman F et al. Efficacy of physical therapeutic modalities in women with proven bladder overactivity. *Eur. Urology* 2002;**6**:581–587.

16 Nygaard I, Kreder K, Lepic M et al. Efficacy of pelvic floor muscle exercises in women with stress, urge, and mixed incontinence. *Am J Obs Gynecol.* 1996;**174**(120):125.

17 Millard R. Clinical efficacy of tolterodine with or without a simplified pelvic floor exercise regimen. *Nerourol Urodyn.* 2004;**23**:48–53.

18 Wang A, Wang Y, Chen M. Single-blind, randomized trial of pelvic floor muscle training, biofeedback-assisted pelvic floor muscle training, and electrical stimulation in the management of overactive bladder. *Urology* 2004; **63**(1):61–66

19 Herbert R, Jamtvedt G, Mead J, Hagen KB. *Practical Evidence-Based Physiotherapy*. Elsevier Butterworth Heinemann: Edinburgh, 2005.

20 Godec C, Cass A, Ayala G. Bladder inhibition with functional electrical stimulation. *Urology* 1975;**6**(6):663–666.

21 De Groat W. A neurologic basis for the overactive bladder. *Urology* 1997;**50**(suppl 6A):36–52.

22 Morrison J. The excitability of the micturition reflex. *Scand J Urol Nephrol.* 1993; **29**(suppl 175):21–25.

23 Berghmans B. Electrical stimulation for OAB. In: Bø K, Berghmans B, Mørkved S van Kampen M (Eds) *Evidence-Based Physical Therapy for the Pelvic Floor – Bridging Science And Clinical Practice*. Butterworth Heinemann, Elsevier, 2007: pp. 222–231.

SECTION 4
Second Line Management

CHAPTER 9

Oral medication for overactive bladder

Roger Dmochowski and Jill Danford

Vanderbilt University Medical Center, Nashville, TN, USA

KEY POINTS

- Overactive bladder (OAB) is a prevalent and bothersome condition.
- A variety of oral agents are available for the therapy of OAB and these should be used in conjunction with behavioral therapy.
- Antimuscarinic agents are the most commonly used agents for the therapy of OAB.
- Antimuscarinic agents are similar in efficacy and tolerability, with the exception that long-acting agents may be associated with less occurrence of dry mouth.
- The Beta 3 agonist mechanism of action has recently been shown to be effective for OAB.
- Beta 3 agonists have similar efficacy to antimuscarinic agents, but less adverse events.
- Persistent OAB symptoms may require more intensive therapies.

Introduction

The prevalence of overactive bladder in the population has propelled the many pharmacologic options currently available to practitioners. It is estimated that 13–17% of women and 16% of men in the US are diagnosed with overactive bladder. [1, 2] Until recently, the first line treatment in oral therapy has been a muscarinic receptor antagonist. With the recent addition of Beta 3 adrenergic receptor agonists, there is another option with a different mechanism of action, available. Classification of medications and dosing is seen in Table 9.1.

Antimuscarinics

Overview

Antimuscarinics are the most frequently prescribed medications for OAB and have been the gold standard of treatment. Despite this, the exact mechanism of action is not completely understood. Traditionally it was thought that these drugs block activity of acetylcholine at the muscarinic receptor sites. This was thought to decrease detrusor muscle contraction. However studies have shown that antimuscarinics also may have an afferent effect on storage phase. [3] Acetylcholine is now thought to directly or

---

Overactive Bladder: Practical Management, First Edition. Edited by Jacques Corcos, Scott MacDiarmid and John Heesakkers.

Table 9.1 Currently available oral agents for therapy of the overactive bladder

Drug	Dose	Special considerations
Antimuscarinics		
Oxybutynin	IR: 2.5–7.5 mg bid-tid	IR with increased CNS effects and
	ER: 5–30 mg qday	dry mouth/constipation
Trospium	IR: 20 mg bid	Renally cleared
	ER: 60 mg qday	
Tolterodine	IR: 1–2 mg bid	
	EF: 2–4 mg qday	
Fesoterodine	4–8 mg qday	
Solifenacin	5–10 mg qday	
Darifenacin	7.5–15 mg qday	
Beta 3 AR Agonist		
Mirabegron	25–50 mg qday	May elevate BP
Antidepressants		
Imipramine	75 mg qday	
Doxepin	25–50 mg qday	
Duloxetine	40 mg bid	

indirectly stimulate afferent activity from the bladder and contribute to OAB and detrusor overactivity. [4] Inhibiting this effect decreases urgency symptoms and increases bladder capacity without affecting actual detrusor contraction.

Important properties

- Some antimuscarinics are tertiary amines while others are quaternary amines. Tertiary amines are well absorbed in the gastrointestinal tract and can theoretically pass the blood–brain barrier. Quaternary amines are not as well absorbed and do not readily cross blood–brain barrier. These have lower CNS side-effects.
- Many are metabolized via the cytochrome P450 system. This can cause significant drug–drug interactions

Adverse effects

Muscarinic receptors are prevalent throughout the body, and these locations correspond to the most common side-effects.

While all five muscarinic receptors, M_1–M_5 have shown RNA activity in detrusor muscle, increased activity of M_2 and M_3 had been demonstrated, with M_2 showing a 3:1 predominance over M_3. M_3 controls detrusor contraction. M_1 receptors are found in salivary glands, nerves, and CNS. In addition to the bladder, M_2 receptors are found in the heart, nerves, and other smooth muscle, especially gastrointestinal. M_3 receptors are present in GI smooth muscle, salivary glands and endothelium. M_4 receptors are found predominantly in the CNS. M_5 are also found in the CNS as well as salivary glands and the eye to control iris sphincter contraction. [5] Dry mouth, headache, constipation, blurry vision, and dizziness are seen most often. Serious side-effects are uncommon, however cardiac effects are possible with this drug class. Increase in heart rate as well as QT prolongation can occur. The CNS side-effects are also uncommon, but those of concern are cognitive dysfunction and memory impairment.

- Contraindications:
  - Untreated narrow-angle glaucoma
  - Gastric retention.
- Relative contraindication:
  - Older patients with dementia.

Evidence for efficacy

There are several antimuscarinic drugs currently approved for OAB. Large meta-analyses have shown the efficacy of these medications over placebo.

- One such study by Novara et al. looked at 50 RCTs and three pooled analyses. They concluded that antimuscarinics are effective and determined that extended release (ER) is preferred over immediate release (IR) due to adverse reactions. They also concluded that there are insufficient studies to determine which medications should be first, second, and third line treatments. [6]
- An analysis by Chapple et al. reviewed 73 trials. They concluded that antimuscarinics are superior over placebo. They too found that once daily dosing is better tolerated and that drugs should be tailored to certain patients. [7]
- Hartmann et al. for the Agency for Healthcare Research and Quality (AHRQ) performed a mixed effects meta-analysis of 273 publications for the treatment of medications in OAB in women. Their conclusions stated that while antimuscarinic drugs were effective, these effects were modest: improved >1 OAB symptom compared to placebo, and depended on patient's subjective complaints. [8]
- Gormley et al. found no compelling evidence for differential efficacy across medications. They concluded that patients with worse symptoms had the most improvement and that patients with lower levels of urge incontinence

were more likely to achieve complete symptomatic relief.

While none of these medications appear to be superior to each other in efficacy, the side-effect profile may differ from one medication to the other. There are also differences in the exact mechanism of action between individual medications in this class that may indicate one is superior to another in a specific patient.

Compliance

A large proportion of patients will discontinue use within the first 30 days and fewer than half refill prescriptions. [9, 10] When patients are asked why they did not continue medication, reasons cited were "did not work as expected" (45%) and "side-effects" (35%). There has not been an increased rate of compliance shown with newer medications.

Oxybutynin

This was the first antimuscarinic to be studied for OAB. It is a tertiary amine with M_3 and M_1 selectivity with both IR and ER formulations. The IR formulation has P450 metabolism, therefore it has increased rates of all side-effects, especially dry mouth. There is also an increased rate of CNS side-effects in the IR formulation manifesting as dizziness, cognitive dysfunction, memory impairment, and fatigue. The most frequent side effects are dry mouth and constipation. The recommended dose for the IR formulation is 2.5 mg 2–3 times a day titrating up to 20 mg per day divided 2–3 times. The ER formulation dosing starts at 5 mg once daily and titrates up to 30 mg once daily.

Trospium

This medication is a quaternary amine, therefore crosses blood–brain barrier only to a limited extent. [11] Previously there was concern that this increased with patient age. However, a recent rodent study showed that penetration does not change in adult mice compared with aged mice. [12] It has both IR and ER formulations. Trospium is the only antimuscarinic that is renally cleared, which means it is not metabolized by P450. Because of this the ER formulation should not be used in patients with severe renal impairment (GFR <30 ml/min). However it may allow for fewer drug–drug interactions. There is no muscarinic receptor selectivity seen. Several randomized controlled trials have been performed comparing trospium with placebo and these proved an increased efficacy over placebo. It has also been compared to oxybutynin, which showed that it has similar efficacy but has a lower side-effect profile. They concluded that trospium might be better tolerated than oxybutynin in most patients. The most frequent side effects are dry mouth and constipation. [13] Dosing for the IR formulation is 20 mg twice daily and for ER is 60 mg once daily.

Tolterodine

This drug is a tertiary amine with no selectivity for muscarinic receptors. It is readily metabolized by P450. Because of its low lipophilicity, there is some cross-over through the blood–brain barrier. While there have been case reports of cognitive adverse events mimicking dementia, this has not been seen in prospective trials. A meta-analysis of tolterodine versus oxybutinin showed that tolterodine was better tolerated. [14] Dosing for the IR formulation is 1–2 mg twice daily and for the ER is 2–4 mg once daily.

Fesoterodine

Fesoterodine is a prodrug that is converted to 5-hydroxymethyl tolterodine. Similarly, it is a non-selective muscarinic receptor and it metabolized by P450. Most common side-effects are dry mouth and constipation. The suggested dosing is 4 and 8 mg once daily. A comparison of the 4 mg versus 8 mg dosing showed significant improvement with several factors of OAB including incontinence episodes, number of incontinent days a week, and urgency with incontinence. [7]

Solifenacin

This drug is a tertiary amine that is a relatively M_3 receptor antagonist. It is metabolized by P450 and readily absorbed through the gastrointestinal epithelium (90% availability). The VECTOR study was a RCT that compared solifenacin to oxybutynin IR. Efficacy was similar; however patients in the solifenacin arm were less likely to report dry mouth than in the oxybutynin arm. [15] Despite this, the most common side-effects are dry mouth and constipation. Dosing is 5–10 mg once daily.

Darifenacin

This medication is a tertiary amine with high selectively to M_3. It also is metabolized by P450 and does not extensively cross the blood–brain barrier. Most common side-effects are dry mouth and constipation without cardiac or CNS effects greater than placebo. Haab et al. performed a RCT comparing darifenacin to placebo and showed significant improvement of OAB symptoms over placebo. While dry mouth and constipation were the most common sid- effects, few participants withdrew from the study for these effects. They did not note any more CNS or cardiac adverse events compared to placebo. [16] The recommended dosing is 7.5–15 mg once daily.

Beta 3 (β_3) adrenergic receptor (AR) agonists

Mirabegron

This is the first β_3 AR agonist and currently the only one approved by the FDA. β_3 adrenergic receptors are found in the urothelium of the bladder wall. These medications are thought to facilitate urine storage through stimulation of β_3 adrenoreceptors thus facilitating bladder relaxation. [17] The most common adverse events are increased BP, nasopharyngitis, UTI, constipation, fatigue, tachycardia, and abdominal pain. Mirabegron is contraindicated in patients with uncontrolled HTN. Three, double blind, placebo controlled studies have been performed that demonstrated a decrease in mean urinary incontinence episodes a day and mean number of voids a day from baseline versus placebo. However, there have not been any trials performed that have a trial period greater than 12 weeks. [18] As this is a newer medication, more studies are currently being performed. Mirabegron's dosing is 25 mg and 50 mg daily. Studies have shown that both doses maintained efficacy.

Antidepressants

Tricyclic antidepressants – Imipramine and Doxepin

These medications are alpha agonists with anticholinergic activity; however, exact mechanism of action of tricyclics in OAB is not understood. There are three proposed mechanisms for activity: (i) they have antimuscarinic activity, (ii) block transport system for reuptake of norephinephrine and serotonin, and (iii) they are sedatives possibly related to their antihistamine properties. Because of these properties they can be used in women with mixed incontinence as well as OAB. The AHCPR Guidelines cite only three RCTs for both medications with a cure rate of 31% and urgency incontinence reduction ranging from 20–77%. [8] These trials were determined to not be of good quality and others have not been performed, however these medications can be useful for patients who cannot tolerate first-line medications. Tricyclic antidepressants should not be used in older patients due to orthostatic hypotension concerns.

Duloxetine

This medication is a serotonin norepinephrine reuptake inhibitor that increases bladder capacity. Studies have shown a slight decrease in leakage episodes in women with mixed urinary incontinence versus placebo; however cure rates are the same as placebo. [19] Duloxetine is not FDA approved for this indication.

References

1 Lawrence JM, Lukacz ES, Nager, et al. Prevalence and co-occurrence of pelvic floor disorders in community-dwelling women. *Obstet Gynecol.* 2008;**111**(3):678–685.

2 Stewart WF, Van Rooyen JB, Cundiff CW, et al. Prevalence and burden of overactive bladder in the United States. *World J Urol.* 2003; **20**(6):327–336.

3 De Laet K, De Wachter S, Wyndaele JJ, et al. Systemic oxybutynin decreases afferent activity of the pelvic nerve of the rat: new insights into

the working mechanism of antimuscarinics. *Neurourol Urodyn.* 2006:**25**:156–161.

4 Iijima K, De Wachter S, Wyndaele JJ, et al. Effects of the M3 receptor selective muscarinic antagonist darifenacin on bladder afferent activity of the rat pelvic nerve. *Eur Urol* 2007;**52**:842–847.

5 Abrams P, Andersson K-E, Buccafusco JJ, et al. Muscarinic receptors: their distribution and function in body systems, and the implications for treating overactive bladder. *Br J Pharmacol.* 2006;**148**:565.

6 Novara G, Galfano A, Secco S, et al. A systematic review and meta-analysis of randomized controlled trials with antimuscarinic drugs for overactive bladder. *Eur Urol.* 2008;**54**(4):740–764.

7 Chapple CR, Khullar V, Gabriel Z, et al. The effects of antimuscarinic treatments of in overactive bladder: an update of a systematic review and meta-analysis. *Eur Urol.* 2008;**54**(3):543–562.

8 Hartmann KE, McPheeters ML, Biller DH, et al. *Treatment of Overactive Bladder in Women. Evidence Report/Technology Assessment No. 187 (Prepared by the Vanderbilt Evidence-based Practice Center under Contract No. 290-2007-10065-I). AHRQ Publication No. 09-E017.* Rockville, MD: Agency for Healthcare Research and Quality. August 2009.

9 Shaya FT, Blume S, Gu A, et al. Persistence with overactive bladder pharmacotherapy in a Medicaid population. *Am J Manag Care* 2005;**11**:S121–S129.

10 Gopal M, Haynes K, Bellamy SL, et al. Discontinuation rates of anticholinergic medications used for the treatment of lower urinary tract symptoms. *Obstet Gynecol.* 2008;**112**(6):1311–1318.

11 Callegari E, Malhotra B, Bungay PJ, et al. A comprehensive non-clinical evaluation of the CNS penetration potential of antimuscarinic agents for the treatment of overactive bladder. *Br J Clin Pharmacol.* 2011;**72**(2):235–246.

12 Kranz J, Petzinger E, Geyer J. Brain penetration of the OAB drug trospium chloride is not increased in aged mice. *World J Urol.* 2013;**31**(1):219–224.

13 Dmochowski, Sand PK, Zinner NR, et al. Trospium 60 mg once daily (qd) for overactive bladder syndrome: results from a placebo-controlled interventional study. *Urol.* 2008;**71**(3):449–454.

14 Harvey MA, Baker K, Wells GA. Tolterodine versus oxybutynin in the treatment of urge urinary incontinence: a meta-analysis. *Am J Obstet Gynecol.* 2001;**185**(1):56.

15 Herschorn, S, Stothers L, Carlson K, et al. Tolerability of 5 mg solifenacin once daily versus 5 mg oxybutynin immediate release 3 times daily: results of the VECTOR Trial. *J Uro* 2010;**183**(5):1892–1898.

16 Haab, Stewart L, Dwyer P. Darifenacin, an M3 selective receptor antagonist, is an effective and well-tolerated once-daily treatment for overactive bladder. *Euro Urol.* 2004;**45**(4):420–429.

17 Tyagi P, Tyagi V. Mirabegron, a β_3-adrenoceptor agonist for the potential treatment of urinary frequency, urinary incontinence or urgency associated with overactive bladder. *IDrugs* 2010;**13**(10);713–722.

18 Nitti VW, Auerbach S, Martin N, et al. Results of a randomized phase III trial of mirabegron in patients with overactive bladder. *J Urol.* 2013;**189**(4):1388–1395.

19 Steers, Wd, Herschorn S, Keder KJ, et al. Duloxetine compared with placebo for treating women with symptoms of overactive bladder. *BJU Int.* 2007;**100**:337.

20 Dmochowski RR, Gomelsky A. Update on the treatment of overactive bladder. *Curr Opin in Urol.* 2011;**21**(4):286–290.

21 Andersson K-E. Antimuscarinic mechanisms and the overactive detrusor: an update. *Euro Urol.* 2011;**59**(3):377–386.

22 Murray S, Lemack GE. Overactive bladder and mixed incontinence. *Curr Urol Rep.* 2011;**11**(6):385–392.

23 Gormley EA, Lightner DJ, Burgio KL, et al. Diagnosis and treatment of overactive bladder (non-neurogenic) in adults: AUA/SUFU guideline. *J Urol.* 2012;**188**:2455–2463.

CHAPTER 10

Patches and gels

L.N. Plowright and G.W. Davila

Cleveland Clinic Florida, Weston/Fort Lauderdale, Florida, FL, USA

KEY POINTS

- The prevalence of OAB increases with age in an essentially linear association from 25 to 75 years, with urge incontinence affecting approximately 12% of women aged 45 to 54 years. [3]

- OAB can severely impair physical and mental wellbeing. Nocturia reduces quality of sleep and OAB symptoms, particularly if accompanied by incontinence, may reduce work productivity and sexual activity, and limit mobility and social interactions. [3–6]

- Once a sufferer's QOL impact is significant, he/she will likely request therapy. Pharmacotherapy represents the mainstay of OAB treatment, but efficacy is frequently limited by undesirable anticholinergic side-effects including dry mouth, constipation, dry eyes, and others.

- Discontinuation rates are quite high as many may feel that "the treatment is worse than the disease."

- Oxybutynin (OXY) is one of the principal anticholinergic agents used for OAB around the world, with high reported efficacy rates, but parallel high rates of anticholinergic side-effects. Due to its molecular size, lipophilicity, and ability to be transferred transdermally, OXY has been identified as an agent particularly appropriate for transdermal (TD) delivery in order to alter its metabolism and reduce the occurrence of undesirable side-effects.

Rationale for TD OXY delivery

The prevalence of OAB increases with age in an essentially linear association from 25 to 75 years, with urge incontinence affecting approximately 12% of women aged 45 to 54 years. [3] OAB can severely impair physical and mental wellbeing. Nocturia reduces quality of sleep and OAB symptoms, particularly if accompanied by incontinence, may reduce work productivity and sexual activity, and limit mobility and social interactions. [3–6] Once a sufferer's QOL impact is significant, he/she will likely request therapy. **Pharmacotherapy represents the mainstay of OAB treatment, but efficacy is frequently limited by undesirable anticholinergic side-effects including dry mouth, constipation, dry eyes, and others.** Discontinuation rates are quite high as many may feel that "the treatment is worse than the disease." Oxybutynin (OXY) is one of the principal anticholinergic agents used for OAB around the

Overactive Bladder: Practical Management, First Edition. Edited by Jacques Corcos, Scott MacDiarmid and John Heesakkers.
© 2015 John Wiley & Sons, Ltd. Published 2015 by John Wiley & Sons, Ltd.

world, with high reported efficacy rates, but parallel high rates of anticholinergic side-effects. Due to its molecular size, lipophilicity, and ability to be transferred transdermally, OXY has been identified as an agent particularly appropriate for transdermal (TD) delivery in order to alter its metabolism and reduce the occurrence of undesirable side-effects. This chapter will discuss the theory, applicability, and experience to date with TD formulations of OXY.

Drug pharmacology

Oxybutynin

Oxybutynin is a tertiary amine with well-known anticholinergic and antispasmodic properties. The mechanisms of action, metabolism, and pharmacokinetics of oxybutynin have been studied extensively. Despite the proven clinical efficacy of the original immediate-release oral formulation of oxybutynin, optimal clinical use of this agent has been limited by its propensity to cause dose-dependent anticholinergic adverse events, particularly dry mouth. **More than 80% of OAB patients taking immediate-release oxybutynin reported dry mouth as an adverse event**. Orally administered oxybutynin is metabolized in the liver and gut by cytochrome P-450 (CYP-450), specifically CYP3A4. As a result, high plasma concentrations of the pharmacologically active metabolite *N*-desethyloxybutynin (DEO) result, which may be up to 10 times that of oxybutynin. Several studies have clearly demonstrated that compared with oxybutynin, DEO has a similar or slightly higher affinity for muscarinic receptors in the salivary gland. Together, these observations suggest that **DEO may be responsible for much of the dry mouth, as well as other anticholinergic side-effects that are associated with oxybutynin.**

Extended-release oral OXY represented the first successful effort to reduce the anticholinergic side-effects of oxybutynin. Comparing extended-release with immediate-release OXY, there is no associated difference in efficacy, but a significant reduction in the incidence of dry mouth. Extended-release oxybutynin showed an improved steady-state pharmacokinetic profile characterized by smaller fluctuations in plasma concentrations of DEO and OXY, with a reduced exposure to DEO. However, moderate to severe dry mouth was observed in 25% of the patients treated with extended-release oxybutynin. It is thus well accepted that DEO levels correlate with dry mouth severity, and reduction in first pass metabolism of OXY results in reduced DEO plasma levels and an improved side-effect profile for OXY administration.

Oxybutynin Transdermal Patch (TD)
Drug preparation
Oxybutynin transdermal system is a 39-cm^2 matrix-type patch which can be applied to the buttocks, abdomen, or hips. [7, 8] It contains 36 mg of racemic oxybutynin and triacetin (a skin permeation enhancer) and is dissolved in an acrylic block-copolymer adhesive. [9] The TD OXY system delivers 3.9 mg/day of oxybutynin at a steady rate delivering continuous oxybutynin for up to 3–4 days, therefore a twice per week regimen is recommended. [7, 8] The patch is comprised of an occlusive backing, the adhesive matrix, and release liner (Figures 10.1, 10.2). The active drug agent (OXY) is

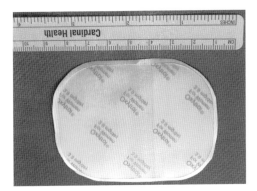

Figure 10.1 The transdermal patch is small in size and can be applied to various sites on the body.

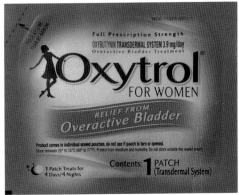

Figure 10.2 The patch is now available over the counter.

dissolved within the adhesive matrix and is thus continuously delivered transdermally, with the amount being determined by various factors including the patch surface area. In order to optimize drug transport, the patch must be appropriately applied to dry skin with the entire surface area firmly in contact with the skin surface.

Efficacy

The clinical efficacy of the transdermal patch in reducing the number of incontinent episodes has been demonstrated in several phase II and phase III studies. [10–12] In a six-week phase II clinical trial, 76 patients with a history of urge and mixed urinary incontinence were randomized to receive TD or oral immediate release oxybutynin. All patients were responders to previous oral immediate-release anticholinergic therapy, with symptomatic improvement during a minimum of 6 weeks of oral oxybutynin. After initiation of treatment, study participants were then assessed after 2, 4, and 6 weeks of therapy. Assessment of incontinent episodes, efficacy, and side-effect severity was accomplished with a three day diary, a visual analog scale, and an anticholinergic index questionnaire, respectively. Urodynamic testing was performed in all subjects at baseline and during therapy. The average number of incontinence episodes was reduced from washout to end of study by approximately five episodes/day in both groups ($p < 0.0001$) with no significant difference between the oral and the TD group. There was no difference in the visual analog score ($p = 0.9$) and there was no significant difference in the average bladder volume at first bladder contraction between groups (TD; 66 ± 126 vs. Oral; 45 ± 163 ml). [10] The Oxybutynin transdermal patch has also demonstrated equivalent efficacy when compared to tolteridine extended release formulations. [11, 12] Quality of life has been studied utilizing validated questionnaires, and has been demonstrated to be significantly improved with TD OXY in a community-based population. [13]

Tolerability

When compared to the oral immediate release formulation, the oxybutynin TD system achieved remarkably improved anticholinergic tolerability. [10] In a 12-week double-blind, double-dummy treatment with TD, tolteridine, and placebo the incidence of dry mouth was 4.1% with TD compared to 1.7% with placebo. [12] This is much lower than the 17–87% reported in previous studies of oral oxybutynin. **The reason for improvement in anticholinergic side-effect profile is thought to be largely due to the avoidance of the first-pass effect leading to steady-state concentrations of oxybutynin and DEO.**

Transdermal application can cause a local reaction at the skin site. [9–11] A phase III pivotal trial revealed 16.8% of patients reported application site pruritus and 8.3% of patients reported application site erythema. [11] These reactions were self-limited and avoidable through the use of multiple application sites. As a follow-up to the above trial, an open label study extension was offered to patients. Prior to doing so patients were given a satisfaction questionnaire. Approximately two-thirds of participants stated that they would prefer a TD system to others if repeat treatment for OAB was needed. The majority of patients (72%) reported that application site erythema and pruritus disappeared within a week. Many users (68%) described the patch as very easy to apply and slightly easier to remember than taking a pill (45 versus 33%). [14]

Oxybutynin Topical Gel (OTG)
Drug preparation
The oxybutynin topical gel-based formulation was developed from efforts to minimize the local skin reactions experienced with the transdermal system. In this preparation the skin acts as the reservoir for continuous release of oxybutynin. The gel is clear, colorless, and fragrance free, and when applied to the skin dries quickly without leaving a residue. Typical sites for applications include the abdomen, arms,

shoulders, or thighs. Each dose consists of a 1 gram sachet, which contains oxybutynin 100 mg (10% gel) in a small application volume (1.14 ml). Alternatively, a multi-dose delivery pump is available with three pumps delivering a standard 1g of OXY which can then be applied to the skin. Unlike the patch, daily application of gel is needed in order to achieve steady-state OXY levels in the circulation. The base of the gel is a mixture of water and alcohol. Other components include hydroxypropyl cellulose as the gelling agent, glycerin as an emollient, and sodium hydroxide for pH adjustment of the gel to mirror the physiologic pH of the skin. [15]

Efficacy
Oxybutynin topical gel has demonstrated clinical efficacy in a double-blind, randomized, multicenter placebo controlled phase III study of OTG in patients with OAB. [16] This was a 12-week study of 789 patients with urge or mixed urinary incontinence who received either OTG (389) or placebo (400). The patients were predominantly women (89.2%) with greater than a third of the participants 65 years or older. One quarter of all patients had previously taken OAB medications. At baseline the mean number of daily urinary incontinence episodes was 5.4, daily nocturia was 2.5, and mean frequency was approximately 12 for both groups indicating that a substantial amount of patients had OAB of the severe form. Patients using OTG demonstrated a great reduction in daily incontinence episodes (mean decrease -3.0 vs. -2.5; $p<0.0001$) and daily urinary frequency episodes (mean decrease -2.7 vs. 2.0; $p=0.0017$) compared with placebo (Table 10.1). A significant decrease in daily nocturia episodes was observed only in patients

Table 10.1 Efficacy variable changes from baseline to study end.

Variables	OTG	Placebo
No. pts*	389	400
No. daily urinary incontinence episodes		
Baseline:		
Mean±SD	5.4±3.3	5.4±3.3
Median	4.7	4.7
p Value [least squares adjusted mean]	0.9946	
Study end:		
Mean±SD	2.4±13	2.9±3.3
Median	1.0	1.7
Change from baseline by study end:		
Mean±SD	−3.0±2.7	−2.5±3.1
Median	−2.7	−2.0
p Value (least squares adjusted mean)	<0.0001	
Daily urinary frequency (No. Episodes)		
Baseline:		
Mean±SD	12.4±3.3	12.2±3.3
Median	11.7	11.3
p Value (least squares adjusted mean)	0.3516	
Study end:		
Mean±SD	9.8±3.5	10.2±3.2
Median	9.3	9.7
Change from baseline by study end:		
Mean±SD	−2.7±3.2	−2.0±2.8
Median	−2.7	−1.7
p Value (least squares adjusted mean)	0.0017	
Voided urinary vol (ml)		
Baseline:		
Mean±SD	163.4±65.8	167.9±68.4
Median	160.1	160.6
p Value (least squares adjusted mean)	0.3543	
Study end:		
Mean±SD	184.2±82.9	171.8±74.8
Median	177.9	165.3
Change from baseline by study end:		
Mean±SD	21.0±65.3	3.8±53.8
Median	11.5	0.0
p Value (least squares adjusted mean)	0.0018	
No. daily nocturia events		
Baseline:		
Mean±SD	2.5±1.6	2.5±1.7
Median	2.3	2.3
p Value (least squares adjusted mean)	0.9484	
Study end:		
Mean±SD	1.7±1.5	1.8±1.5

(*Continued*)

Table 10.1 (Continued)

Variables	OTG	Placebo
Median	1.3	1.7
Change from baseline by study end:		
Mean ± SD	−0.75 ± 1.4	−0.65 ± 1.3
Median	−0.7	−0.7
p Value (least squares adjusted means)	0.1372	

*No significant differences were observed in end point findings between patients who completed the study and those who withdrew (last observation carried forward).
Source: Staskin 2009 [16]. Reproduced with permission of Elsevier.

younger than 65 years (mean decrease −0.91 vs. 0.72; $p=0.363$) There was also a significant increase in voided volume for those treated with OTG (placebo 3.8 Ml; $p=0.0018$). At the conclusion of the study, 28% of the patients treated with OTG and 17% of those receiving placebo achieved complete continence.

The clinical efficacy has also been demonstrated specifically by a *post hoc* analysis of the phase III study data. [17] In this study 352 received the topical gel while 352 received a placebo treatment. Mean age was 59 years. Baseline demographic and urinary symptom values for the female subgroup were very similar to those for the total study population. After 12 weeks of treatment the female patients treated with OTG achieved greater improvements in daily urinary incontinence episodes (−3.0 vs. placebo, −2.5; $p<0.0001$), daily urinary frequency (−2.8 vs. placebo, −2.0; $p=0.0013$), and voided volume (mean increase 22.7 ml vs. 4.0 ml; $p=0.0002$). At study end, 27.0% of women treated with OTG compared with 15.6% of those receiving placebo had achieved complete continence.

Safety

No treatment-related serious adverse events were observed during the phase III study of OTG. [11] Dry mouth was the most commonly reported adverse event at 6.9 vs. 2.8% ($p=0.0060$) (Table 10.2). This incidence was similar to that seen for the transdermal patch but substantially smaller than the incidences of dry mouth reported in comparable studies of oral oxybutynin. [6, 7, 15] Other treatment related anticholinergic adverse events include the following: constipation (1.3%), dizziness (1.5%), nausea (0.3%), dry eye (0.5%), dysuria (0.3%), and somnolence (0.3%) (Table 10.2). [18]

Effects on skin

Skin tolerability of the topical gel has also been demonstrated in clinical studies. As there is minimal absorption of light by the gel at wavelengths of 290–700 nm the gel is unlikely to cause phototoxic skin reactions. In addition, a study in albino guinea pigs further suggested that the topical gel does not elicit dermal reactions or delayed contact sensitization. These findings were confirmed by two placebo- controlled phase I dermatological studies in healthy subjects. In the cumulative skin irritation study the scale of Berger and Bowman was used to score 41 subjects after being treated with three weeks of daily topical gel and gel placebo on contralateral sites of the back. [19] The mean scores obtained with the topical gel

Table 10.2 Treatment related anticholinergic AEs reported during double-blind study treatment.

AE	No. OTG (%)	No Placebo (%)	p Value
No. pts	389	400	
Dry mouth	27 (6.9)	11 (2.8)	0.0060 (chi-square test)
Constipation	5 (1.3)	4 (1.0)	0.7494 (Fisher's exact test)
Dizziness	6 (1.5)	2 (0.5)	0.1719 (Fisher's exact test)
Nausea	1 (0.3)	2 (0.5)	1.0000 (Fisher's exact test)
Dry eye	2 (0.5)	1 (0.3)	0.6194 (Fisher's exact test)
Dysuria	1 (0.3)	1 (0.3)	1.0000 (Fisher's exact test)
Somnolence	1 (0.3)	0	0.4930 (Fisher's exact test)
Urinary retention	0	1 (0.3)	1.0000 (Fisher's exact test)

Source: Staskin 2009 [16]. Reproduced with permission of Elsevier.

and placebo were 35 and 24. Both scores were substantially less than 50, which is the lowest score considered as evidence of cumulative irritation. Excellent skin tolerability of OTG also was observed during the phase III trial. [16] Application site skin reactions as adverse events were reported by 5.4% of patients who received topical gel and by 1% of those who received placebo. Eight of 389 patients (2.1%) treated with topical gel and 3 of 400 patients (0.8%) receiving placebo reported application site pruritus as an adverse event. The incidence of application site erythema was similar among patients treated with topical gel (1.3% per visit) and those who received placebo (0.9% per visit). At study end, inspection of application sites by the investigator revealed no erythema on 97.4 and 98.7% of patients receiving topical and placebo, respectively. Among the few patients receiving topical gel who had application site erythema, none had severe symptoms. Three patients (0.8%) in the topical group and one patient (0.3%) in the placebo group discontinued treatment because of application site reactions. [16]

Patient experience
Impact on quality of life
In a subgroup analysis of the phase III study, quality of life effects of topical gel versus placebo were evaluated using the five-item Incontinence Impact Questionnaire (IIQ) and the 10-item King's Health Questionnaire (KHQ). [15] Topical gel demonstrated significant improvement in total scores and in all IIQ domains, including travel ($p=0.0021$), physical activity ($p=0.003$), social relationships ($p=0.0005$), and emotional health ($p<0.0001$). Topical gel use also promoted significant HRQoL improvements in 6 of 10 King's Health Questionnaire domains, including incontinence impact ($p=0.0002$), symptom severity ($p=0.0003$), role limitations ($p=0.004$), personal relationships ($p=0.0161$), sleep/energy ($p=0.008$), and severity (coping) measures ($p=0.0021$). [20]

Future prospects
Future transdermal drug delivery options for OXY include usage of other skin sites. Transvaginal delivery via a vaginal ring delivery system is in development and early data has been reported. [21] Patches

with reduced skin occlusive properties have also been evaluated and may be available in the future. As with other pharmacologic agents amenable to TD delivery, such as hormonal agents and antihypertensives, we can expect new technology to provide us with new skin-based drug administration options.

Conclusion/expert opinion

The efficacy of oxybutynin for treatment of OAB has been proven in many clinical trials. Due to the anticholinergic side-effects associated with oral delivery, in particular dry mouth, patient adherence is problematic. The development of a transdermal oxybutynin delivery system has improved the side-effect profile while maintaining drug efficacy. Application site reactions for the transdermal patch are minimal and short lived and are less prevalent for the gel formulation. **This technology is seen more favorably by many OAB patients and may improve medication adherence and treatment persistence.**

References

1 Chapple CR, Khullar V, Gabriel Z, et al. The effects of antimuscarinic treatments in overactive bladder: an update of a systematic review and meta-analysis. *Eur Urol.* 2008;**54**(3):543–562.

2 D'Souza AO, Smith MJ, Miller LA, et al. Persistence, adherence, and switch rates among extended-release and immediate-release overactive bladder medications in a regional managed care plan. *J Manag Care Pharm.* 2008;**14**(3):291–301.

3 Stewart WF, Van Rooyen JB, Cundiff GW, et al. Prevalence and burden of overactive bladder in the United States. *World J Urol.* 2003; **20**(6):327–336.

4 Coyne KS, Payne C, Bhattacharyya SK, et al. The impact of urinary urgency and frequency on health-related quality of life in overactive bladder: results from a national community survey. *Value Health.* 2004;**7**(4):455–463.

5 Coyne KS, Sexton CC, Irwin DE, et al. The impact of overactive bladder, incontinence and other lower urinary tract symptoms on quality of life, work productivity, sexuality and emotional well-being in men and women: results from the EPIC study. *BJU Int.* 2008;**101** (11):1388–1395.

6 Sexton CC, Coyne KS, Vats V, et al. Impact of overactive bladder on work productivity in the United States: results from EpiLUTS. *Am J Manag Care.* 2009;**15**(4 Suppl):S98–S107.

7 Sahai A, Mallina R, Dowson C, et al. Evolution of transdermal oxybutynin in the treatment of over-active bladder. *Int J Clin Pract.*2008; **62**(1):167–170.

8 Caramelli KE, Staskin DR, Volinn W. Steady-state pharmacokinetics of an investigational oxybutynin topical gel in comparison with oxybutynin transdermal system. *J Urol.* 2008;**179**(4, suppl.):513–514.

9 Davila GW. Transdermal oxybutynin in the treatment of overactive bladder. *Clin Interven Aging* 2006;**1**(2):99–105.

10 Davila GW, Daugherty CA, Sanders SW. Transdermal Oxybutynin Study Group. A short-term, multicenter, randomized double-blind dose titration study of the efficacy and anticholinergic side effects of transdermal compared to immediate release oral oxybutynin treatment of patients with urge urinary incontinence. *J Urol* 2001;**166**(1):140–145.

11 Dmochowski RR, Sand PK, Zinner NR, et al. Transermal Oxybutynin Study Group. Comparitive efficacy and safety of transdermal oxybutynin and oral tolterodine versus placebo in previously treated patients with urge and mixed urinary incontinence. *Urology* 2003;**62**(2):237–242.

12 Domochowski RR, Davila GW, Zinner NR, et al. For The Transdermal Oxybutyinin Study Group. Efficacy and safety of transdermal oxybutyin in patients with urge and mixed urinary incontinence. *J Urol.* 2002;**168**(2):580–586.

13 Sand PK, Zinner N, Newman D, et al. Oxybutynin transdermal symstem improves the quality of life in adults with overactive

bladder: A multicentre, community-based, randomized study. *BJU Int.* 2007;**99**(4): 836–844.

14 Newman DK. 2003. Patient perception on new therapeutic options for the control of overactive bladder. Poster presented at the 34th Annual Conference of SUNA, March 26–30, San Antonio, TX USA.

15 Staskin DR, Salvatore S. Oxybutynin topical and transdermal formulations: an update. *Drugs of Today*, 2010;**46**(6):417–425.

16 Staskin DR, Dmochowski RR, Sand PK, et al. Efficacy and safety of Oxybutynin chloride topical gel in women with overactive bladder: A randomized, double-blind, placebo controlled, multi-center-study. *J Urol* 2009;**81**(4):1764–1772

17 Dmochwski RR, Staskin DR, Macdiarmid AS et al. Efficacy and safety of oxybutynin topical gel for overactive bladder: A randomized, double-blind study (abstract). *J Urol.* 2009;**181**:589.

18 Starkman JS, Dmochowski RR. Management of overactive bladder with transdermal oxybutynin. *Rev Urol.* 2006;**8**(3):93–103.

19 Berger RS, Bowman JP. A reappraisal of the 21-day cumulative irritation test in man. *J Toxicol Cutaneous Ocul Toxicol.*1982;**1**(2):109–115.

20 Sand PK, Davila GW, Lucente VR, et al. Efficacy and Safety of oxybutynin chloride topical gel for women with overactive bladder syndrome. *Am J Obstet Gynecol.* 2012;**206**:168.e1–6.

21 Nelken RS, Ozel BZ, Leegant AR, et al. Randomized trial of estradiol vaginal ring versus oral oxybutynin for the treatment of overactive bladder. *Menopause* 2011;**18**(9): 962–966.

CHAPTER 11

Promising experimental drugs and drug targets

Karl-Erik Andersson

Faculty of Health, Institute for Clinical Medicine, University of Arhus, Arhus, Denmark

---

KEY POINTS

- Due to the multifactorial pathophysiology, lower urinary tract symptoms (LUTS), including overactive bladder syndrome (OAB), still offer therapeutic challenges.

- Although the efficacy of β_3-adrenoceptor agonists (mirabegron), PDE5 inhibitors (tadalafil), and onabotulinum toxinA have recently been demonstrated, these drugs are not suitable for all patients, and new drugs with theoretically interesting profiles are being developed.

- Among the different new targets being investigated, the most promising seem to be the purinergic and cannabinoid systems and the different members of the TRP channel family.

Introduction

The overactive bladder (OAB), defined symptomatically as OAB syndrome (OAB) or urodynamically as detrusor overactivity (DO), is a condition that can have major effects on quality of life and social functioning. Antimuscarinic drugs are still first-line pharmacological treatment. These drugs often have good initial response rates, but adverse effects and decreasing efficacy cause long-term compliance problems and alternatives are needed. The recognition of the functional contribution of the urothelium, the spontaneous myocyte activity during bladder filling, and the diversity of nerve transmitters involved in bladder activation has sparked interest in both peripheral and central modulation of OAB/DO pathophysiology. Three drugs, mirabegron, tadalafil, and onabotulinum toxinA have recently been approved for treatment of OAB/DO; however, other drugs with theoretically interesting profiles are being investigated (Table 11.1). For example, NGF and other neurotrophins have been suggested to be interesting targets for treatment and biomarkers for diagnosis and evaluation of treatment outcomes. [1–3] However, the adverse effects found in non-bladder studies with the humanized NGF antibody tested clinically

---

Overactive Bladder: Practical Management, First Edition. Edited by Jacques Corcos, Scott MacDiarmid and John Heesakkers.

Table 11.1 Future drugs and targets

- *Purinergic receptors – Antagonists*
- *Cannabinoid*
  system – Agonists – Antagonists – Inhibitors
- *TRP channels – Antagonists*
- *Prostanoid receptors – Antagonists*
- *Nerve growth factor – Inhibitor*
- *Rho-kinase – Inhibitors*
- *Vitamin D$_3$ receptor – Agonists*
- *K+ channels – K+ channel openers*
- *Centrally acting drugs*

(tanezumab) stopped further development. Prostanoids are synthesized in the bladder wall (COX I and II), and PGE2, which stimulates bladder contractile activity by sensitization of afferent nerves, is increased in urine from patients with lower urinary tract symptoms (LUTS)/OAB. PGE2 acts via different EP receptors. [4] Despite promising results in animal experiments, it seems that EP1-receptor antagonism is not an effective therapeutic approach. The efficacy and safety of an EP-1 receptor antagonist was examined in a randomized, double-blind, placebo-controlled phase II study which concluded that the role of EP1 receptor antagonist in the management of OAB syndrome is minimal. A theoretically interesting principle is Rho-kinase inhibition. [5] Upregulation of the Rho-kinase pathway has been associated with bladder changes in diabetes, outflow obstruction, and idiopathic DO. The vitamin D3 agonist, elocalcitol, was shown to have an inhibitory effect on the RhoA/Rho kinase pathway, [6, 7] and showed some promising effects in female patients with OAB. However, whether or not vitamin D3 receptor agonism (monotherapy or in combination) will be a useful alternative for the treatment of LUTS/OAB, requires further RCTs. The opening of bladder K+ channels has shown great promise in preclinical

experiments. [8] Many of the K-channel openers have been studied clinically – all so far with disappointing results. Maxi-K therapy (injection of "naked" Maxi-K DNA directly into detrusor) is an interesting future possibility. [9] Several proof of principle studies on drugs with an action on the CNS have been performed. [10] However, it seems that the currently used drugs have low efficacy and/or unacceptable side-effects. On the other hand, here may be a great potential for further developments.

Presently, the most promising targets seem to be the purinergic and cannabinoid systems and different members of the TRP channel family. P2X receptors are considered important in OAB pathophysiology, and P2X3 receptor antagonists have a good preclinical rationale. [11, 12] Clinical observations have indicated that cannabinoid receptor agonists offer a promising therapeutic approach, but interference with endogenous cannabinoid generation may offer additional possibilities. [13, 14] Studies of the lower urinary tract (LUT) have indicated that several TRP channels, including TRPV1, TRPV2, TRPV4, TRPM8, and TRPA1, are expressed in the bladder and urethra, and may act as sensors of stretch and/or chemical irritation. [15] However, the roles of these individual receptors for normal LUT function and in LUTS/OAB have not been established.

This chapter is focused on the purinergic and cannabinoid systems and some of the members of the TRP channel family.

P2X$_3$-receptors and P2X$_3$ receptor antagonists

P2X receptors are ligand-gated ion channels. Seven P2X receptor subunits for these ionotropic ATP receptors have been identified from molecular studies and characterized functionally and pharmacologically. [11, 16, 17]

Sensory nerve fibers expressing $P2X_3$ immunoreactivity have been found projecting into the lamina propria, urothelium, and detrusor smooth muscle, [11] where this and several other P2X receptors are functionally expressed. [11, 18] These findings suggest that $P2X_3$ receptors have a role in regulating bladder sensory functions. Numerous studies have shown that ATP is released from the bladder urothelium in response to distension [19–21] and studies using an isolated bladder-pelvic nerve preparation in rodents have shown that distension leads to increased afferent nerve activity that is mimicked by ATP and/or α,β-meATP. [22, 20, 23] Intravesical infusion of ATP or α,β-meATP can directly stimulate bladder overactivity in conscious rats, in a manner that is concentration-dependent and sensitive to the ATP receptor antagonist TNP-ATP.

In bladder urothelial cells from patients with bladder pain syndrome/interstitial cystis (BPS/IC), $P2X_3$ receptor expression appears to be abnormally u-regulated in response to stretch. [24, 25] An increased density of $P2X_3$ and TRPV1-expressing nerve fibers has been observed in the bladders of patients with neurogenic detrusor overactivity, and following treatment with resiniferatoxin patients responding to treatment showed diminished levels of both TRPV1 and $P2X_3$ immunoreactivity. [26]

A mechanosensory transduction pathway within the micturition reflex involving ATP has been suggested. ATP released from the urothelium activates $P2X_3$ and/or $P2X_{2/3}$ receptors on suburothelial primary afferents. ATP and α,β-meATP have been shown to not only activate low- and high-

threshold bladder afferents directly, but also to sensitize their mechanosensory responses. [20, 23] Bladder inflammation can also sensitize and enhance P2X receptor function on pelvic visceral and hypogastric splanchnic afferents in the lumbosacral and thoracolumbar DRG. [27] Thus, $P2X_3$ and $P2X_{2/3}$ receptors may be important in sensing volume changes during normal bladder filling, and may participate in lowering the threshold for C-fiber activation under pathophysiological conditions.

P2X receptors, and in particular $P2X_3$ receptors, have been of interest for treatment of LUT disorders for a long time. [11, 12, 28, 29]: Selective $P2X_3$ antagonists, such as A-317491, were shown to effectively improve the signs of cyclophosphamide-induced cystitis, [30] and to improve bladder function in a rat spinal cord injury (SCI) model [31]; A-317491 produced a dose-dependent inhibition of non-micturition bladder contractions, increased inter-micturition intervals and bladder capacity without influencing the amplitude of voiding contractions. The diaminopyrimidine, AF-353[32] was studied in SCI rats with neurogenic bladder overactivity. [33] SCI rats had significantly higher frequencies for field potentials and non-voiding contractions than normal rats. Intravesical ATP increased field potential frequency in control, but not SCI, rats while systemic AF-353 significantly reduced this parameter in both groups. AF-353 also reduced the inter-contractile interval in control, but not in SCI rats; however, the frequency of non-voiding contractions in SCI rats was significantly reduced. AF-353 was also studied in a closed cystometric model ("refill VIBC") in a urethane anesthetized rat with a dose-dependent increase in volume threshold by up to 50–70%, with frequency slightly reduced, but no appreciable change in amplitude. [11] As AF-353 penetrates the blood–brain barrier, [32] it was not clear whether these effects resulted from $P2X_3$ antagonism at peripheral terminals within the bladder wall, or alternatively at central terminals in the spinal cord dorsal horn. It has been suggested that ATP can be released and act on spinal $P2X_3$ and $P2X_{2/3}$ receptors to affect afferent signals originating from the bladder. [29] Spinal ATP may then constitute an endogenous central presynaptic purinergic mechanism to regulate visceral sensory transmission. Further characterization of this spinal purinergic control in visceral activities may help the development of $P2X_3$ and $P2X_{2/3}$ antagonist to treat urological dysfunction, such as overactive bladder. [29]

The cannabinoid system

The endocannabinoid system comprises the cannabinoid (CB) receptors, their endogenous ligands, and related enzymes for biosynthesis and degradation. [34]. Plant-derived cannabinoids (phytocannabinoids) can be extracted from the cannabis plant (marijuana), the main psychoactive compounds being Δ9-tetrahydrocannabinol (Δ9-THC), cannabidiol, and cannabinol. Based on the effects of these compounds, two G-protein coupled cannabinoid (CB) receptors type 1 (CB1) and type 2 (CB2) have been defined. A third receptor, the G-protein coupled receptor 55 (GPR55) has been described, but what pharmacological effect it mediates is incompletely known. These receptors can interact with endocannabinoids and "exocannabinoids," such as phytocannabinoids and synthetic cannabinoids, and some associated endogenous

fatty acid amides (FAA). The endocannabinoid system contains at least two major arachidonate-derived ligands, anandamide and 2-arachidonoylglycerol (2-AG), that mediate their effects by binding to CB1 and CB2 receptors. [34–36]

In the nervous system, anandamide and 2-arachidonoylglycerol are primarily metabolized by the serine hydrolase enzymes fatty acid amide hydrolase (FAAH) and monoacylglycerol lipase (MAGL), respectively. [37] Preventing their degradation with inhibitors of these enzymes can enhance their endogenous actions. Anandamide and several exogenous CB receptor agonists are known to also act at other receptors such as the vanilloid TRPV1 channel. [38] Most cannabinoids have the capacity to pass the blood–brain barrier.

Distribution of cannabinoid receptors

Both CB1 and CB2 receptors are expressed in the LUT, and cannabinoid-related functions have been amply demonstrated in isolated tissues and in experimental *in vivo* models of normal micturition and bladder dysfunction. [39–46] In the rat bladder, both CB1 and CB2 receptors have been demonstrated, particularly on the urothelium. [39] Also in human whole bladders obtained from male organ donors, both CB1 and CB2 receptor were found to be expressed – twice as much in the urothelium as in the detrusor. Overall the expression of CB1 was higher than that of CB2 receptors. [44] Bladders of humans and rats were found to express CB1 receptors, TRPV1 channels, and FAAH. [47] CB2 receptors were expressed in higher densities in rat, monkey, and human bladder mucosa (urothelium and surburothelium) than in the detrusor, and were also colocalized with TRPV1 and CGRP. [40] In the detrusor wall, CB2 immunoreactive fibers were identified on cholinergic nerves. [41] CB1 immunoreactive fiber density was significantly increased in the suburothelium of bladder specimen from patients with painful bladder syndrome and idiopathic detrusor overactivity (IDO). In patients with IDO, the density correlated with their symptom scores, as compared to control. [46]

CB1 and CB2 receptors were identified in the spinal cord and dorsal root ganglia of rats. [43, 48–51], At the spinal level, several studies have located CB receptors in areas involved in modulation of afferent activity. [49] Both CB1 and CB2 receptor mRNA and protein were detected in the lumbosacral spinal cord and in L5-L6/S1 dorsal root ganglia (DRG). Interestingly, the expression in the DRG or spinal cord was not affected by acute or chronic inflammation of the bladder. [43]

Supraspinally, high densities of CB1 receptors were found in the cingulate gyrus and the medial frontal cortex, in moderate densities in the periaqueductal gray matter, thalamus, and insula, and in low densities in the pons. [52] A high density of CB2 receptors was found in the thalamus and a moderate density in the periaqueductal gray matter and pons. [52] Unforunately, the functional role of both spinal and supraspinal CB receptors in the control of micturition is incompletely known.

Cannabinoids in micturition

There are many studies both in isolated bladder tissue and *in vivo* showing that cannabinoids can affect bladder function. In general, these studies have shown a lack of direct effect of cannabinoid receptor agonists on bladder contractility, but results

are not always consistent, partly due to species differences and experimental techniques. The actions of the endocannabinoid – anandamide – is complicated since it is known to also activate TRPV1 receptors, potentially via the release of CGRP. [53] Thus in rat detrusor muscle strips, anandamide application produced slowly developing contractions which were attenuated by previous capsaicin sensitization, suggesting involvement of TRPV1 receptors. [54]. Neither anandamide nor CP55,940 (CB1 and CB2 receptor agonist) affected carbachol induced contractions in rat, monkey, or human bladder preparations; however, anandamide increased EFS induced contractions while CP55,940 decreased them at all frequencies. [40] ACEA, a selective CB1 receptor agonist, attenuated the EFS and carbachol-induced contractions of rat bladder, whereas GP1A, a selective CB2 receptor agonist, only decreased carbachol-induced contractions in rat bladder. [47]

The effect *N*-acylethanolamides, anandamide (via CB1 receptors) and palmitoylethanolamide (putative endogenous CB2 receptor agonist), caused analgesia in models of bladder overactivity induced by inflammation. [55, 56] Intraperitoneal administration of GP1A decreased the mechanical sensitivity in a mouse model of acrolein induced cystitis, possibly by preventing phosphorylation of ERK1/2 via MAPK activation. [57] Treatment with another selective CB2 receptor agonist (O-1966) following spinal cord injury improved bladder recovery in rats by modifying the inflammatory response. [58] CB2 receptor agonism appears to decrease viscera-visceral pain caused by bladder inflammation, possibly by modulating afferent signaling in the spinal cord and promoting an anti-inflammatory effect. CB2 receptor activation has immuno-modulatory functions that can limit the endothelial inflammatory response, chemo-taxis, and inflammatory cell adhesion and activation in atherosclerosis and reperfusion injury. [59]

Cannabinor, a highly selective CB2 agonist, increased micturition intervals and threshold pressures during conscious cystometry. [41] Chronic administration of this compound over two weeks following partial urethral obstruction in rats decreased post void residual and the number of non-voiding contractions and increased bladder compliance as compared to controls. [42]

Overall, exocannabinoid agonists seem to have an inhibitory effect on micturition, by increasing threshold pressure and decreasing frequency, possibly through inhibition of afferent signaling.

In 2012, Stritmatter et al. [60] demon-strated that FAAH is expressed in the bladder of rats, mice, and humans. They also dem-onstrated that systemic or intravesical administration of a FAAH inhibitor, oleoyl ethyl amide, during awake cystometry sig-nificantly increased intercontraction inter-vals, micturition volume, bladder capacity, and threshold pressure in rats. These effects were abolished with the concomitant use of SR144528, a CB2 receptor antagonist, showing that FAAH inhibition mediated its effect on micturition via CB2 receptors.

Clinical trials

Early reports showing that patients with multiple sclerosis (MS) could have a positive on their urinary tract symptoms [61] were followed by a small number of open-label and placebo-controlled studies demonstrating that orally administered cannabinoid modulators may alleviate

neurogenic OAB symptoms. [62–64] The effects of whole plant cannabis extracts (containing delta-9- tetrahydrocannabinol and/or cannabidiol) have been mostly studied in patients with advanced MS and severe LUTS, and a significant decrease in urinary urgency, the number and volume of incontinence episodes, frequency, and nocturia has been demonstrated. [62–64] However, this symptomatic improvement was not well reflected urodynamically. [63, 64]

Side-effects from cannabinoids, such as dizziness, light-headedness, attention deficit, fatigue, and disorientation, have been reported [62, 64, 65] and are an obvious disadvantage with exocannabinoid therapy. Efforts to avoid the CNS-related side-effects of the cannabinoids have led to the development of alternative drug approaches with peripheral CB subtype receptor–selective compounds, or drugs that target the turnover of endocannabinoids or FAA. Amplification of endocannabinoid activity by FAAH inhibitors may be a novel, attrac-tive drug principle that has therapeutic potential in specific regions of the lower urinary tract or in sensory regulatory path-ways of micturition that are involved in the development of LUTS.

TRP channels

Studies of the LUT have shown that several TRP channels – including TRPV1, TRPV2, TRPV4, TRPM8, and TRPA1 – are expressed in both the bladder and the urethra and may act as sensors of stretch and/or chemical irritation. [66–68] However, the roles of these individual receptors for normal LUT function and in LUTS/DO/OAB have not been definitely established.

They are highly expressed in, but not restricted to, primary afferent neurons. Thus the urothelium, some interstitial cells, and detrusor muscle also express several TRP channels. [66–68]

TRPV1 and bladder function

TRPV1 is the best-characterized member of the TRPV subfamily TRPV1-6 in terms of expression pattern, properties, and clinical translation of its manipulation. [69] It is a non-selective cationic channel with high Ca2+ permeability allowing the passage of cations, mainly calcium, upon activation by vanilloids, noxious heat, and low pH. [70] Despite extensive information on morphology and function in animal models, the role of TRPV1 in normal human bladder function is still controversial. However, its role in the pathophysiology and treatment of particularly neurogenic DO (NDO) is well established.

In single-unit bladder nerve recordings, low-threshold neuronal responses were attenuated in TRPV1 knockout mice compared with their TRPV1 littermates, whereas high-threshold sensitivity was unchanged. [71] This suggested that the neuronal TRPV1 channels in the suburothelium were needed for normal excitability of low-threshold bladder fibers. TRPV1 knock out mice showed enhanced intermicturition spotting, whereas normal micturitions seemed to be unaffected. [66] This was reflected in the cystometrograms by an increase in the frequency of non-voiding contractions and a regular pattern of voluntary voiding contractions. Urethane anesthetized TRPV1 knock out mice displayed increases in mean bladder capacity and reductions in spinal cord c-fos induction in response to bladder distension. [72] In conscious mice, the micturition frequency

was unaffected in these knock outs, suggesting that TRPV1-mediated mechanisms are responsible for setting the micturition threshold under anesthesia, whereas non-TRPV1-mediated mechanisms set the threshold in voluntary conditions.

The clinical application of TRPV1 agonists has been extensively reviewed elsewhere. [66, 73–75] Maggi et al. [76], instilling capsaicin intravesically to patients with bladder hypersensitivity disorders, found the drug to produce a concentration-related reduction of the first desire to void, bladder capacity, and pressure threshold for micturition, suggesting the occurrence of capsaicin-sensitive structures in the human bladder. The neuronal TRPV1 channel was suggested to have pathophysiological roles, contributing to overactive bladder and pain. [77] Patients with NDO were found to have an increased immunoreactivity of PGP9.5 (nerve stain) and TRPV1 in the suburothelium and an increased TRPV1 reactivity in the basal layers of the urothelium compared to control patients. In addition, patients with NDO clinically responding to intravesical instillations of RTX showed a significant decrease of this TRPV1 immunoreactivity in both the suburothelium and the basal urothelial layers compared to non-responders, suggesting a role for TRPV1 in the pathophysiology of NDO. [78–80] The effects of vanilloids (capsaicin, RTX) on urothelial TRPV1 indicate that vanilloid actions are more complex than simple C-fiber desensitization. The exact effect of capsaicin or its analogs on the different TRPV1 positive structures (urothelium, afferent nerve fibers, interstitial cells) still needs further elucidation.

Patients with OAB symptoms without demonstrable DO, but an early first sensation during bladder filling due to sensory discomfort (sensory urgency), showed an increased TRPV1 mRNA expression in the trigonal mucosa. In these patients, TRPV1 expression levels in the trigone were inversely correlated to the volume at first sensation during bladder filling. In patients with IDO, on the other hand, there were no changes in TRPV1 expression levels, suggesting a distinct molecular basis between sensory urgency and IDO. [81]

The primary defect in DO may be found in the urethra. [82]. In females, it has been reported that a rapid pattern of urethral pressure variation ("unstable urethra") is closely associated with DO. [83–85] The presence of TRPV1-IR nerves in the urethra, and the effects of capsaicin on both urethral and striated muscles [66], raise the question whether this channel is involved in urethral functions that can be linked to DO/OAB.

TRPV2 channels and bladder function

TRPV2 is a nonselective cation channel with high Ca2+ permeability; it acts as a heat sensor with a temperature threshold of 50–52 °C, and is activated by agonists such as 2-aminoethoxydiphenyl borate and D9-tetrahydrocannabinol (THC). [86] In vascular smooth muscle cells TRPV2 is stretch-activated channel and can increase stretch-induced [Ca2+]i. [87]

In rat urinary bladders, TRPV2 mRNA is expressed in urothelial and smooth muscle cells, [72] and the channel is also functionally expressed in mouse urothelial cells. [88] Ost et al. [89] found immunostaining for TRPV2 in small nerve fibers, suburothelial cells and smooth muscle cells in the human bladder, but the specificity of the antibodies was uncertain. [66] In the

human bladder, Caprodossi et al. [90] found TRPV2 expression in normal human urothelial cells and bladder tissue specimens. The TRPV2 channel is also highly expressed in sensory DRG neurons. Even if TRPV2 channels are expressed in different parts of the bladder, its functional significance is still unclear. It has been suggested that TRPV2 has a role as a sensor of urothelium stretch and a pivotal role in bladder cancer development. [68]

TRPV4 and bladder function

TRPV4 is a Ca^{2+}-permeable stretch-activated cation channel, which is expressed in rat and mouse urothelial and detrusor muscle cells. The activation of TRPV4 induces significant increases in [Ca2+]i in rat urothelial cells, leading to ATP release. TRPV4 has been suggested to be an important urothelial mechanosensor for bladder distension. [68, 91] TRPV4 knock out mice showed an altered micturition pattern, having significantly more intermicturition spotting, whereas micturitions seemed to be normal. Continuous cystometrograms revealed an increase of the intermicturition intervals and an increased number of non-micturition contractions. [92] The amplitude of the spontaneous contractions in bladder strips from TRPV4 knock out mice was significantly reduced, and there was a decreased intravesical stretch-evoked ATP release in isolated whole bladders from these animals. Gevaert et al. [92] raised the possibility that TRPV4 plays a critical role in urothelium-mediated transduction of intravesical mechanical pressure. This suggestion was supported by the results of Mochizuki et al. [93] observing functional expression of TRPV4 in urothelial cells using a selective agonist, 4a-PDD, in Ca2+-imaging experiments. In *in vitro* mechanical stretch stimulation of urothelial cells activated TRPV4, leading to increased [Ca2+]i and ATP release. Mochizuki et al. [93] suggested that the TRPV4 channel participates in the mechanosensory pathway in the urinary bladder and that mechanical stimulus-dependent activation of TRPV4 in urothelial cell layers is a key event for ATP signaling in the micturition reflex pathway.

As mentioned, TRPV4 receptors seem to be located to detrusor muscle. Thus, TRPV4 activation with a potent TRPV4 activator GSK1016790A contracted normal mouse bladders *in vitro*, both in the presence and absence of the urothelium; this effect was undetected in bladders from TRPV4 knock out mice. [94] Direct infusion of GSK1016790A into the bladders of normal mice induced DO with no effect in TRPV4 knock out mice. In another study, the amplitude of the spontaneous contractions in bladder strips from TRPV4 knock out mice was significantly reduced. [92]

In vivo, the TRPV4 channels in the urothelium and in the bladder smooth muscle could cooperatively play important roles in urinary bladder function that include not only the urothelium-mediated transduction of intravesical mechanical pressure, but also an ability to contract the bladder. As pointed out by Everaerts et al. [66], another possible role for TRPV4 might be the detection of urine flow in the urethra, thereby activating the urethra-to-bladder reflex, promoting bladder emptying. [95, 96] Once micturition is started, bladder emptying is facilitated by contraction of the detrusor. The mechanisms responsible for these detrusor contractions are still poorly understood, but bladder-to-bladder and urethra-to-bladder reflexes seem to play an important role. In the awake ewe, urethra-to-bladder reflexes

are stimulated by urethral infusion saline at body temperature, but not at temperatures below the physiological rate. [96] As TRPV4 is activated by shear stress at body temperature, it is a candidate for mediating the urethra-to-bladder reflex.

Even if, as Mochizuki et al. [93] suggest, the TRPV4 channel participates in the mechanosensory pathway by stimulus dependent activation of TRPV4 channels in urothelial cell layers with consequent release of ATP, this may not be the only way to initiate the micturition reflex via stimulation of TRPV4 channels. TRPV4 proteins were found to be located in mouse sensory neurons, [97] and this is in good agreement with the RT-PCR and *in situ* hybridization data of Yamada et al. [98] These findings suggest that the TRPV4 channels may be expressed on the bladder sensory terminals themselves and that the channels may be mechanically gated by bladder distension without any release of chemical mediators from the urothelium.

TRPA1 and bladder function

TRPA1 is the only mammalian member of the Ankyrin TRP subfamily. It is known to be present on capsaicin-sensitive primary sensory neurons and can be activated by plant-derived irritants such as allylisothiocyanate (AI), cinnamonaldehyde (CA), [99–101] hydrogen sulfide (H_2S), [102] menthol, [103] and formalin. [104] Streng et al. [102] investigated the effects of H_2S and known TRPA1 activators on micturition in conscious rats. Cystometric investigations were performed in conscious animals subjected to intravesical administration of sodium hydrogen sulfide (NaHS, donor of H_2S), AI, and CA. Fluorometric calcium imaging was used to study the effect of NaHS on human and mouse TRPA1 expressed in

CHO cells. AI increased micturition frequency and reduced voiding volume. CA and NaHS produced similar changes in urodynamic parameters after disruption of the urothelial barrier with protamine sulfate. NaHS also induced calcium responses in TRPA1-expressing CHO cells, but not in untransfected cells. The finding that intravesical TRPA1 activators initiate detrusor overactivity indicates that TRPA1 may have a role in sensory transduction in this organ. The study also highlights H_2S as a TRPA1 activator potentially involved in inflammatory bladder disease.

TRPA1-agonists had no contractile effect in human urethral preparations. [40] However, after precontraction with phenylephrine, AI, CA, and NaHS caused concentration-dependent relaxations of urethral strip preparations. These relaxations seemed to work in cooperation with TRPV1 mediated signals, were negatively coupled via cannabinoid receptor activation, and involved cyclooxygenase products. [105] Even if urothelial TRPA1 signals are not important in regulating normal human urethral smooth muscle tone, [105] this does not exclude a role in the initiation of afferent activity normally and in disease states. Since the bladder and urethra work in concert, it is likely that urethral effects mediated via TRPA1 channels can influence bladder activity. It may also be speculated that TRPA1 together with TRPV4 channels may be involved in the urethra-to-bladder reflex.

TRPM8 and bladder function

TRPM8 is a cool receptor expressed in the urothelium and suburothelial sensory fibers. It may be implicated in the bladder cooling reflex (BCR) and in patients with idiopathic DO. [15, 68] The positive corre-lation between the density of TRPM8 in the bladder mucosa and voiding frequency in IDO, and also increased TRPM8 expression in bladder pain patients, led to the suggestion that this channel was involved in the symptomatology and pathophysiology of these disorders. [106] Mukerji et al. [107] also studied the BCR in patients with IDO and NDO. In both conditions a BCR could be elicited (IDO 6/22: 27%; NDO 4/4: 100%). The authors suggested that the BCR in DO reflects loss of central inhibition, which is necessary to elicit this reflex.

The BCR was studied in guinea pigs before and after pretreatment with menthol. [108] It was found that the BCR is observed if the animals were pretreated with menthol. Since the reflex was sensitive to capsaicin treatment, it was speculated that it was mediated by C-fibres via TRPM receptors. Nomoto et al. [109] evaluated the effect of intravesical menthol in conscious rats. They found a facilitation of the micturition reflex, which was not affected by capsaicin pretreatment. It was suggested that menthol could act on capsaicin-resistant afferents, hypothetically via TPRM8 receptors in the urothelium and on suburothelial nerve endings.

However, Du et al. [110] questioned the role of urothelial TRPM8 in human bladder sensory function, finding extremely low expression of TRPM8 mRNA in the bladder mucosa compared to its expression in the prostate. Furthermore, they found that BPH or BOO did not significantly affect the expression of TRPM8, and they suggested that TRPM8 may play an essential role in survival and proliferation of prostate epithelial cells, as suggested by Zhang and Barritt. [111]

Lashinger et al. [112] evaluated a selective TRPM8 channel blocker, AMTB, and used it as a tool to assess the effects of this class of ion channel blocker on volume-induced bladder contraction and nociceptive reflex responses to noxious bladder distension in the rat. In the anesthetized rat, intravenous administration of AMTB decreased the frequency of volume-induced bladder contractions, without reducing the amplitude of contraction. The nociceptive response was measured by analyzing both visceromotor reflex (VMR) and cardiovascular (pressor) responses to urinary bladder distension (UBD) under 1% isoflurane. AMTB significantly attenuated reflex responses to noxious UBD. The authors suggest that their results demonstrate that TRPM8 channel blocker can act on the bladder afferent pathway to attenuate the bladder micturition reflex and nociceptive reflex responses in the rat, and they suggested that targeting the TRPM8 channel may provide a new therapeutic opportunity for DO/OAB and painful bladder syndromes.

A sudden drop in environmental temperature may change micturition patterns in conscious rats, and these changes are mediated, at least in part, through a RTX-sensitive (C-fiber) nervous pathways. [113] Interestingly, when menthol was applied to the skin from the leg and back in conscious rats, DO was induced. [114] TRPM8 was expressed in the skin, and it was speculated that menthol – via stimulation of these receptors – was able to initiate that activity.

TRP channel antagonists

Development of TRP antagonists may be useful for a number of conditions. Some such antagonists have been tested preclinically on normal LUT function and in models of disease, but information on

effects on the LUT in humans is scarce or lacking.

TRPV1

The first molecule to be used as a competitive TRPV1 antagonist was capsazepine, but its low potency and lack of specificity in high concentrations led to the development of several new TRPV1 antagonists. [115, 116] A potent TRPV1 antagonist, GRC 6211, decreased bladder overactivity in a dose-dependent manner. [117] when tested in two models of bladder inflammation, either acute, induced by acetic acid, or prolonged, induced by LPS. [117] The application of the same antagonist was also found to be effective in the reduction of detrusor overactivity in chronic spinalized rats. [118] In low doses, GRC 6211 had no effect on bladder reflex activity of normal rats and WT mice. [117] However, in high doses, it transiently blocked bladder contractions. This effect was specifically mediated by TRPV1, as the same dose did not produce any effect on TRPV1 KO mice.

One serious side-effect of TRPV1 antagonists is hyperthermia following systemic administration, which is well described in both animals and humans. [116] However, it has been suggested that that TRPV1 antagonists with a classic polymodal inhibition profile can be identified where the analgesic action is separated from the effects on body temperature. [119]

TRPV4

Several experimental novel TRPV4 antagonists have been described, [120] and it has been suggested that these compounds will likely shed some light on the potential of TRPV4 inhibition for the treatment of inflammatory and neuropathic pain, bladder and urinary tract disorders. In normal mice and rats with cystitis, HC-067047, a potent and selective TRPV4 antagonist, increased functional bladder capacity and reduced micturition frequency in normal mice and rats with cystitis. Experiences in humans do not seem to be available.

TRPM8

As mentioned previously, AMTB, a selectiveTRPM8 channel blocker, was shown to act on the bladder afferent pathway to attenuate the bladder micturition reflex and nociceptive reflex responses in the rat. [112] Targeting the TRPM8 channel has been suggested as providing a new therapeutic opportunity for OAB and BPS/IC, but clinical experiences have not been published.

OAB and TRP channels

Available information suggests that some members of the TRP superfamily may be involved in both normal bladder function and dysfunction, including DO/OAB. However, the information for some of the members is fragmentary and cannot be adequately assessed. Importantly, there may be significant differences between species, meaning it is questionable to make extrapolations from animal to human data.

The role of TRPV1 channel in the pathophysiology of different types of bladder dysfunction such as NDO and IDO is well documented. However, its role in normal bladder function still remains to be established. Since a majority of IDO patients also have OAB symptoms, it would be expected that drugs like capsaicin and RTX may be effective in the treatment of the OAB syndrome. However such studies do not seem to have been performed. It would be interesting to find out whether or not some of the selective, small molecule

TRVPV1 channel antagonists [115–117] would be of benefit for OAB patients.

The distribution of TRPV4 channels in the bladder, and the involvement of these channels in preclinical effects of bladder (and urethral) function, seem to make them candidate targets for drugs aimed at treatment of DO/OAB. This may be the case also for TRPA1 channels. However, based on available information, it is not possible to assess the pathophysiological links between TRPV4 and TRPA1 channels and DO/OAB, nor to make predictions on the importance of these channels as targets for future drugs. The channels are not limited to the LUT, and systemic effects of future drugs acting on these channels have to be considered.

The studies by Stein et al. [121] and Mukerji et al. [106, 107] initiated an interest in TRPM8 channels not only for the pathophysiology of the BCR, but also for the potential of these channels as targets for future DO/OAB drugs. The correlation between the density of TRPM8 channels in the bladders of IDO and voiding frequency was very suggestive. However, the findings of Du et al. [110] that the channel was mainly localized to the prostate, cast some doubts on a direct relation between the TRPM8 channels in the bladder and IDO with associated OAB symptoms. Even if there may be gender differences in the channel distribution, the differences in results indicate that possible relations may be complicated. In this context, the data of Lashinger et al. [112] with the selective TRPM8 antagonist, AMTB, clearly showing an involvement of the channels in the micturition reflex and nociceptive signaling in the rat, suggests that further exploration of the TRPM8 channels in the pathophysiology of LUTS/

DO/OAB may be motivated. Targeting of this receptor may still provide a new opportunity for treatment of these disorders.

The possible role of the urethral TRP channel in the pathophysiology of DO/OAB should not be disregarded. It may be speculated that urothelial TRP receptors in the proximal urethra, activated by urine flow, may stimulate detrusor contraction. In addition, the relaxant effect on urethral muscle obtained by TRP receptor activation may be involved in the "unstable urethra," which at least in women may be linked to DO.

There are thus several links between activation of different members of the TRP superfamily and DO/OAB (several of them admittedly hypothetical), and further exploration of the involvement of these channels in LUT function – normally and in dysfunction – may be rewarding.

References

1 Ochodnicky P, Cruz CD, Yoshimura N, Cruz F. Neurotrophins as regulators of urinary bladder function. *Nat Rev Urol.* 2012 Nov;**9**(11): 628–637

2 Cruz CD. Neurotrophins in bladder function: What do we know and where do we go from here? Neurourol Urodyn. 2013 Jun 17. doi: 10.1002/nau.22438. [Epub ahead of print]

3 Seth JH, Sahai A, Khan MS, et al. Nerve growth factor (NGF): a potential urinary biomarker for overactive bladder syndrome (OAB)? *BJU Int.* 2013 Mar;**111**(3):372–380.

4 Rahnama'i MS, van Kerrebroeck PE, de Wachter SG, van Koeveringe GA. The role of prostanoids in urinary bladder physiology. *Nat Rev Urol.* 2012 Mar 13;**9**(5):283–290.

5 Christ GJ, Andersson KE. Rho-kinase and effects of Rho-kinase inhibition on the lower urinary tract. *Neurourol Urodyn.* 2007 Oct;**26** (6 Suppl):948–954.

6 Morelli A, Vignozzi L, Filippi S, et al.BXL-628, a vitamin D receptor agonist effective in benign prostatic hyperplasia treatment, prevents RhoA activation and inhibits RhoA/Rho kinase signaling in rat and human bladder. *Prostate.* 2007 Feb 15;**67**(3):234–247.

7 Penna G, Fibbi B, Amuchastegui S, et al. The vitamin D receptor agonist elocalcitol inhibits IL-8-dependent benign prostatic hyperplasia stromal cell proliferation and inflammatory response by targeting the RhoA/Rho kinase and NF-kappaB pathways. *Prostate.* 2009 Apr 1; **69**(5):480–493.

8 Petkov GV. Role of potassium ion channels in detrusor smooth muscle function and dysfunction. *Nat Rev Urol.* 2011 Dec 13;**9**(1): 30–40.

9 Christ GJ, Day NS, Day M, et al. Bladder injection of "naked" hSlo/pcDNA3 ameliorates detrusor hyperactivity in obstructed rats in vivo. *Am J Physiol Regul Integr Comp Physiol.* 2001 Nov;**281**(5):R1699–1709.

10 Andersson KE. LUTS treatment: future treatment options. *Neurourol Urodyn.* 2007 Oct;**26**(6 Suppl):934–947

11 Ford AP, Cockayne DA. ATP and P2X purinoceptors in urinary tract disorders. *Handb Exp Pharmacol.* 2011;(**202**):485–526.

12 North RA, Jarvis MF. P2X receptors as drug targets. *Mol Pharmacol.* 2013 Apr;**83**(4):759–769.

13 Tyagi P, Tyagi V, Yoshimura N, Chancellor M. Functional role of cannabinoid receptors in urinary bladder. *Indian J Urol.* 2010 Jan-Mar; **26**(1):26–35.

14 Ruggieri MR Sr. Cannabinoids: potential targets for bladder dysfunction. *Handb Exp Pharmacol.* 2011;(**202**):425–451.

15 Andersson KE, Gratzke C, Hedlund P. The role of the transient receptor potential (TRP) superfamily of cation-selective channels in the management of the overactive bladder. *BJU Int.* 2010 Oct;**106**(8):1114–1127.

16 North RA, Surprenant A. Pharmacology of cloned P2X receptors. *Annu Rev Pharmacol Toxicol.* 2000;**40**:563–580

17 Gever JR, Cockayne DA, Dillon MP, et al. Pharmacology of P2X channels. *Pflugers Arch.* 2006 Aug;**452**(5):513–537

18 Shabir S, Cross W, Kirkwood L, et al. Functional expression of purinergic p2 receptors and

transient receptor potential channels by human urothelium. Am J Physiol Renal Physiol. 2013 May 29. [Epub ahead of print]

19 Ferguson DR, Kennedy I, Burton TJ. ATP is released from rabbit urinary bladder epithelial cells by hydrostatic pressure changes–a possible sensory mechanism? *J Physiol.* 1997 Dec 1;**505** (Pt 2):503–511.

20 Vlaskovska M, Kasakov L, Rong W, et al. P2X3 knock-out mice reveal a major sensory role for urothelially released ATP. *J Neurosci.* 2001 Aug 1;**21**(15):5670–5677.

21 Wang EC, Lee JM, Ruiz WG, et al. ATP and purinergic receptor-dependent membrane traffic in bladder umbrella cells. *Clin Invest.* 2005 Sep;**115**(9):2412–2422.

22 Namasivayam S, Eardley I, Morrison JF. Purinergic sensory neurotransmission in the urinary bladder: an in vitro study in the rat. *BJU Int.* 1999 Nov;**84**(7):854–860.

23 Rong W, Spyer KM, Burnstock G. Activation and sensitisation of low and high threshold afferent fibres mediated by P2X receptors in the mouse urinary bladder. *J Physiol.* 2002 Jun 1;**541**(Pt 2):591–600.

24 Sun Y, Chai TC. Up-regulation of P2X3 receptor during stretch of bladder urothelial cells from patients with interstitial cystitis. *J Urol.* 2004 Jan;**171**(1):448–452.

25 Sun Y, Keay S, Lehrfeld TJ, Chai TC. Changes in adenosine triphosphate-stimulated ATP release suggest association between cytokine and purinergic signaling in bladder urothelial cells. *Urology.* 2009 Nov;**74**(5):1163–1168

26 Brady CM, Apostolidis A, Yiangou Y, et al. P2X3-immunoreactive nerve fibres in neurogenic detrusor overactivity and the effect of intravesical resiniferatoxin. *Eur Urol.* 2004 Aug;**46**(2):247–253.

27 Dang K, Lamb K, Cohen M, et al. Cyclophosphamide-induced bladder inflammation sensitizes and enhances P2X receptor function in rat bladder sensory neurons. *J Neurophysiol.* 2008 Jan;**99**(1):49–59

28 Ford AP, Gever JR, Nunn PA, et al. Purinoceptors as therapeutic targets for lower urinary tract dysfunction. *Br J Pharmacol.* 2006 Feb;**147** Suppl 2:S132–143

29 Ford AP. In pursuit of P2X3 antagonists: novel therapeutics for chronic pain and afferent sensitization. *Purinergic Signalling* 2012; **8** (Suppl 1):S3–S26.

30 Ito K, Iwami A, Katsura H, Ikeda M. Therapeutic effects of the putative P2X3/P2X2/3 antagonist A-317491 on cyclophosphamide-induced cystitis in rats. *Naunyn Schmiedebergs Arch Pharmacol.* 2008 Jun;**377**(4-6):483–490.

31 Lu SH, Groat WC, Lin AT, et al. Evaluation of purinergic mechanism for the treatment of voiding dysfunction: a study in conscious spinal cord-injured rats. *J Chin Med Assoc.* 2007 Oct;**70**(10):439–444.

32 Gever JR, Soto R, Henningsen RA, et al. AF-353, a novel, potent and orally bioavailable P2X3/P2X2/3 receptor antagonist. *Br J Pharmacol.* 2010 Jul;**160**(6):1387–1398.

33 Munoz A, Somogyi GT, Boone TB, et al. Modulation of bladder afferent signals in normal and spinal cord-injured rats by purinergic P2X3 and P2X2/3 receptors. *BJU Int.* 2012 Oct;**110**(8 Pt B):E409–414.

34 Pacher P, Bátkai S, Kunos G. The endocannabinoid system as an emerging target of pharmacotherapy. *Pharmacol Rev* 2006;**58**:389–462

35 Howlett AC, Barth F, Bonner TI, et al. International Union of Pharmacology. XXVII. Classification of cannabinoid receptors. *Pharmacol Rev* 2002;**54**:161–202.

36 Pertwee RG, Howlett AC, Abood ME, et al. International Union of Basic and Clinical Pharmacology. LXXIX. Cannabinoid receptors and their ligands: beyond CB_1 and CB_2. *Pharmacol Rev* 2010;**62**:588–631.

37 Blankman JL, Cravatt BF. Chemical probes of endocannabinoid metabolism. *Pharmacol Reviews.* 2013 April 1, 2013;**65**:849–871.

38 van der Stelt M, Di Marzo V. Endovanilloids. *Eur Biochem.*2004;**271**:1827–1834.

39 Hayn MH, Ballesteros I, de Miguel F, et al. Functional and immunohistochemical characterization of CB1 and CB2 receptors in rat bladder. *Urology* 2008;**72**:1174–1178.

40 Gratzke C, Streng T, Park A, et al. Distribution and function of cannabinoid receptors 1 and 2 in the rat, monkey and human bladder. *J Urol* 2009;**181**:1939–1948.

41 Gratzke C, Streng T, Stief CG, et al. Effects of cannabinor, a novel selective cannabinoid 2 receptor agonist, on bladder function in normal rats. *Eur Urol* 2010;**57**:1093–1100.

42 Gratzke C, Streng T, Stief CG, et al. Cannabinor, a selective cannabinoid-2 receptor agonist, improves bladder emptying in rats with partial urethral obstruction. *J Urol* 2011;**185**:731–736.

43 Merriam FV, Wang ZY, Guerios SD, Bjorling DE. Cannabinoid receptor 2 is increased in acutely and chronically inflamed bladder of rats. *Neurosci Lett* 2008;**445**:130–134.

44 Tyagi V, Philips BJ, Su R, et al. Differential expression of functional cannabinoid receptors in human bladder detrusor and urothelium. *J Urol* 2009;**181**:1932–1938.

45 Walczak JS, Price TJ, Cervero F. Cannabinoid CB1 receptors are expressed in the mouse urinary bladder and their activation modulates afferent bladder activity. *Neuroscience* 2009;**159**:1154–1163.

46 Mukerji G, Yiangou Y, Agarwal SK, Anand P. Increased cannabinoid receptor 1-immunoreactive nerve fibers in overactive and painful bladder disorders and their correlation with symptoms. *Urology* 2010;**75**:e15–e20.

47 Bakali E, Elliott RA, Taylor AH, et al. Distribution and function of the endocannabinoid system in the rat and human bladder. *Int Urogynecol J.* 2013 May;**24**(5):855–863

48 Bridges D, Rice AS, Egertová M, et al. Localisation of cannabinoid receptor 1 in rat dorsal root ganglion using in situ hybridisation and immunohistochemistry. *Neuroscience* 2003;**119**:803–812.

49 Guindon J, Hohmann AG. The endocannabinoid system and pain. *CNS Neurol Disord Drug Targets* 2009;**8**:403–421.

50 Brownjohn PW, Ashton JC. Spinal cannabinoid CB2 receptors as a target for neuropathic pain: an investigation using chronic constriction injury. *Neuroscience* 2012;**203**:180–193.

51 Veress G, Meszar Z, Muszil D, et al. Characterisation of cannabinoid 1 receptor expression in the perikarya, and peripheral and spinal processes of primary sensory neurons. *Brain Struct Funct.* 2013 May;**218**(3):733–750

52 Svízenská I, Dubový P, Sulcová A. Cannabinoid receptors 1 and 2 (CB1 and CB2), their distribution, ligands and functional involvement in nervous system structures--a short review. *Pharmacol Biochem Behav.* 2008;**90**:501–511.

53 Zygmunt PM, Petersson J, Andersson DA, et al. Vanilloid receptors on sensory nerves mediate the vasodilator action of anandamide. *Nature* 1999 Jul 29;**400**(6743):452–457.

54 Saitoh C, Kitada C, Uchida W, et al. The differential contractile responses to capsaicin and anandamide in muscle strips isolated from the rat urinary bladder. *Eur J Pharmacol.* 2007;**570**:182–187.

55 Jaggar SI, Hasnie FS, Sellaturay S, Rice AS. The anti-hyperalgesic actions of the cannabinoid anandamide and the putative CB2 receptor agonist palmitoylethanolamide in visceral and somatic inflammatory pain. *Pain* 1998;**76**:189–199.

56 Farquhar-Smith WP, Rice AS. Administration of endocannabinoids prevents a referred hyperalgesia associated with inflammation of the urinary bladder. *Anesthesiology* 2001;**94**: 507–513.

57 Wang ZY, Wang P, Bjorling DE. Activation of cannabinoid receptor 2 inhibits experimental cystitis. *Am J Physiol Regul Integr Comp Physiol.* 2013 May 15;**304**(10):R846–853.

58 Adhikary S, Li H, Heller J, et al. Modulation of inflammatory responses by a cannabinoid-2-selective agonist after spinal cord injury. *J Neurotrauma* 2011 Dec;**28**(12):2417–2427

59 Pacher P, Steffens S. The emerging role of the endocannabinoid system in cardiovascular disease. *Semin Immunopathol.* 2009 Jun;**31**(1): 63–77.

60 Strittmatter F, Gandaglia G, Benigni F, et al. Expression of fatty acid amide hydrolase (FAAH) in human, mouse, and rat urinary bladder and effects of FAAH inhibition on bladder function in awake rats. *Eur Urol.* 2012;**61**:98–106.

61 Consroe P, Musty R, Rein J, et al. The perceived effects of smoked cannabis on patients with multiple sclerosis. *Eur Neurol.* 1997;**38**:44–48.

62 Brady CM, DasGupta R, Dalton C, et al. An open-label pilot study of cannabis-based extracts for bladder dysfunction in advanced multiple sclerosis. *Mult Scler.* 2004;**10**: 425–433.

63 Freeman RM, Adekanmi O, Waterfield MR, et al. The effect of cannabis on urge incontinence in patients with multiple sclerosis: a multicentre, randomised placebo controlled trial (CAMS-LUTS). *Int Urogynecol J Pelvic Floor Dysfunct.* 2006;**17**:636–641.

64 Kavia R, De Ridder D, Constantinescu S, et al. Randomised controlled trial of Sativex to treat detrusor overactivity in multiple sclerosis. *Mult Scler.* 2010;**16**:1349–1359

65 Wade DT, Makela P, Robson P, et al. Do cannabis-based medicinal extracts have general or specific effects on symptoms in multiple sclerosis? A double-blind, randomized, placebo-controlled study on 160 patients. *Mult Scler.* 2004;**10**: 434–441.

66 Everaerts W, Gevaert T, Nilius B, De Ridder D. On the origin of bladder sensing: Tr(i)ps in urology. *Neurourol Urodyn.* 2008;**27**(4): 264–273.

67 Andersson KE, Gratzke C, Hedlund P. The role of the transient receptor potential (TRP) superfamily of cation-selective channels in the management of the overactive bladder. *BJU Int.* 2010 Oct;**106**(8):1114–1127.

68 Avelino A, Charrua A, Frias B, et al. Transient receptor potential channels in bladder function. *Acta Physiol (Oxf).* 2013 Jan;**207**(1):110–122

69 Vennekens R, Owsianik G, Nilius B. Vanilloid transient receptor potential cation channels: an overview. *Curr Pharm Des.* 2008;**14**(1):18–31.

70 Caterina MJ, Schumacher MA, Tominaga M, et al. The capsaicin receptor: a heat-activated ion channel in the pain pathway. *Nature* 1997 Oct 23;**389**(6653):816–824.

71 Daly D, Rong W, Chess-Williams R, et al. Bladder afferent sensitivity in wild-type and TRPV1 knockout mice. *Physiol.* 2007 Sep 1;**583**(Pt 2):663–674.

72 Birder LA, Nakamura Y, Kiss S, et al. Altered urinary bladder function in mice lacking the vanilloid receptor TRPV1. *Nat Neurosci.* 2002 Sep;**5**(9):856–860.

73 Cruz F, Dinis P. Resiniferatoxin and botulinum toxin type A for treatment of lower urinary tract symptoms. *Neurourol Urodyn.* 2007 Oct;**26**(6 Suppl):920–927.

74 MacDonald R, Monga M, Fink HA, Wilt TJ. Neurotoxin treatments for urinary incontinence in subjects with spinal cord injury or multiple sclerosis: a systematic review of effectiveness and adverse effects. *J Spinal Cord Med.* 2008;**31**(2):157–165.

75 Andersson KE, Chapple CR, Cardozo L, et al. Pharmacological treatment of overactive bladder: report from the International Consultation on

Incontinence. *Curr Opin Urol.* 2009 Jul;**19**(4): 380–394.

76 Maggi CA, Barbanti G, Santicioli P, et al. Cystometric evidence that capsaicin-sensitive nerves modulate the afferent branch of micturition reflex in humans. *J Urol.* 1989 Jul;**142**(1):150–154.

77 Avelino A, Cruz F. TRPV1 (vanilloid receptor) in the urinary tract: expression, function and clinical applications. *Naunyn Schmiedebergs Arch Pharmacol.* 2006 Jul;**373**(4):287–299.

78 Brady CM, Apostolidis AN, Harper M, et al. Parallel changes in bladder suburothelial vanilloid receptor TRPV1 and pan-neuronal marker PGP9.5 immunoreactivity in patients with neurogenic detrusor overactivity after intravesical resiniferatoxin treatment. *BJU Int.* 2004 Apr;**93**(6):770–776.

79 Apostolidis A, Brady CM, Yiangou Y, et al. Capsaicin receptor TRPV1 in urothelium of neurogenic human bladders and effect of intravesical resiniferatoxin. *Urology.* 2005a Feb;**65**(2):400–405.

80 Apostolidis A, Popat R, Yiangou Y, et al. Decreased sensory receptors P2X3 and TRPV1 in suburothelial nerve fibers following intradetrusor injections of botulinum toxin for human detrusor overactivity. *J Urol.* 2005b Sep;**174**(3): 977–982.

81 Liu L, Mansfield KJ, Kristiana I, et al. The molecular basis of urgency: regional difference of vanilloid receptor expression in the human urinary bladder. *Neurourol Urodyn.* 2007;**26**: 433–438, discussion 439, 451–453.

82 Hindmarsh JR, Gosling PT, Deane AM. Bladder instability. Is the primary defect in the urethra? *Br J Urol.* 1983 Dec;**55**(6):648–651.

83 Low JA, Armstrong JB, Mauger GM. The unstable urethra in the female. *Obstet Gynecol.* 1989 Jul;**74**(1):69–74.

84 Farrell SA, Tynski G. The effect of urethral pressure variation on detrusor activity in women. *Int Urogynecol J Pelvic Floor Dysfunct.* 1996;**7**(2):87–93.

85 McLennan MT, Melick C, Bent AE. Urethral instability: clinical and urodynamic characteristics. *Neurourol Urodyn.* 2001;**20**(6):653–660.

86 Neeper MP, Liu Y, Hutchinson TL, et al. Activation properties of heterologously expressed mammalian TRPV2: evidence for

species dependence. *J Biol Chem.* 2007 May 25;**282**(21):15894–15902.

87   Muraki K, Iwata Y, Katanosaka Y, et al. TRPV2 is a component of osmotically sensitive cation channels in murine aortic myocytes. *Circ Res.* 2003 Oct 31;**93**(9):829–838.

88   Everaerts W, Vriens J, Owsianik G, et al. Functional characterization of transient receptor potential channels in mouse urothelial cells. *Am J Physiol Renal Physiol.* 2010 Mar;**298**(3):F692–701.

89   Ost D, Roskams T, Van Der Aa F, De Ridder D. Topography of the vanilloid receptor in the human bladder: more than just the nerve fibers. *J Urol.* 2002 Jul;**168**(1):293–297.

90   Caprodossi S, Lucciarini R, Amantini C, et al. Transient receptor potential vanilloid type 2 (TRPV2) expression in normal urothelium and in urothelial carcinoma of human bladder: correlation with the pathologic stage. *Eur Urol.* 2008 Sep;**54**(3):612–620.

91   Everaerts W, Nilius B, Owsianik G. The vanilloid transient receptor potential channel TRPV4: from structure to disease. *Prog Biophys Mol Biol.* 2010 Sep;**103**(1):2–17.

92   Gevaert T, Vriens J, Segal A, et al. Deletion of the transient receptor potential cation channel TRPV4 impairs murine bladder voiding. *J Clin Invest.* 2007 Nov;**117**(11):3453–3462.

93   Mochizuki T, Sokabe T, Araki I, et al. The TRPV4 cation channel mediates stretch-evoked Ca2+ influx and ATP release in primary urothelial cell cultures. *J Biol Chem.* 2009 Aug 7;**284**(32):21257–21264.

94   Thorneloe KS, Sulpizio AC, Lin Z, et al. N-((1S)-1-{[4-((2S)-2-{[(2,4-dichlorophenyl)-sulfonyl]amino}-3-hydroxypropanoyl)-1-piperazinyl]carbonyl}-3-methylbutyl)-1-benzothiophene-2-carboxamide (GSK1016790A), a novel and potent transient receptor potential vanilloid 4 channel agonist induces urinary bladder contraction and hyperactivity: Part I. *J Pharmacol Exp Ther.* 2008 Aug;**326**(2):432–442.

95   Robain G, Combrisson H, Mazières L. Bladder response to urethral flow in the awake ewe. *Neurourol Urodyn.* 2001;**20**(5):641–649.

96   Combrisson H, Allix S, Robain G. Influence of temperature on urethra to bladder micturition reflex in the awake ewe. *Neurourol Urodyn.* 2007;**26**(2):290–295.

97   Suzuki M, Watanabe Y, Oyama Y, et al. Localization of mechanosensitive channel TRPV4 in mouse skin. *Neurosci Lett.* 2003 Dec 26;**353**(3):189–192.

98   Yamada T, Ugawa S, Ueda T, et al. Differential localizations of the transient receptor potential channels TRPV4 and TRPV1 in the mouse urinary bladder. *J Histochem Cytochem.* 2009 Mar;**57**(3):277–287.

99   Jordt SE, Bautista DM, Chuang HH, et al.Mustard oils and cannabinoids excite sensory nerve fibres through the TRP channel ANKTM1. *Nature* 2004;**427**:260–265.

100   Bautista DM, Movahed P, Hinman A, et al. Pungent products from garlic activate the sensory ion channel TRPA1. *Proc Natl Acad Sci USA* 2005;**102**:12248–12252.

101. Bautista DM, Jordt SE, Nikai T, et al. TRPA1 mediates the inflammatory actions of environmental irritants and proalgesic agents. *Cell* 2006;**124**: 1269–1282.

102   Streng T, Axelsson HE, Hedlund P, et al. Distribution and function of the hydrogen sulfide-sensitive TRPA1 ion channel in rat urinary bladder. *Eur Urol.* 2008 Feb;**53**(2):391–399.

103   Karashima Y, Damann N, Prenen J, et al. Bimodal action of menthol on the transient receptor potential channel TRPA1. *J Neurosci.* 2007 Sep 12;**27**(37):9874–9884.

104   McNamara CR, Mandel-Brehm J, Bautista DM, et al. TRPA1 mediates formalin-induced pain. *Proc Natl Acad Sci USA* 2007 Aug 14;**104**(33):13525–13530.

105   Weinhold P, Gratzke C, Streng T, et al. TRPA1 receptor induced relaxation of the human urethra involves trpv1 and cannabinoid receptor mediated signals, and cyclooxygenase activation. *J Urol.* 2010 May;**183**(5):2070–2076.

106   Mukerji G, Yiangou Y, Corcoran SL, et al. Cool and menthol receptor TRPM8 in human urinary bladder disorders and clinical correlations. *BMC Urol.* 2006 Mar 6;**6**:6.

107   Mukerji G, Waters J, Chessell IP, et al. Pain during ice water test distinguishes clinical bladder hypersensitivity from overactivity disorders. *BMC Urol.* 2006 Dec 27;**6**:31.

108   Tsukimi Y, Mizuyachi K, Yamasaki T, et al. Cold response of the bladder in guinea pig: involvement of transient receptor potential channel, TRPM8. *Urology.* 2005 Feb;**65**(2): 406–410.

109   Nomoto Y, Yoshida A, Ikéda S, et al. Effect of menthol on detrusor smooth-muscle contraction and the micturition reflex in rats. *Urology* 2008 Sep;**72**(3):701–705.

110   Du S, Araki I, Kobayashi H, et al. Differential expression profile of cold (TRPA1) and cool (TRPM8) receptors in human urogenital organs. *Urology* 2008 Aug;**72**(2):450–455.

111   Zhang L, Barritt GJ. TRPM8 in prostate cancer cells: a potential diagnostic and prognostic marker with a secretory function? *Endocr Relat Cancer.* 2006 Mar;**13**(1):27–38.

112   Lashinger ES, Steiginga MS, Hieble JP, et al. TB, a TRPM8 channel blocker: evidence in rats for activity in overactive bladder and painful bladder syndrome. *Am J Physiol Renal Physiol.* 2008 Sep;**295**(3):F803–810.

113   Imamura T, Ishizuka O, Aizawa N, et al. Cold environmental stress induces detrusor overactivity via resiniferatoxin-sensitive nerves in conscious rats. *Neurourol Urodyn.* 2008;**27**(4):348–352.

114   Chen Z, Ishizuka O, Imamura T, et al. Stimulation of skin menthol receptors stimulates detrusor activity in conscious rats. *Neurourol Urodyn.* 2009;**28**(3):251–256.

115   Cefalu JS, Guillon MA, Burbach LR, et al. Selective pharmacological blockade of the TRPV1 receptor suppresses sensory reflexes of the rodent bladder. *J Urol.* 2009 Aug;**182**(2):776–785.

116   Khairatkar-Joshi N, Szallasi ATRPV1 antagonists: the challenges for therapeutic targeting. *Trends Mol Med.* 2009 Jan;**15**(1): 14–22

117   Charrua A, Cruz CD, Narayanan S, et al. GRC-6211, a new oral specific TRPV1 antagonist, decreases bladder overactivity and noxious bladder input in cystitis animal models. *J Urol.* 2009 Jan;**181**(1):379–386.

118   Santos-Silva A, Charrua A, Cruz CD et al. Rat detrusor overactivity induced by chronic spinalization can be abolished by a transient receptor potential vanilloid 1 (TRPV1) antagonist. *Auton Neurosci.* 2012 Jan 26;**166**(1-2):35–38.

119   Nash MS, McIntyre P, Groarke A, et al. 7-tert-Butyl-6-(4-chloro-phenyl)-2-thioxo-2,3-dihydro-1H-pyrido[2,3-d]pyrimidin-4-one, a classic polymodal inhibitor of transient receptor potential vanilloid type 1 with a reduced liability for hyperthermia, is analgesic and ameliorates visceral hypersensitivity. *J Pharmacol Exp Ther.* 2012 Aug;**342**(2):389–398.

120   Vincent F, Duncton MA. TRPV4 agonists and antagonists. *Curr Top Med Chem.* 2001; **11**(17):2216–2226.

121   Stein RJ, Santos S, Nagatomi J, et al. Cool (TRPM8) and hot (TRPV1) receptors in the bladder and male genital tract. *J Urol.* 2004 Sep;**172**(3):1175–1178.

CHAPTER 12

The role of co-medication in the treatment of OAB

Nadir I. Osman and Christopher R. Chapple

Department of Urology, Royal Hallamshire Hospital, Sheffield, UK

KEY POINTS

- Current combination therapy aims to relieve storage LUTS/OAB by targeting the bladder or its neural control as well a relieving voiding LUTS by ameliorating bladder outlet obstruction (BOO).

- The most established combination regimen for men with OAB is an alpha-adrenoreceptor antagonists (α-AA) with an antimuscarinic agent (anti-M).

- Well-designed prospective randomized studies have demonstrated clear advantages in storage LUTS/OAB efficacy endpoints for an α-AA + anti-M over an α-AA alone, when treatment is commenced with both agents simultaneously, or when the anti-M is given as an add-on.

- There does not appear to be a significantly increased risk of acute urinary retention with combination of α-AA + anti-M, although studies excluded men at greatest risk (low flows, PVRs > 200 ml and previous urinary retention) and extended only to three months.

- α-AA with phosphodiesterase (PDE5) inhibitor is a newer, less well-studied combination regimen, predominately investigated in small pilot studies.

- α-AA + PDE5 inhibitor therapy has demonstrated improvement in LUTS and flow rates, which in some cases has been greater than improvements observed with α-AA alone.

- There is a need for studies with longer follow-up to determine the long term safety and efficacy of α-AA + anti-M, whereas larger prospective randomized placebo controlled studies are required to establish the efficacy of α-AA + PDE5 inhibitor combination over either agent alone.

- In future it will be important to define the clinical features that determine which patients are most likely to benefit from current or new combination regimens.

Introduction

Pharmacotherapy is the mainstay of the treatment of overactive bladder (OAB) after the failure of conservative measures. Over the past two decades there has been an increasing recognition that the pathogenesis of storage lower urinary tract symptoms (LUTS) may have its basis in bladder function or its neural control mechanisms rather than simply arising due to bladder outlet obstruction (BOO)

Overactive Bladder: Practical Management, First Edition. Edited by Jacques Corcos, Scott MacDiarmid and John Heesakkers.

© 2015 John Wiley & Sons, Ltd. Published 2015 by John Wiley & Sons, Ltd.

secondary to benign prostate hyperplasia (BPH), as was traditionally thought. With this, there has been a growing emphasis on using classes of agents that target the pathophysiologies that underlie specific symptoms. OAB represents an important and highly bothersome subgroup of storage LUTS. Voiding LUTS, such as weak stream and intermittency, frequently coexist with storage LUTS and OAB in men and are normally attributed to BOO due to BPH. Thus the possibility of using one agent to relieve BOO and another to target OAB symptoms arose. The earliest and most established combination regimen for this indication is an antimusacarinic (anti-M) with an α-adrenoreceptor antagonists (α-AA). More recently the development of novel agents and the recognition of new indications for established agents has opened up the possibility of entirely novel combinations that allow treatment to be tailored to an individual patient's symptoms. We discuss the evidence for the different combination regimens for the treatment of OAB symptoms with a focus on the two combinations that have been investigated most in the contemporary literature.

Antimuscarinics and α-adrenoreceptor antagonists

Most men with LUTS have a combination of both voiding and storage symptoms. Anti-Ms were traditionally avoided in men due to the perception that they precipitated urinary retention (UR). Chapple and Smith first alluded to the theoretical possibility of using an anti-M with an α-AA in 1994. [1] In 1999, Saito et al. were the first to publish a clinical study assessing this combination, administering propiverine and tamsulosin to men with BPH and urinary frequency (including neuropathic patients). Subsequently a series of well-designed, mostly 12-week, randomized controlled trials (RCTs) were published which demonstrated the short term safety and efficacy of anti-M monotherapy in men with LUTS and low PVR. Several of these studies included an arm that combined treatment with an anti-M and α-AA, most commonly with the anti-M being given as an add-on therapy. We review the pivotal studies in Table 12.1.

The tolterodine and tamsulosin for treatment of men with lower urinary tract symptoms and overactive bladder (TIMES) study

The TIMES study was designed to assess the efficacy and safety of the anti-M tolterodine either alone or in combination with the α-AA tamsulosin, as initial pharmacotherapy in men with LUTS/BPH and significant OAB symptoms. It is unique as it is the only study to prospectively separately compare an anti-M, a α-AA, and combination therapy to placebo. The study included a total of 879 subjects randomized into four groups: tolterodine ER 4 mg, tamsulosin 0.4 mg, a combination, or placebo for a period of 12 weeks. [2] Subjects were over the age of 40 yr and met entry criteria for both LUTS and OAB trials. Men suspected of having BOO (Qmax <5 ml/s, post-void residual (PVR) >200 ml) or a history of acute urinary retention (AUR) were excluded. At 12 weeks, combination treatment resulted in the highest patient reported treatment benefit on the patient perception of bladder condition questionnaire (PPBC) with 80%

Table 12.1 Landmark studies of combination antimuscarinics and α-adrenoreceptor antagonists

Study	No of patients	Study length (weeks)	Efficacy endpoints	Treatment arms	AUR requiring catheterization (%)
Kaplan et al.	879	12	PPBC Bladder diary IPSS	Tolterodine Tamsulosin Tolterodine + Tamsulosin placebo	0 0 <1 <1
Chapple et al.	652	12	IPSS Symptom bother Bladder diary Flow rate PVR	Tolterodine ER + α-AA Placebo + α-AA	<1 <1
MacDiarmid et al.	420	12	IPSS QoL Flow rate PVR	Oxybutynin + Tamsulosin Placebo + Tamsulosin	0 0
Kaplan et al.	398	12	Bladder diary IPSS Flow rate PVR	Solifenacin + Tamsulosin Placebo + Tamsulosin	1.5 0
Lee et al.	211	8	Bladder diary IPSS PVR	Propiverine + Doxazosin Doxazosin	0 0

of patients reporting benefit by week 12 in comparison to placebo, tamsulosin, and tolterodine ER groups where 62, 71, and 65% reported benefit respectively. At 12 weeks, tolterodine monotherapy significantly reduced urgency urinary incontinence (UUI) episodes versus placebo but no other parameters. By contrast combination treatment led to significant improvements in several efficacy endpoints including UUI episodes (-0.88 vs. −0.31, $p = 0.005$), urgency without incontinence episodes (−3.33 vs. −2.54, $p = 0.03$), number of voids/24 h (−2.54 vs. −1.41, $p < 0.001$), nighttime voids (−0.59 vs. −0.39, $p = 0.02$), IPSS score (−8.02 vs. −6.19, $p = .003$), and IPSS QoL score (−1.61 vs. −1.17, $p = .003$). In *post hoc* analysis, combination therapy demonstrated a significant reduction in terms of IPSS storage subscores as well as frequency, urgency, and nocturia items (all $p < 0.001$). By contrast, the monotherapy group was not significantly different from placebo. [3] However further *post hoc* analyses, showed that tolterodine monotherapy did improve IPSS storage subscores in men with smaller prostates (vol. < 30 ml and PSA < 1.3 ng/ml) but not in men with larger prostates (vol. > 30 ml and PSA > 1.3 ng/ml). [4, 5] This suggested that in men with smaller prostates an anti-M alone may be justified. There was no significant difference in Qmax or PVR between the groups. Overall there was a low incidence of AUR that with no significant differences between groups; tamsulosin 0, tolterodine 0.5, combination 0.4, and placebo 0%.

The detrusitol LA "add-on" to α-blocker in men (ADAM) study

Tolterodine ER 4 mg as an add-on to an α-AA in men with persistent storage LUTS was also assessed in the ADAM study. [6] Included subjects were over 40 yr with urinary urgency and frequency, moderate to severe symptoms on the PPBC questionnaire, and had been on an α-AA for over a month. Men with PVRs above 200 ml were excluded. At 12 weeks, add-on tolterodine led to a significant reduction in total voids per 24 hrs (-1.8 vs. -1.2; $p = 0.0079$) and daytime voids (-1.3 vs. -0.8; $p = 0.0123$), compared to placebo. Moreover, significantly greater improvements in 24 h urgency episodes (-2.9 vs. -1.8; $p = 0.0010$) were observed with tolterodine add-on compared to placebo. IPSS storage subscore (-2.6 vs. -2.1; $p = 0.0370$); and OABq symptom bother scale (-17.9 vs. -14.4; $p = 0.0086$) were also significantly reduced compared to placebo. AUR occurred in $<1\%$ of each group and there was no clinically significant increase in PVR or decrease in Qmax. There was no significant difference in improvements in PPBC between add-on tolterodine and placebo.

The solifenacin in combination with tamsulosin in overactive bladder residual symptoms (VICTOR) study

The VICTOR study assessed add-on solifenacin 5 mg in men with persistent storage LUTS after being on tamsulosin (400 mcg) in comparison to placebo. [7] Subjects were 45 yr or older and complained of frequency ≥ 8, urgency ≥ 1, had a total IPSS score ≥ 13, PPBC ≥ 3, PVR ≤ 200 ml, and Qmax ≥ 5 ml/randomized. There was a significant reduction in urgency episodes with add-on solifenacin compared to

placebo (-2.18 vs. -1.10, $p < 0.001$) whilst total number of voids/24 h was similar between the groups. In terms of patient reported outcomes, there were significant differences between the two groups. Three percent of the add-on solifenacin group experienced AUR compared to none of the placebo group.

Oxybutynin as add-on to tamsulosin

MacDiarmid et al. studied 420 men older than 45 yr with a total IPSS ≥ 13 and storage subscore of ≥ 8. Subjects were randomized to receive oxybutynin 10 mg extended release formulation or placebo as add-on to therapy with tamsulosin 400 mcg. [8] Exclusion criteria included a Qmax < 8 ml/s and a PVR > 150 ml on two occasions. Total IPSS scores were noted to show a significantly greater improvement with add-on oxybutynin compared to placebo ($p = 0.006$) as did IPSS storage subscores ($p < 0.01$). The IPSS QoL score also improved to a significantly greater extent with oxybutynin ($p < 0.01$). In 2.9% of patients receiving tamsulosin + oxybutynin, a PVR of > 300 ml occurred compared to 0.5% in the tamsulosin + placebo group.

Propiverine and doxazosin

Lee et al. conducted an eight-week multi-center study of propiverine 20 mg plus doxazosin controlled release gastrointestinal therapeutic system formulation 4 mg in urodynamically obstructed patients (Abrams-Griffiths number > 20). The study included a total of 211 patients, 142 randomized to α-AA plus anti-M and 69 to α-AA alone. Combination treatment demonstrated significantly greater improvements in frequency (23.5% vs.

14.3%, $p = 0.004$) and IPSS storage sub-score (41.3% vs. 32.6%, $p = 0.029$) than doxazosin alone. Patient satisfaction was significantly higher with combination treatment ($p = 0.002$). The study failed to demonstrate a significant increase risk of AUR with propiverine despite a small rise in PVR (from mean 28.8 to 49.6 ml, $p = 0002$).[9]

Summary

From the available literature it appears that co-medication with an anti-M and an α-AA in men with storage symptoms/OAB concomitant with LUTS suggestive of BPH is a safe and efficacious treatment option. There are, however, several important caveats when extrapolating the data to clinical practice. Most studies excluded the men who would be at the greatest risk of AUR (high PVRs – usually above 200 ml – and low flow rates) as a consequence of reduced detrusor contractility or more severe BOO. Similarly prostatic volumes, when measured, were towards the low end of the spectrum. The majority of studies lasted three months or less, and although the incidence of AUR was very low, this length of time may not be long enough to determine accurately the long-term risk of AUR which is known to increase with the length of follow-up. In applying this data, the current American urological association guidelines (AUA) (2010) suggest co-medication is an "appropriate and effective treatment alternatives for the management of LUTS secondary to BPH in men without an elevated post-void residual and when LUTS are predominantly irritative." Similarly, the European association of Urology (EAU) states that co-medication "might be considered in patients with moderate to severe LUTS if symptom relief has been insufficient with the monotherapy of either drug" (Table 12.2). A simplified clinical algorithm for the male with storage LUTS/OAB is presented in Figure 12.1.

Phosphodiesterase-5 inhibitors and α-adrenoreceptor antagonists

Both LUTS and erectile dysfunction (ED) are common conditions in aging men. The epidemiological data suggest a strong correlation between ED and LUTS. [10] It has

Table 12.2 Current guidance by AUA and EUA

Guideline	α-adrenoreceptor antagonists + Antimuscarinics	α-adrenoreceptor antagonists + PDE5 inhibitors
AUA (2010)	Appropriate and effective treatment alternatives for the management of LUTS secondary to BPH in men without an elevated post-void residual and when LUTS are predominantly irritative.	No guidance
EAU (2013)	Might be considered in patients with moderate to severe LUTS if symptom relief has been insufficient with the monotherapy of either drug.	Reduce moderate to severe male LUTS. Currently restricted to men with erectile dysfunction, pulmonary arterial hypertension, or to those who have lower urinary tract symptoms and participate in clinical trials.

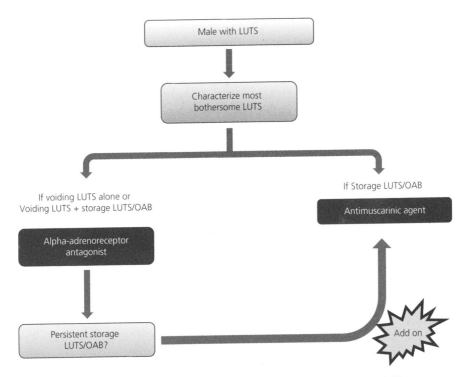

Figure 12.1 Simplified clinical algorithm for the management of male storage LUTS/OAB.

been proposed that an alteration in the NO/cGMP signaling pathway may be an important common underlying mechanism in the pathogenesis of both LUTS and ED. [11] Siaram et al., in 2002, reported that PDE5 inhibition improved LUTS in men being treated for ED. Subsequently, evidence from RCTs of PDE5 inhibitor monotherapy in men with LUTS has shown significant reductions in IPSS scores versus placebo without a concomitant improvement in Qmax, suggesting the mechanism of action is not simply the relief of BOO. [12] Certainly, PDE5 gene and protein expression has been demonstrated throughout the entire lower urinary tract in men [13] as well as the pelvic blood vessels, whilst PDEF inhibition was shown to induce relaxation of strips of detrusor muscle, prostate, and pelvic blood vessels.

[14] *In vivo* studies also suggest that PDE5 inhibition reduces afferent signaling. [15, 16] Thus, it is possible that PDE5 inhibition improves LUTS through a predominant bladder related mechanism and/or through an improvement in blood flow to the lower urinary tract.

Although the efficacy of PDE5 inhibitors for OAB in women remains to be established, their efficacy in treating LUTS in men is now widely accepted and recently tadalafil monotherapy was approved for this indication. Combination therapy of PDE5 inhibitors with an α-AA is less well studied, mainly in several small pilot studies. The rational for combination therapy would be to optimize LUTS related efficacy and treat concomitant ED. We review the evidence relating to LUTS in the key studies.

Sildenafil and alfuzosin

Kaplan et al. conducted the first prospective randomized study to compare the combination of an α-AA (alfuzosin 10 mg) with a PDE5 inhibitor (sildenafil 25 mg). A total of 62 subjects who had both LUTS suggestive of BPH and ED and aged 50 or over were included. [17] Men were randomized to the three groups; alfuzosin alone, sildenafil alone, or combination treatment. There were significant improvements in IPSS scores across all groups. The greatest improvement, however, was with combination treatment (24.1%), significantly greater than both sildenafil alone (16.9%) and alfuzosin alone (15.6%) groups. Changes in IPSS storage subscores were not presented; however, frequency and nocturia episodes were significantly improved only with combination and alfuzosin, not sildenafil alone.

Sildenafil and tamsulosin

Tuncel et al. conducted an eight-week study after randomizing a total of 60 men with LUTS suggestive of BPH to treatment with sildenafil 25 mg, tamsulosin 400 mcg, or a combination of both. [18] The combination group demonstrated the greatest improvement in total IPSS scores at 40.1%, although this was not significantly different from tamsulosin monotherapy (36.2%). Sildenafil alone also led to an improvement in IPSS to a significantly lesser degree at 28.2%. Separate IPSS storage subscores were not presented. Both tamsulosin alone and combination treatment led to similar changes in Qmax.

Tadalafil and tamsulosin

Bechara et al. performed a crossover study, randomizing 30 men over the age of 50 with LUTS suggestive of BPH to receive either tamsulosin 400 mcg or tamsulosin 400 mcg + tadalafil 20 mg for 45 days before switching to the alternate treatment for another 45 days. [19] Whilst both treatments led to equivalent improvements in Q max and PVR, combination therapy led to significantly greater improvements in IPSS score as well as the IPSS QoL score. As with the previous studies, outcomes in terms of IPSS storage subscores were not presented.

Tadalafil and alfuzosin

An open label study prospectively comparing treatment with alfuzosin (10 mg), monotherapy, tadalafil (20 mg), monotherapy, or combination therapy in men with LUTS suggestive of BPH was reported by Liquori et al. [20]. IPSS improved significantly in the alfuzosin group (27.2%) and to a greater extent in the combination group (41.6%) with a non-significant increase in the tadalafil monotherapy group (8.4%). The greatest increase in Qmax was observed in the combination group (29.6%) compared to alfuzosin (21.7%) and tadalafil (9.5%). The difference between combination therapy and alfuzosin was non-significant. Nocturia improved significantly with both alfuzosin and combination but not with sildenafil alone.

Vardenafil and tamsulosin

More recently Gacci et al. reported a 12-week placebo controlled study, comparing treatment with tamsulosin 400 mcg plus vardenafil with tamsulosin 400 mcg plus placebo. [21] The study included subjects who had ongoing storage LUTS (based upon an IPSS storage subscore > 8) after a four-week washout period and a two-week run-in period with tamsulosin. Combination therapy showed greater, though not statistically significant, improvements in total IPSS, IPSS bother score, and OAB-q than tamsulosin with placebo. In terms of IPSS storage subscore, combination treatment improved scores to a significantly greater extent than tamsulosin with placebo (-3.11 vs. 1.67, $p=0.039$). Interestingly, this study showed significant advantage in terms of Qmax with combination therapy compared to tamsulosin plus placebo ($+2.56$ vs. $+0.07$, $p=0.034$).

Summary

Gacci and colleagues recently preformed a meta-analysis of the studies of combination of α-AA with PDE5 inhibitors [12] including 202 patients; 99 receiving α-AA and 103 receiving combination. Total IPSS scores were reduced in both groups to a significantly a greater extent with combination treatment than α-AA alone (-1.8 [-3.7 to 0.0] $p=0.05$). There was also a significant advantage for combination therapy in improvement of Qmax (1.5 ml/s [$+0.9$ to $+2.2$]; $p<0.0001$), which is surprising given that PDE5 inhibitors alone do not increase Qmax. In terms of safety, the AE rate was similar for the two regimens (6.8% for combination and 5.1% with α-AA alone).

Clearly, in view of the small numbers, the use of varying agents at varying dosages, as well as lack of blinding in some cases, the evidence base for the combination of an α-AA with PDE5 inhibitor is substantially weaker than α-AA with an anti-M. Moreover, most studies lack an adequate assessment of storage LUTS/OAB using total IPSS score as the primary subjective efficacy endpoint. Nevertheless, taken together these small studies suggest that combining an α-AA with PDE5 inhibitor

may be an efficacious option in some men with LUTS. The combination is not yet recommended for use in routine clinical practice (Figure 12.1). How PDE5 inhibitors improve LUTS is unclear, even less is known regarding the mechanism of LUTS improvement when combined with an α-AA. *In vitro*, combination alfuzosin with tadalafil was shown to more effectively inhibit electrical-induced human prostate and bladder contractions than either agent alone, suggesting a synergistic effect may perhaps explain the improved efficacy when the agents are used in combination. [22]

Other combination regimens

Combined medication with two different anti-M agents is an alternative approach that has been studied by few investigators. The aim is to optimize the efficacy of anti-M. Amend et al. studied the co-medication with two anti-Ms in 27 patients wiith neurogenic DO who had not responded to dose escalation with a single agent. Instances of urgency urinary incontinence decreased and bladder capacity increased after add-on therapy with another anti-M, consequently 85% of participants reported satisfaction with the treatment. [23] Two patients discontinued combination treatment. More recently, Yi et al. assessed addition of a second anti-M in patients with idiopathic OAB who failed to obtain sufficient symptomatic improvement with a single anti-M after dose escalation in a retrospective series that included 49 patients. [24] Following the addition of a second anti-M, mean urgency episodes decreased from 3.8 to 1.9 ($p<0.001$) whilst day frequency reduced from 10.4 to 7.4

($p<0.001$) after a mean duration of treatment of 9.3 months. There was no difference in efficacy between patients receiving two non-selective agents and those receiving a non-selective agent and an M3 selective agent. In total, 22.4% patients discontinued combination treatment due to poor efficacy or dry mouth. Theoretically, any efficacy derived from co-medicating with two anti-M agents may be related to a dose dependent effect, differences in receptor selectivity of two agents, or perhaps a synergistic effect. Further prospective randomized studies would be required to establish the efficacy and tolerability of this approach.

Other combination regimens for the treatment of storage LUTS/OAB are at present largely experimental or theoretical and have not been investigated in the setting of prospective randomized clinical studies. With the availability of new agent classes, such as the beta-3 agonist and PDE5 inhibitors, there will be in the future the opportunity to assess the efficacy and safety of these agents in combination with generic formulations of α-AA and anti-Ms that are becoming available.

Future directions

Combination therapies for the concomitant alleviation of both voiding LUTS and storage LUTS/OAB are now emerging. Anti-M with α-AA is the most established combination in men and although the three-month studies provide strong safety and efficacy data there is a need for studies with extended follow-up to determine the long-term outcomes. Additionally the inclusion of men with PVRs > 200 ml would help inform whether it is safe to use anti-M

in men with higher residuals. A PDE5 inhibitor with an α-AA is an emerging combination with a smaller, weaker evidence base – larger placebo controlled studies are needed to establish the efficacy and safety of this combination. There is particular a need for more comprehensive assessment of storage LUTS/OAB using more specific outcome measures. Moreover, given the expense of PDE5 inhibitors in many regions of the world, analysis of the cost-effectiveness of their use in men with LUTS is required. Other combination regimens are at present largely theoretical or studied in only a handful of pilot or retrospective clinical studies. In future, it will be important to establish the characteristics of patients who have the greatest chance of deriving benefit from any given combination regimen. It will be essential to consider any cost implications as well as the risk of further side-effects in using two agents. With generic formulations of agents in several pharmacological classes now available, there is an opportunity to comparatively evaluate new combinations.

References

1 Chapple CR, Smith D. The pathophysiological changes in the bladder obstructed by benign prostatic hyperplasia. *Br J Urol.* 1994 Feb;**73**: 117–123.

2 Kaplan SA, Roehrborn CG, Rovner ES, et al. Tolterodine and tamsulosin for treatment of men with lower urinary tract symptoms and overactive bladder: a randomized controlled trial. *JAMA* 2006 Nov 15;**296**:2319–2328.

3 Kaplan SA, Roehrborn CG, Chancellor M, et al. Extended–release tolterodine with or without tamsulosin in men with lower urinary tract symptoms and overactive bladder: effects on urinary symptoms assessed by the International

Prostate Symptom Score. *BJU I* 2008 Nov;**102**: 1133–1139.

4 Roehrborn CG, Kaplan SA, Jones JS, et al. Tolterodine extended release with or without tamsulosin in men with lower urinary tract symptoms including overactive bladder symptoms: effects of prostate size. *Eur Urol.* 2009 Feb; **55**:472–479.

5 Roehrborn CG, Kaplan SA, Kraus SR, et al. Effects of serum PSA on efficacy of tolterodine extended release with or without tamsulosin in men with LUTS, including OAB. *Urology* 2008 Nov;**72**:1061–1067; discussion 7.

6 Chapple C, Herschorn S, Abrams P, et al. Tolterodine treatment improves storage symptoms suggestive of overactive bladder in men treated with alpha–blockers. *Eur Urol.* 2009 Sep;**56**:534–541.

7 Kaplan SA, McCammon K, Fincher R, et al. Safety and tolerability of solifenacin add–on therapy to alpha–blocker treated men with residual urgency and frequency. *J Urol.* 2009 Dec;**182**:2825–2830.

8 MacDiarmid SA, Peters KM, Chen A, et al. Efficacy and safety of extended–release oxybutynin in combination with tamsulosin for treatment of lower urinary tract symptoms in men: randomized, double–blind, placebo–controlled study. *Mayo Clin Proc.* 2008 Sep;**83**:1002–1010.

9 Lee KS, Choo MS, Kim DY, et al. Combination treatment with propiverine hydrochloride plus doxazosin controlled release gastrointestinal therapeutic system formulation for overactive bladder and coexisting benign prostatic obstruction: a prospective, randomized, controlled multicenter study. *J Urol.* 2005 Oct;**174**: 1334–1338.

10 Gacci M, Eardley I, Giuliano F, et al. Critical analysis of the relationship between sexual dysfunctions and lower urinary tract symptoms due to benign prostatic hyperplasia. *Eur Urol.* 2011 Oct;**60**:809–825.

11 McVary K. Lower urinary tract symptoms and sexual dysfunction: epidemiology and pathophysiology. *BJU Int.* 2006 Apr: **97** Suppl 2:23–28; discussion 44–45.

12 Gacci M, Corona G, Salvi M, et al. A systematic review and meta–analysis on the use of phosphodiesterase 5 inhibitors alone or in combination with alpha–blockers for lower

urinary tract symptoms due to benign prostatic hyperplasia. *Eur Urol.* 2012 May;**61**: 994–1003.

13 Fibbi B, Morelli A, Vignozzi L, et al. Characterization of phosphodiesterase type 5 expression and functional activity in the human male lower urinary tract. *J Sex Med.* 2010 Jan;**7**:59–69.

14 Giuliano F, Uckert S, Maggi M, et al. The mechanism of action of phosphodiesterase type 5 inhibitors in the treatment of lower urinary tract symptoms related to benign prostatic hyperplasia. *Eur Urol.* 2012;**64**:118–140.

15 Minagawa T, Aizawa N, Igawa Y, Wyndaele JJ. Inhibitory effects of phosphodiesterase 5 inhibitor, tadalafil, on mechanosensitive bladder afferent nerve activities of the rat, and on acrolein–induced hyperactivity of these nerves. *BJU Int.* 2012 Sep;**110**:E259–266.

16 Behr-Roussel D, Oger S, Caisey S, et al. Vardenafil decreases bladder afferent nerve activity in unanesthetized, decerebrate, spinal cord–injured rats. *Eur Urol.* 2011 Feb;**59**: 272–279.

17 Kaplan SA, Gonzalez RR, Te AE. Combination of alfuzosin and sildenafil is superior to monotherapy in treating lower urinary tract symptoms and erectile dysfunction. *Eur Urol.* 2007 Jun;**51**:1717–1723.

18 Tuncel A, Nalcacioglu V, Ener K, et al. Sildenafil citrate and tamsulosin combination is not superior to monotherapy in treating lower urinary tract symptoms and erectile dysfunction. *World J Urol.* 2010 Feb;**28**:17–22.

19 Bechara A, Romano S, Casabe A, et al. Comparative efficacy assessment of tamsulosin vs. tamsulosin plus tadalafil in the treatment of LUTS/BPH. Pilot study. *J Sex Med.* 2008 Sep;**5**:2170–2178.

20 Liguori G, Trombetta C, De Giorgi G, et al. Efficacy and safety of combined oral therapy with tadalafil and alfuzosin: an integrated approach to the management of patients with lower urinary tract symptoms and erectile dysfunction. *Preliminary report. J Sex Med.* 2009 Feb; **6**:544–552.

21 Gacci M, Vittori G, Tosi N, et al. A randomized, placebo–controlled study to assess safety and efficacy of vardenafil 10 mg and tamsulosin 0.4 mg vs. tamsulosin 0.4 mg alone in the

treatment of lower urinary tract symptoms secondary to benign prostatic hyperplasia. *J Sex Med.* 2012 Jun;**9**:1624–1633.

22 Oger S, Behr-Roussel D, Gorny D, et al. Combination of alfuzosin and tadalafil exerts an additive relaxant effect on human detrusor and prostatic tissues in vitro. *Eur Urol.* 2010 Apr; **57**:699–707.

23 Amend B, Hennenlotter J, Schafer T, et al. Effective treatment of neurogenic detrusor dysfunction by combined high–dosed anti-muscarinics without increased side-effects. *Eur Urol.* 2008 May;**53**:1021–1028.

24 Yi J, Jeong SJ, Chung MS, et al. Efficacy and tolerability of combined medication of two different antimuscarinics for treatment of adults with idiopathic overactive bladder in whom a single agent antimuscarinic therapy failed. *Can Urol Assoc J.* 2013 Jan–Feb; **7**:E88–92.

CHAPTER 13

Other non-surgical approaches for the treatment of overactive bladder

Geneviève Nadeau[1] and Sender Herschorn[2]

[1] Division of Urology, CHU de Québec, Université Laval, Québec, QC, Canada
[2] Sunnybrook Health Sciences Centre, University of Toronto, Toronto, ON, Canada

---

KEY POINTS

- Overactive bladder (OAB) treatment follows a well-defined and accepted stepped approach with lifestyle modifications, pelvic floor exercises, pharmacologic agents (antimuscarinics, β3-agonists), and lastly more invasive interventions (botulinum toxin, neuromodulation, surgery) as necessary.

- When those standard options fail or cannot be applied to a specific patient, one can become familiar with various ancillary treatments that have been studied and proposed for management of OAB.

- Herein we will review the rationale and results to be expected from bladder training, acupuncture, naturopathic and herbal remedies, magnetic stimulation, catheters, and tissue engineering.

Introduction

Overactive bladder (OAB) treatment follows a well-defined and accepted stepped approach with lifestyle modifications, pelvic floor exercises, pharmacologic agents (antimuscarinics, β3-agonists), and lastly more invasive interventions (botulinum toxin, neuromodulation, surgery) as necessary.

When those standard options fail or cannot be applied to a specific patient, one can become familiar with various ancillary treatments that have been studied and proposed for management of OAB. Herein we will review the rationale and results to be expected from bladder training, acupuncture, naturopathic and herbal remedies, magnetic stimulation, catheters, and tissue engineering.

Bladder training

This can be initiated in the primary care setting with other lifestyle interventions. The goal is to reduce voiding frequency, potentially increasing bladder capacity and reducing the need to void in response to urgency. Timed voiding or a scheduled voided regimen involves urinating at

---

regularly set intervals that disregard the normal urge to void. [1] With the urge suppression strategy, patients are instructed to delay urination by gradually increasing the interval from when the urge is felt to when they actually void. Distraction (counting backwards) or relaxation (deep breathing) may help patients to hold long enough. A Cochrane review examined the effect of bladder training for treatment of urinary incontinence. It included data from eight trials involving 858 participants. Despite lack of long-term follow-up and statistical significance, bladder training was slightly favored compared to no training but there was not enough evidence to determine whether it was useful as a supplement to another therapy. [2] There are many variations in bladder training parameters and it is not clear what the most appropriate protocol would be. [3] These are quite innocuous but time-consuming techniques that require a highly motivated patient since a minimum of six-week trial is required to see any benefit. [4]

Acupuncture

Acupuncture is a traditional Chinese modality that has been used for more than 2000 years to treat many conditions, including urinary incontinence. The exact mechanism of action is not quite understood but many are convinced that it is primarily mediated through the nervous system through activation of cutaneo-visceral effects. [5] Traditionally, acupuncturists use the concepts of "qi" (life-force, pronounced "chee"), "yang," and "yin." Different from Western medicine, the kidneys' qi plays a role in holding the urine in the bladder. Urinary incontinence typically involves the kidney's

qi energy being weak or deficient. [6] Acupuncture focuses on correcting those body's imbalances by inserting fine needles into specific points of the body, called "acupoints."[6] Interestingly, most of the acupoints traditionally used to treat urinary incontinence are located within the nerve segments or dermatomes targeted by neuromodulation methods. Treatment sessions typically last between 30–60 minutes, with the needles being retained for 15 minutes or so, and are performed once or twice per week for 10–12 sessions. [7] To enhance the efficacy of the treatment, the acupuncturist may manually stimulate the needles or use electrical stimulation or moxibustion (heating the needle using moxa, a therapeutic herb). [5]

Most of the scientific literature concerning acupuncture for treatment of urgency urinary incontinence includes small, uncontrolled studies. We identified five full-text articles of reasonable quality involving 126 patients from 1988 to 2000. [8–12] Despite considerable variation across the studies, all demonstrated significant improvements in subjective outcome measures such as quality of life, while results from objective measures (pad weights, number of micturitions, voided volumes, etc.) were more diminished, precluding meaningful conclusions.

Of note, Chang et al., who reported the longest follow-up study (up to five years), described no cumulative effect and usefulness of intermittent treatments for maintenance of symptom relief over time, with 4 out of 26 women dropping out due to lack of efficacy. [10]

Recently, a systematic review based on the Cochrane criteria identified three RCTs addressing the topic. [13] From 1994 to 2011, a total of 203 participants were involved in these studies, with protocols that varied in terms of control groups (sham acupuncture, oxybutynin), acupoints used, stimulation method, outcome measures (bladder diary, questionnaires, urodynamic assessment), and duration of treatment (4–6 weeks) and follow-up (2–12 weeks). [14–17] The results from the selected RCTs failed to demonstrate any statistically significant improvements in urinary incontinence, although acupuncture or acupressure did exhibit favorable effects on overactive bladder symptoms and quality of life in comparison with other conventional therapies.

Overall, studies have shown that it is well tolerated with very few and minor side-effects, such as drowsiness, minor bleeding, bruising or discomfort from needle placement. [13] Despite globally supporting higher continence rates with acupuncture, the results were not statistically significant for all four trials, [14–17] as expected from the low numbers of participants, making the clinical evidence insufficient to conclude on the effectiveness of acupuncture in OAB.

The use of acupuncture as an adjunct to Western medicine is a safe modality that seems to offer beneficial effects on OAB symptoms. Nevertheless, not all patients will respond to acupuncture treatments. [18] Inconsistencies in protocols across the studies and scarcity of data warrant some caution before making definitive recommendations, and higher quality and rigorous trials with longer-term follow-up are required.

Naturopathic and herbal remedies

Patients may seek complementary and alternative medicines for various reasons: dissatisfaction with the results or side-effects of conventional agents such as antimuscarinics, need for personal control over their treatment, perception that natural/herbal remedies are more innocuous, or dissatisfaction from interactions with physicians. [19, 20] Despite the lack of randomized controlled trials (RCTs), the frequent and empirical use of some over-the-counter traditional herbal medicines warrants some basic knowledge on the part of the physician to counsel patients appropriately.

Gosha-jinki-gan (GJG), a traditional Asian medicine composed of 10 different herbs, has been the most studied of the commonly used herbal medications for OAB. Kajiwara and Mutaguchi reported on a prospective study among 44 Japanese females with OAB treated for eight weeks. Significant improvements in International Prostate Symptom Scores (IPSS) (from 14.2 to 10.0), QoL (from 4.2 to 3.1), and reduction in daily frequency of micturitions (from 9.3 to 7.8/d) were observed. Adverse reactions occurred in 9.1% of patients, mostly gastrointestinal symptoms of mild intensity. [21] Ogushi and Takahashi followed 30 men with OAB who were administered GJG over six weeks with similar results. [22] The mechanism of action of GJG remains unclear but it is thought to be associated not with anticholinergic action but with inhibition of spinal κ opioid receptors, resulting in decreased bladder sensation and reduced urinary frequency. [23]

An extract of Ba-Wei-Die-Huang-Wan has also been studied by Andersson and co-workers demonstrating its effect in inhibiting ATP-induced detrusor overactivity in rats, but so far this has not been translated into human studies. [24] Other herbal remedies frequently used for OAB have been reviewed by Chughtai et al. and include Hachi-mi-jio-gan, Buchu (*Barosma betulina*), Cornsilk (*Zea mays*), Cleavers (*Galium aparine*), *Ganoderma lucidum*, and horsetail (*Equisetum*). [25]

Bearing in mind that these preparations are not regulated by medical regulatory bodies – such as the FDA – for safety, consistency of labeling, and ingredients, considerably more research is required to support their use.

Magnetic stimulation

Extracorporeal magnetic innervation or magnetic stimulation (MStim) can be applied at the sacral or perineal levels for treatment of urinary incontinence. Surface coils produce pulsed electromagnetic rapidly changing fields which result in nerve stimulation and probable neuromodulation, in a similar manner to electrical stimulation. [26]

Treatment sessions typically last 20 to 30 minutes and are performed twice a week for a 6–8 week period. [27] Advantages to this technique include its non-invasiveness, no need for the patient to undress as the magnetic fields pass through clothing, and lower current (compared to electrical stimulation) is delivered at the surface body to achieve the same current at the nerve root since the magnetic field is unaffected by tissue impedance. This results in less discomfort for the patients. [27] MStim can be chair-based or home-based. The Neocontrol chair (Neotonus Inc., Marietta, Georgia, USA) was approved by the FDA in 1998 and appeared initially as a promising alternative treatment for OAB. Reported side-effects of MStim include leg pain, abdominal pain, cystitis, bowel symptoms, backache, tingling sensation, perineal pain, neck pain,

and potential exacerbation of pre-existing lumbar ischialgia. [28]

Five trials examined MStim in men and women with UI, mixed UI, or predominant urgency UI, [29–33] comparing it to sham or electrical stimulation. Interestingly, short-term data showed encouraging results with objective inhibition of provoked detrusor contractions for both idiopathic and neurogenic detrusor overactivity in patients in a number of studies, [34–37] although the exact mechanism of action is not fully understood. Limitations of those studies included small patient populations, lack of control groups, lack of long-term results, and inconsistencies in procedural protocol (various stimulation parameters in intensity and duration). For the long-term, compliance may be an issue as the effects appear to be temporary and patients need to continue to attend twice weekly for their treatment sessions, which might be costly. [26, 27]

MStim has fallen out of favor, probably because it has not been proved to increase continence more than sham stimulation. [38] It is now considered an experimental and/or investigational modality for the treatment of UI due to insufficient long-term data of quality available to assess its safety and/or efficacy. [3]

Containment products

Products are available for intractable incontinence: pads or protective garments, indwelling catheters, condom (male external sheath) catheters, and so on. They should be considered as a last resort alternative when other options have failed or proved to be insufficient. Catheters in particular should be reserved for patients who are cognitively impaired, with poor hand function, those who have limited assistance from caregiver for other types of bladder management (such as intermittent catheterization), [39] or when protection of wounds that need to be kept clean of urine is required. [40] A catheter can be used sporadically or on a long-term basis. For long-term use, a supra pubic catheter might be the preferred option, with advantages such as less risk of urethral trauma, less interference with sexual activity, and greater comfort and easier access for those who are chair bound. [41] However, this is not evidence-based as a Cochrane review concluded that there are a lack of data regarding the use of different types of catheters for long-term bladder management. Indeed, it was not possible to address conclusively whether external sheath catheters are better than indwelling, and whether indwelling urethral are better or worse than supra pubic catheters. [42] Catheters carry risks of blockage, infections, stones, and even bladder carcinoma due to chronic irritation of the bladder mucosa and, therefore, patients with indwelling catheterization still require periodic monitoring.

One should bear in mind that for recalcitrant OAB symptoms, catheters alone are often unhelpful as uninhibited contractions might lead to leakage around the catheter. In selected cases where no other treatment is feasible, appropriate, or satisfactory, urinary retention needs to be induced pharmacologically combined with indwelling catheterization. [43] This often happens with detrusor hyperactivity with impaired contractility (DHIC), a variety of OAB frequently encountered in the elderly. It presents with a seemingly paradoxical set of findings, as the bladder is

overactive but empties ineffectively [44] in the absence of bladder outlet obstruction. It is a challenging condition to treat, especially considering the numerous limitations to consider in a frail population. Combination of an antimuscarinic with an indwelling catheter might be the only solution.

The debilitating symptoms of OAB shatter the quality of life and, in some people, the only possible feasible management might be to control urinary incontinence through containment products such as pads, external sheath catheters, or indwelling catheters. An excellent source of information on products can be found on the combined ICI (International Consultation on Incontinence) ICS (International Continence Society) website entitled "Continence Product Advisor" (http://www.continenceproductadvisor. org).

Future: tissue engineering and gene therapy

Since current interventional therapies have limitations, cell-based and gene therapies are emerging as new treatment concepts. The field of tissue engineering has made tremendous progress in many areas since its beginning in the early 1990s. [45] The ultimate goal of regenerative medicine for OAB would be the implantation of tissue-engineered autologous bladders or urinary conduits in patients as an alternative to augmentation cystoplasty or cystectomy. [46] With encouraging results from preclinical and clinical phase I studies, Joseph et al. recently reported the first phase II prospective study performed on a total of 11 children and adolescents with spina bidifa. Autologous urothelial and smooth muscle cells were grown and seeded on biodegradable scaffolds and then implanted in patients for use as bladder augmentation. Bladders were cycled postoperatively to promote regeneration. Unfortunately, no significant improvement in clinical parameters and a rate of adverse events higher than expected were observed. [47] The theory behind using stem cell therapy for bladder regeneration or replacement is exciting, but it is expected that meaningful advances in this field will take a long time and the ultimate cost of technology will also determine whether it becomes a viable alternative.

Various applications of gene therapy for the treatment of OAB have been described. Yokoyama et al. reported the effects of herpes simplex virus (HSV) vectors mediating expression of encephalin on bladder overactivity and pain. [48] Kashyap and his team showed that blocking nerve growth factor overexpression in bladder urothelium by antisense oligonucelotides would suppress bladder overactivity. [49] Other studies involving injecting adipose-derived stem cells or bone-marrow-derived mesenchymal stem cells in animal models with OAB showed bladder remodeling and improved bladder function. [50, 51] Taken together, these preliminary data support gene therapy as a potentially useful modality in the future for the treatment of OAB.

Despite major expansion and progress in the field of regenerative and personalized medicine in the last two decades, many challenges remain to be addressed and it is too early to comment on their future usefulness and applicability.

Conclusion

OAB symptoms can be devastating on quality of life and, when more traditional modalities appear insufficient to relieve symptoms, other non-surgical approaches might be considered, either bladder training, acupuncture, herbal remedies, magnetic stimulation or, as a last-resort option, containment products such as pads or catheters. Given the high placebo rate and substantial heterogeneity among many studies addressing treatment of urinary incontinence, more RCTs are required to strengthen the evidence regarding effectiveness of these modalities. Healthcare providers should be knowledgeable about alternative options for OAB and keep their eyes open for emerging strategies, such as tissue engineering and gene therapy.

Abbreviations

DHIC: detrusor hyperactivity with impaired contractility
FDA: Food and Drug Administration
GJG: gosha-jinki-gan
MStim: magnetic stimulation
OAB: overactive bladder
PFMT: pelvic floor muscle physiotherapy
RCTs: randomized controlled trials
UI: urinary incontinence

Financial and competing interests disclosure

Geneviève Nadeau: Advisory board for AMS, Astellas, Pfizer. Speaker for Allergan, Astellas, Pfizer. Sender Herschorn: Grant funding for clinical trials from Astellas,

Pfizer, AMS, Allergan, and Contura. Advisory boards for Pfizer, Allergan, Astellas, and AMS. Speaker for Astellas, Pfizer, AMS.

References

1 Burgio KL, Locher JL, Goode PS. Combined behavioral and drug therapy for urge incontinence in older women. *J Am Geriatr Soc.* Apr 2000;**48**(4):370–374.

2 Wallace SA, Roe B, Williams K, Palmer M. Bladder training for urinary incontinence in adults. *Cochrane Database Syst Rev.* 2004(**1**): CD001308.

3 Smith JH BB, Burgio K, Dumoulin C, et al. *Adult Conservative Management. Incontinence – 4th International Consultation 2009 edn.* Paris: Health Publications, 2009.

4 Arnold J MN, Thani-Gasalam R, Rashid P. Overactive bladder syndrome – Management and treatment options. *Aus Fam Physician* 2012; **41**(11):878–883.

5 Kreder K, Acupuncture for Treatment of Overactive Bladder. In: Kreder K DR, ed. *The Overactive Bladder: Evaluation and Management.* London: Informa HealthCare; 2007: 277–281.

6 Maciocia G. *The Foundations of Chinese Medicine: A Comprehensive Text for Acupuncturists and Herbalists.* 2 edn. New York, 2005.

7 Addison A. Acupuncture and Chinese Herbs for the Benefit of OAB. 2010; http://www.nafc.org/library/articles/acupuncture–and–chinese–herbs–for–the–benefit–of–oab/. Accessed April 2nd 2014.

8 Philp T, Shah PJ, Worth PH. Acupuncture in the treatment of bladder instability. *Br J Urol.* Jun 1988;**61**(6):490–493.

9 Chang PL. Urodynamic studies in acupuncture for women with frequency, urgency and dysuria. *J Urol. Sep* 1988;**140**(3):563–566.

10 Chang PL, Wu CJ, Huang MH. Long–term outcome of acupuncture in women with frequency, urgency and dysuria. *Am J Chin Med.* 1993;**21**(3–4):231–236.

11 Honjo H, Naya Y, Ukimura O, et al. Acupuncture on clinical symptoms and urodynamic measurements in spinal-cord-injured

patients with detrusor hyperreflexia. *Urol Int.* 2000;**65**(4):190–195.

12 Bergström K, Carlsson CP, Lindholm C, Widengren R. Improvement of urge– and mixed–type incontinence after acupuncture treatment among elderly women – a pilot study. *J Auton Nerv Syst.* Mar 2000;**79**(2–3): 173–180.

13 Paik SH, Han SR, Kwon OJ, et al. Acupuncture for the treatment of urinary incontinence: A review of randomized controlled trials. *Exp Ther Med.* Sep 2013;**6**(3):773–780.

14 Kelleher C FJ, Khullar V, Cardozo L. Acupuncture and the treatment of irritative bladder symptoms. *Acupunct Med.* 1994;**12**:9–12.

15 Emmons SL, Otto L. Acupuncture for overactive bladder: a randomized controlled trial. *Obstet Gynecol.* Jul 2005;**106**(1):138–143.

16 Engberg S, Cohen S, Sereika SM. The efficacy of acupuncture in treating urge and mixed incontinence in women: a pilot study. *J Wound Ostomy Continence Nurs.* 2009 Nov–Dec 2009; **36**(6):661–670.

17 Chang KK, Wong TK, Wong TH, et al. Effect of acupressure in treating urodynamic stress incontinence: a randomized controlled trial. *Am J Chin Med* 2011;**39**(6):1139–1159.

18 Graham O. CT. Acupuncture for the treatment of overactive bladder. *J Assoc Chartered Physiother Women's Health Spring* 2008;**102**:53–58.

19 Siapush M. Postmodern values, dissatisfaction with conventional medicine and popularity of alternative therapies. *J Sociol.* 1998;**34**(1): 58–70.

20 Eisenberg DM, Kessler RC, Van Rompay MI, et al. Perceptions about complementary therapies relative to conventional therapies among adults who use both: results from a national survey. *Ann Intern Med.* Sep 2001;**135**(5): 344–351.

21 Kajiwara M, Mutaguchi K. Clinical efficacy and tolerability of gosha-jinki-gan, Japanese traditional herbal medicine, in females with overactive bladder. *Hinyokika Kiyo.* Feb 2008;**54**(2):95–99.

22 Ogushi T, Takahashi S. Effect of Chinese herbal medicine on overactive bladder. *Hinyokika Kiyo.* Dec 2007;**53**(12):857–862.

23 Gotoh A, Goto K, Sengoku A, et al. Inhibition mechanism of Gosha-jinki-gan on the micturition

reflex in rats. *J Pharmacol Sci.* Oct 2004;**96**(2): 115–123.

24 Imamura T, Ishizuka O, Zhong C, et al. An extract (THC–002) of Ba-Wei-Die-Huang-Wan inhibits expression of tachykinins, and P2X3 and TRPV1 receptors, and inhibits ATP-induced detrusor overactivity in spontaneously hypertensive rats. *Neurourol Urodyn.* 2009;**28**(6): 529–534.

25 Chughtai B, Kavaler E, Lee R, et al. Use of herbal supplements for overactive bladder. *Rev Urol.* 2013;**15**(3):93–96.

26 Quek P. A critical review on magnetic stimulation: what is its role in the management of pelvic floor disorders? *Curr Opin Urol.* Jul 2005;**15**(4):231–235.

27 Takahashi S, Kitamura T. Overactive bladder: magnetic versus electrical stimulation. *Curr Opin Obstet Gynecol.* Oct 2003;**15**(5):429–433.

28 UCare. Extracorporeal Magnetic Stimulation for Urinary Incontinence – Medical Policy. 2014; https://http://www.ucare.org/providers/Resources–Training/Medical–Policy/Documents/Extracorporeal Magnetic Stimulation for Urinary Incontinence.pdf. Accessed April 2nd 2014.

29 Yamanishi T, Sakakibara R, Uchiyama T, et al. Comparative study of the effects of magnetic versus electrical stimulation on inhibition of detrusor overactivity. *Urology Nov* 2000;**56**(5): 777–781.

30 But I. Conservative treatment of female urinary incontinence with functional magnetic stimulation. *Urology Mar* 2003;**61**(3):558–561.

31 But I, Faganelj M, Sostaric A. Functional magnetic stimulation for mixed urinary incontinence. *J Urol. May* 2005;**173**(5):1644–1646.

32 Morris AR, O'Sullivan R, Dunkley P, Moore KH. Extracorporeal magnetic stimulation is of limited clinical benefit to women with idiopathic detrusor overactivity: a randomized sham controlled trial. *Eur Urol.* Sep 2007;**52**(3): 876–881.

33 Fujishiro T, Takahashi S, Enomoto H, et al. Magnetic stimulation of the sacral roots for the treatment of urinary frequency and urge incontinence: an investigational study and placebo controlled trial. *J Urol. Sep* 2002;**168**(3): 1036–1039.

34 Bradshaw HD, Barker AT, Radley SC, Chapple CR. The acute effect of magnetic stimulation of the pelvic floor on involuntary

detrusor activity during natural filling and overactive bladder symptoms. *BJU Int.* Jun 2003;**91**(9):810–813.

35 Sheriff MK, Shah PJ, Fowler C, et al. Neuromodulation of detrusor hyper–reflexia by functional magnetic stimulation of the sacral roots. *Br J Urol.* Jul 1996;**78**(1):39–46.

36 McFarlane JP, Foley SJ, de Winter P, et al. Acute suppression of idiopathic detrusor instability with magnetic stimulation of the sacral nerve roots. *Br J Urol.* Nov 1997;**80**(5):734–741.

37 McFarlane JP FS, De Winter P, et al. Suppression of detrusor instability by magnetic stimulation of the sacral nerve roots. *Br J Urol.* 1997;**80**:164–165.

38 Shamliyan T, Wyman J, Kane RL. Nonsurgical Treatments for Urinary Incontinence in Adult Women: Diagnosis and Comparative Effectiveness. Comparative Effectiveness Review No. 36. (Prepared by the University of Minnesota Evidence-based Practice Center under Contract No. HHSA 290-2007-10064-I.) AHRQ Publication No. 11(12)-EHC074- EF. Rockville, MD. Agency for Healthcare Research and Quality. April 2012. Available at: www.effectivehealthcare.ahrq.gov/reports/final.cfm. Accessed April 2nd 2014.

39 Consortium for Spinal Cord Medicine – Clinical Practice Guidleines. Bladder Management Following Spinal Cord Injury: What You Should Know. Paralyzed Veterans of America; 2010, 29 p.: http://www.themiamiproject.org/Document.Doc?id=210. Accessed April 2nd 2014.

40 Kuchel G.A. DCE. Chapter 30: Urinary Incontinence in the Elderly. Online Curricula: Geriatric Nephrology: American Society of Nephrology; 2009: https://http://www.asn–online.org/education/distancelearning/curricula/geriatrics/Chapter30.pdf. Accessed April 2nd 2014.

41 Geng V. C–BH, Farrell J., Gea–Sánchez M., et al. Catheterisation : Indwelling catheters in adults. Evidence–based Guidelines for Best Practice in Urological Health Care. February 2012. http://www.uroweb.org/fileadmin/EAUN/guidelines/EAUN_Paris_Guideline_2012_LR_online_file.pdf. Accessed April 2nd 2014.

42 Jamison J, Maguire S, McCann J. Catheter policies for management of long term voiding problems in adults with neurogenic bladder

disorders. *Cochrane Database Syst Rev.* 2013;**11**: CD004375.

43 Goldman L. Incontinence. In: *Goldman L SAI, ed. Goldman's Cecil Medicine. Vol 1.* 24th edn. Saint Louis, MO: Elsevier Saunders; July 2011: 110–114.

44 Resnick NM, Yalla SV. Detrusor hyperactivity with impaired contractile function. An unrecognized but common cause of incontinence in elderly patients. *JAMA.* Jun 1987; **257**(22):3076–3081.

45 Stanasel I, Mirzazadeh M, Smith JJ. Bladder tissue engineering. *Urol Clin North Am.* Nov 2010;**37**(4):593–599.

46 Atala A. Regenerative bladder augmentation using autologous tissue–when will we get there? *J Urol. May* 2014;**191**(5):1204–1205.

47 Joseph DB, Borer JG, De Filippo RE, Hodges SJ, McLorie GA. Autologous cell seeded biodegradable scaffold for augmentation cystoplasty: phase ii study in children and adolescents with spina bifida. *J Urol. May* 2014;**191**(5): 1389–1395.

48 Yokoyama H, Oguchi T, Goins WF, et al. Effects of herpes simplex virus vector–mediated enkephalin gene therapy on bladder overactivity and nociception. *Hum Gene Ther.* Feb 2013;**24**(2):170–180.

49 Kashyap M, Kawamorita N, Tyagi V, et al. Down–regulation of nerve growth factor expression in the bladder by antisense oligonucleotides as new treatment for overactive bladder. *J Urol. Aug* 2013;**190**(2):757–764.

50 Huang YC, Shindel AW, Ning H, et al. Adipose derived stem cells ameliorate hyperlipidemia associated detrusor overactivity in a rat model. *J Urol. Mar* 2010;**183**(3):1232–1240.

51 Woo LL, Tanaka ST, Anumanthan G, et al. Mesenchymal stem cell recruitment and improved bladder function after bladder outlet obstruction: preliminary data. *J Urol. Mar* 2011;**185**(3):1132–1138.

SECTION 5
Third Line Management

CHAPTER 14

Maximizing the treatment of overactive bladder with sacral nerve stimulation

Scott MacDiarmid

Alliance Urology Specialists Bladder Control and Pelvic Pain Center, Greensboro, NC, USA

What is neuromodulation?

The International Neuromodulation Society defines therapeutic neuromodulation as "the alteration of nerve activity through the delivery of electrical stimulation or chemical agents to targeted sites of the body." [1] By altering neurotransmission processes and restoring neural balance, neuromodulation can have profound effects on pain relief, restoration of normal bowel and bladder control, tremor control, and many other things. [2]

The clinical need for neuromodulation?

The clinical need for sacral nerve stimulation (SNS), percutaneous tibial nerve stimulation (PTNS), and onabotulinum toxin type A is enormous. In order for us to raise the level of care we are currently providing we must liberally offer all three therapies to our OAB patients. It is important to remember that OAB is common, it significantly impacts quality of life, and the treatment of OAB with conservative therapy does not reach the patient's treatment goal in the majority of cases.

KEY POINT

- In order to elevate care we must liberally offer all three neuromodulation therapies to our OAB patients.

OAB is common

According to the National Overactive Bladder Evaluation (NOBLE) Study, the prevalence of OAB in adult Americans is 16.9% in women and 16.0% in men, approaching 34 million sufferers. [3] In a recent Internet survey the prevalence of "at least somewhat bothersome" OAB in the United Kingdom and Sweden was 22.5

Overactive Bladder: Practical Management, First Edition. Edited by Jacques Corcos, Scott MacDiarmid and John Heesakkers.

© 2015 John Wiley & Sons, Ltd. Published 2015 by John Wiley & Sons, Ltd.

and 33.7% for women, and 10.9 and 14.6% for men, respectively. [4] Its prevalence increases with age, with estimates of 30% in women 65 years of age and older. Based on patient volume and other factors, OAB might be one of the most important populations urologists care for.

KEY POINT

- The millions with OAB represent a very important population to urologists.

The impact of OAB

The negative impacts of OAB on quality of life include impaired mobility, social isolation, impaired work-related productivity, depression, disturbed sleep, and impaired domestic and sexual function. [5] A QOL survey in a US community-based sample using the Medical Outcomes Study Short-Form 20 demonstrated that the OAB patients had significantly lower QOL scores on every domain than controls. [6]

Recurrent urinary tract infections and perineal skin breakdown are more prevalent among patients with urge incontinence. [7] The risk of falls and associated non-spine fractures is also significantly increased. [8]

The economic cost associated with OAB is substantial both to the individual patient and to the healthcare system. The total economic cost of urinary incontinence in the US in 1995 for persons aged 65 years and older has been estimated at $26.3 billion, or $3565 per person affected. [9] More recently, Ganz estimated that the average annual per capita costs of OAB were $1925. The total estimated national costs were $65.9 billion. [10]

The limitations of conservative therapies

The mainstay of OAB therapy consists of non-pharmacologic and pharmacologic approaches, either as monotherapy or in combination. Non-pharmacologic treatment includes dietary and fluid modifications, behavioral therapy, and pelvic floor muscle rehabilitation. [11] The antimuscarinics – darifenacin, fesoterodine, oxybutynin, solifenacin, tolterodine, and trospium chloride – are recommended as second-line therapy. [12] Myrbetriq, a newly approved Beta-3 agent, is an alternative for both the treatment naïve and for those who have failed antimuscarinics.

Unfortunately, the majority of patients do not reach their treatment goal with conservative therapies. Although published improvements in urgency incontinence episodes with behavioral therapy range from 50 to 80%, these were achieved in highly motivated patients treated by experts using strict behavioral protocols. [12] Such improvement in daily practice may be unrealistic and many offices do not offer non-pharmacological treatments. Many patients benefit from antimuscarinics but the data and clinical experience support a low adherence rate to them. Brostrom reported continuation rates with OAB agents of less than 50% at 6 months, less than 25% at 1 year, and less than 10% at 2 years or longer. [13]

KEY POINT

- Conservative therapies fail to meet the patient's treatment goal in the majority of cases.

These patients with refractory OAB I have coined as having ROAB. If one critically evaluates the current usage of refractory treatments it is obvious that the vast majority of ROAB patients are left untreated. As experts we must do better.

KEY POINT

- Unfortunately the majority of ROAB patients are left untreated. As experts we must do better.

Refractory OAB

The American Urological Association (AUA) guideline panel [12] defines the refractory OAB patient as one who has failed appropriate behavioral therapy and who has failed a trial of at least one antimuscarinic medication administered for 6 to 12 weeks. Failure may include lack of efficacy and/or inability to tolerate adverse drug effects. The panel notes that it is important to combine behavioral and medical therapy and to try alternative antimuscarinics before calling the patient refractory.

In daily practice, the definition of ROAB is much more encompassing. ROAB patients have likely failed two or more antimuscarinics, and more recently a Beta-3 agonist. They may not be able to afford their medications, have contraindications to them, or perhaps prefer not to take a pharmaceutical. Third-party payers often define ROAB before they will pay for a refractory neuromodulation therapy. And if one includes partial responders to medication still experiencing bothersome symptoms, the number of ROAB patients is tremendous.

There have been approximately 150 000 sacral nerve stimulators placed worldwide since 1997, with 25 000 implanted in the USA in 2012. Approximately 15 000 and 35 000 were treated with PTNS and onbotulinum toxin, respectfully. Estimating 10 000 US Urologists and Urogynecologists, we are each treating on average 7–8 ROAB patients annually. Clearly we are not treating ROAB.

KEY POINT

- ROAB is markedly undertreated with neuromodulation.

Sacral nerve stimulation

Sacral nerve stimulation by the Interstim® (Medtronic, Minneapolis, MN) device is an innovative neuromodulation treatment for lower urinary tract symptoms. Originally approved by the FDA in 1997, it is indicated for the treatment of non-obstructive urinary retention and the symptoms of OAB when more conservative treatments fail or have intolerable side-effects.

In 2011, InterStim® received FDA approval for the treatment of chronic fecal incontinence in patients who have failed or who are not candidates for more conservative therapies. In addition, SNS has gained popularity for the treatment of a number of other indications in clinical practice including neurogenic detrusor overactivity, chronic pelvic pain syndrome, voiding dysfunction following sling cystourethropexy, and pediatric voiding dysfunction.

It appears that the mechanism of action of SNS is through activation of the somatic pudendal nerve afferent inflow at the sacral root level that in turn affects bladder storage and emptying by modifying bladder and central nervous system reflexes. [14, 15] Pudendal nerve afferent stimulation can modulate and inhibit sensory outflow from the bladder to the pontine micturition center, thereby preventing bladder overactivity. In addition, it is believed that SNS can restore voiding in patients with urinary retention by inhibition of the spinal guarding reflex.

Outcomes of SNS

The data supporting the efficacy and safety of SNS in the treatment of OAB is plentiful and robust. Despite the fact that there is no true FDA-approved indication for a number of select populations, many groups are managed based on their symptoms of urinary frequency, urgency, and/or urgency incontinence.

KEY POINT

- The data supporting the efficacy and safety of SNS in the treatment of OAB is plentiful and robust.

In 1999, Schmidt et al. evaluated SNS in 34 patients and compared them to a delayed therapy group of 42 as a control. [16] At six months the number of daily incontinence episodes, severity of incontinence, and pad usage were significantly reduced in the stimulation group vs. the delay group ($p < 0.0001$); 46% of the SNS patients were dry and an additional 29% were greater than 50% improved. The most common complications included implantable pulse generator site pain in 15.9%, implant site pain 19.1%, lead migration in 7.0%, and a surgical revision rate due to complications of 32.5%.

In a six-month multicenter trial, SNS was statistically superior to the control with respect to the number of daily voids (16.9 ± 9.7 to 9.3 ± 5.1), volume per void (118 ± 74 to 226 ± 124 ml), and degree of urgency (rank 2.2 ± 0.6 to 1.6 ± 0.9). Improvements in quality of life were demonstrated and efficacy was sustained at 24 months. [17]

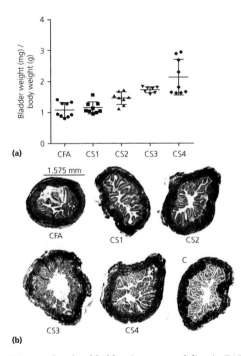

(a)

(b)

Figure 2.4 Clinical score (CS) is correlated to bladder tissue remodeling in EAE mice. (a) The bladder-weight-to-body-weight ratio increase correlates with increasing clinical score (CS) in EAE mice compared to CFA-immunized mice. (b) Histological examination showed bladder hypertrophy and lumen dilation in the EAE mice relative to the CFA control mice, corresponding with increasing CS.

Overactive Bladder: Practical Management, First Edition. Edited by Jacques Corcos, Scott MacDiarmid and John Heesakkers.

© 2015 John Wiley & Sons, Ltd. Published 2015 by John Wiley & Sons, Ltd.

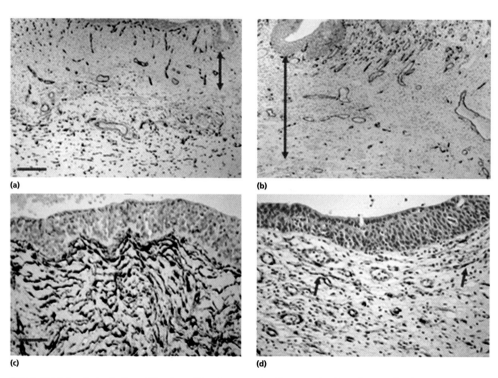

Figure 2.5 Morphological modification of lamina propria. Characterization of upper lamina propria interstitial cells in bladders from control (a) and (c) and MS patients (b) and (d) with CD34 (a) and (b) and SMA (c) and (d). Scale bar: 50 μm. Adapted from Gevaert 2011 [52]. Source: Reproduced with permission of John Wiley & Sons Ltd.

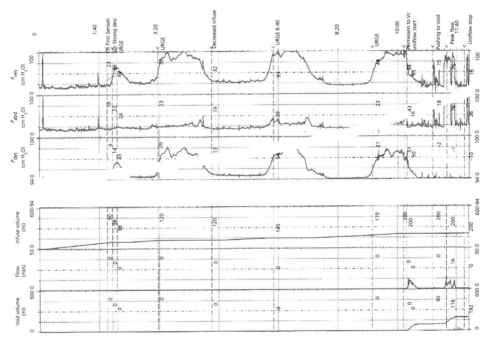

Figure 5.1 Detrusor overactivity without urinary incontinence. Note the rise in detrusor pressure (P_{det}) and vesical pressure (P_{ves}) without a rise in intra-abdominal pressure (P_{abd}). Increased sensation and urgency are noted at low fill volumes. This tracing also illustrates terminal DO.

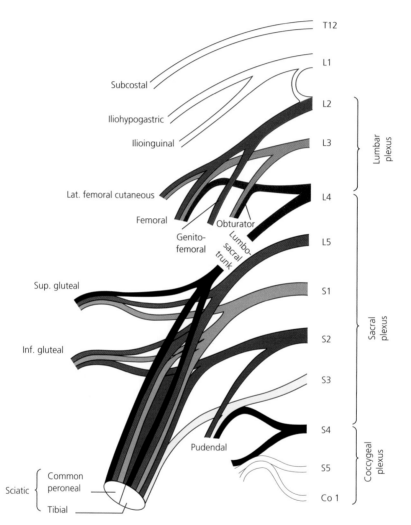

Figure 15.1 Organization of the lower lumbar, sacral, and coccygeal nerve plexus, the merger of the various roots and the most important nerves that branch from the merged nerve plexus. The tibial nerve has it's offspring in the sacral roots of mainly S2 and S3. Source: Basic Human Anatomy: A Regional Study of Human Structure. Source: http://www.dartmouth.edu/~humananatomy/figures/chapter_30/30-6. HTM#top. Reproduced with permission of Ronan O'Rahilly, MD.

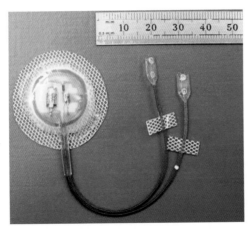

Figure 15.3 The Urgent-SQ implant consisting of an internal electromagnetic pulse receiver, the body with two leads, and monopolar platinum electrodes.

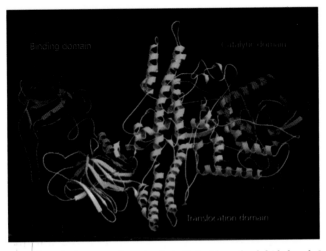

Figure 15.4 Site of implantation during surgery. The two electrodes are placed on tow opposite sides of the tibial nerve just proximal to the medial malleolus.

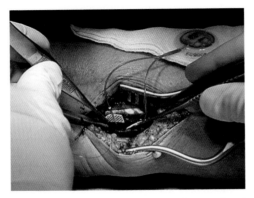

Figure 16.1 BoNT/A consists of a heavy and a light chain linked by a disulphide bond. Source: Lacy, D.B., Tepp, W., Cohen, A.C., DasGupta, B.R., Stevens, R.C. (PDB-Bild 3BTA) [CC-BY-SA-2.0-de (http://creativecommons.org/licenses/by-sa/2.0/de/deed.en)], via Wikimedia Commons.

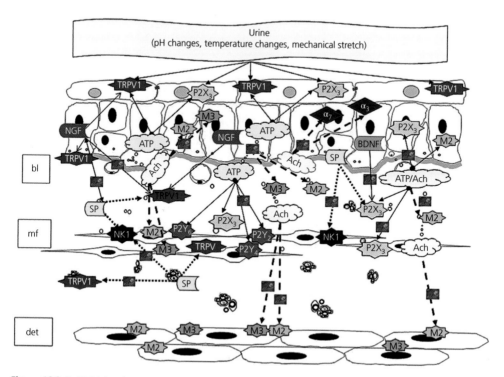

Figure 16.2 BoNT/A has been proposed to affect at multiple levels the complex system of interactions between the release of neurotransmitters and actions on receptors located on the bladder pathways which are thought to be involved in mechanosensation. This cartoon representation of the human bladder wall with known or proposed location of receptors and sites of release of neuropeptides and growth factors has been updated from the relevant Figure in reference [5]. Abbreviations: bl = basal lamina of urothelium, mf = myofibroblast layer, det = detrusor muscle. All connections identified by arrows (see reference [5] for arrow identification) are thought to be upregulated in detrusor overactivity. Apostolidis 2006 [5]. Source: Reproduced with permission of Elsevier.

Abbreviations:

TRPV1:	Transient Receptor Potential Vanilloid 1
$P2X_3$:	ionotropic purinergic receptor type 3
$P2Y_2/P2Y_4/P2Y_6$:	metabotropic purinergic receptors types 2, 4 and 6
M2/M3:	muscarinic acetylcholine receptors types 2 and 3
α_3, α_7:	nicotinic acetylcholine receptors types 3 and 7
NK1:	Neurokinin receptor type 1 (SP receptor)
SP:	Substance P
NGF:	Nerve Growth Factor
BDNF:	Brain Derived Neurotrophic Factor
ACh:	Acetylcholine, ATP - Adenosine Triphosphate

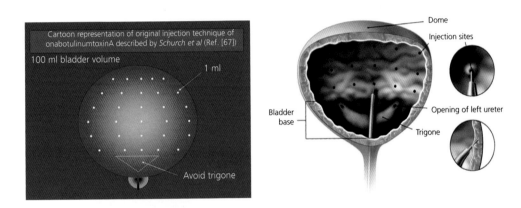

Figure 16.3 2D (left) and 3D (right) cartoon representation of the onabotulinumtoxinA bladder injection technique in NDO/OAB patients. According to the original description by Schurch et al. [68], each 100 U toxin vial was diluted in 10 ml normal saline, and 1 ml of the dilute was delivered at each injection site. The bladder wall is virtually mapped by the surgeon and injection sites should be at a distance of ≥1 cm from each other and exclude the trigone in a half-full bladder. The injection needle should be adequately inserted (up to 4mm) to achieve a detrusor muscle delivery, minimizing at the same time the risk of injecting outside a thinned bladder wall by overdistension. Schurch 2000 [68]. Source: Reproduced with permission of Elsevier.

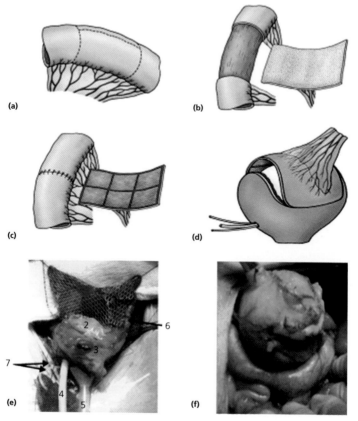

Figure 17.5 The different stages of composite cystoplasty. (a) To develop a vascularized, de-epithelialized seromuscular segement, a Foley catheter was inserted rectally and the balloon filled with sterile water within the portion of sigmoid bowel to be dissected. The dissection limits of the bowel and mesentery were defined. (b) Using the balloon as a support, the seromuscular layer of the bowel was incized and separated from the lamina propria deep to the mucosa. (c) The vascularized, deepithelialized patch was isolated and received the autologous tissue-engineered urothelial cell sheet in complex with the Vicryl mesh. The mesenteric fenestration was closed to prevent internal hernia. (d) The bladder was opened widely and augmented with the composite bowel segment. Gentle distension of the augmented bladder was maintained with a silicone vesical conformer. Urine was diverted post-operatively with ureteric stents and a Malecot suprapubic catheter. Stages (c) and (d), respectively, are illustrated in (e) and (f) during an actual composite cystoplasty operation. (e1) Patches of Vicryl mesh supporting urothelial cell sheets against de-epithelialized colon; (e2) vesical conformer (collapsed); (e3) opened native bladder; (e4) Malecot suprapubic catheter; (e5) filling tube for vesical conformer; (e6) detubularized colon; (e7) ureteric catheters. Turner A, Subramanian R, Thomas DF, Hinley J, Abbas SK, Stahlschmidt J, Southgate J. Transplantation of Autologous Differentiated Urothelium in an Experimental Model of Composite Cystoplasty *J. Eur Urol.* 2011 Mar;59(3):447–54. Source: Reproduced with permission of Elsevier.

van Kerrebroeck et al. reported on the durability of SNS for varying indications in a worldwide series of 152 patients with good success achieved in all groups. [18] For patients with urgency incontinence, mean leaking episodes per day decreased from 9.6±6.0 to 3.9±3.0 at five years.

Similarly, in a single-center study in 60 women, the success rate of SNS was 62% at five years and complete continence was reported in 15%. [19] Leong assessed long-term satisfaction with SNS and reported that 90% of 207 patients were satisfied with the therapy. [20]

KEY POINT

- Sacral nerve stimulation offers patients with OAB a durable treatment option.

Special populations

Patients with neurogenic detrusor overactivity may be managed with SNS. Potential relative contraindications include bony abnormalities of the spine or sacrum, severe functional or mental limitations, and most importantly, their future need for Magnetic Resonance Imaging. The primary concern surrounding MRI is heating of the leads and potential for nerve damage. In addition, the magnetic field may alter the implantable pulse generator. Recently, non-clinical testing demonstrated that the more recent sacral nerve stimulators are MRI conditional and MRI examinations of the head are safe to perform under strict guidelines. [21]

There are no prospective randomized trials evaluating the efficacy and safety of SNS in patients with multiple sclerosis, but a number of small studies exist. Chartier-Kastler et al. evaluated SNS in nine patients with spinal disease (myelitis (1), MS (5), spinal cord injury (2)) and with a mean follow-up of

48.6 months all patients experienced clinically significant improvements in incontinence and five were completely dry. [22]

A number of studies support the use of SNS in the treatment of interstitial cystitis (IC) and painful bladder syndrome, often recommended in combination with other treatments. Comiter demonstrated a success rate of the PNE and staged procedure in 40 and 87% of IC patients, respectively. [23] There was a 73% reduction in mean pain scores with a follow-up of 14 months and the mean daytime frequency and nocturia improved from 17.1 to 8.7 and 4.5 to 1.1, respectfully ($p<0.01$).

Peters evaluated the benefit of SNS on narcotic use in 18 patients who were on chronic pain medication prior to implantation. [24] At 15.4 months the mean in morphine dose equivalents decreased from 81.6 to 52.0 mg daily ($p=0.015$); 22% of patients discontinued narcotics and the majority reported moderate to marked improvement in pain.

KEY POINT

- The symptoms of painful bladder syndrome can be effectively managed by sacral nerve stimulation.

Patients experiencing OAB symptoms following cystourethropexy can be a therapeutic challenge, especially when the timing of events is questionable or the time passed since surgery is lengthy. Sherman et al. evaluated the efficacy of SNS in the management of 34 patients with refractory worsening or *de novo* urgency incontinence following stress incontinence surgery; [25] 65% responded to test stimulation and successfully underwent implantation.

KEY POINT

- Patients with voiding dysfunction following cystourethropexy may be good candidates for sacral nerve stimulation.

Humphreys treated 23 pediatric patients aged 6 to 15 years with dysfunctional elimination syndrome with SNS and reported on 13.3 months follow-up. [26] Of 19 patients with urinary incontinence, 3 (16%) were dry and 12 (68%) were improved. Of the 16 patients with nocturnal enuresis, 2 (13%) had resolution, 9 (56%) improved, and 4 (25%) were unchanged. Constipation improved in 80% of cases. SNS is not FDA-approved in children, perhaps due to lack of data on what the sacral lead would do with concomitant growth of the spinal cord, foramen, and nerve roots.

Despite its efficacy, SNS is associated with a surgical revision rate in up to 30 to 40% of cases, most commonly for loss of efficacy. Lenis et al. reported on the patterns of hardware-related electrode failures in 565 patients between 2003 and 2011 [27]: 72 (12.7%) experienced a total of 86 abnormal impedance events – 66.2% were open circuits and 32.5% were short circuits. Short circuits presented earlier and required surgical intervention more often.

As may be the case with other therapies, increased patient preparedness for SNS outcomes appears to improve patient reported outcomes despite unchanged objective measures. In a study of 36 women, significantly more women in the shared appointment group than controls felt completely prepared (78.9 vs. 29.4%, $p = 0.003$) and completely satisfied (78.9 vs. 17.6%, $p = 0.002$). [28]

A recent randomized trial compared SNS and medical therapy in 142 patients who failed at least one OAB medication. [29] At six months, 61% of patients receiving SNS achieved success compared to 42% in the medication group ($p = 0.016$). Improvements in quality of life were also greater in the SNS patients. Device-related adverse events occurred in 23.7% of SNS patients and 26% of the medication patients experienced an adverse event.

A number of studies have evaluated the PNE versus.the tined lead as the test stimulation. In 30 women, 15 (88%) of the tined lead patients had a successful test compared to 6 (46%) of the PNE group. [30] In a similar study, 46 and 69% of the PNE and tined lead patients, respectively, were successfully tested. Of the 41 PNE failures, 44% successfully tested and went on to implant with the tined lead. [31]

Table 14.1 Motor and sensory responses to stimulation of the sacral nerve plexus.

Nerve Innervation	Response		Sensation
	Pelvic floor	Foot/calf/leg	
S2 Primary somatic contributor of pudendal nerve for external sphincter, leg, foot	"Clamp"* of anal sphincter	Leg/hip rotation, plantar flexion of entire foot, contraction of calf	Contraction of base of penis, vagina
S3 Virtually all pelvic autonomic functions and striated muscle (levator ani)	"Bellows"** of perineum	Plantar flexion of great toe, occassionally other toes	Pulling in rectum, extending forward to scrotum or labia
S4 Pelvic autonomic and somatic no leg or foot	"Bellows"**	No lower extremity motor stimulation	Pulling in rectum only

* Clamp: contraction of anal sphincter and, in males, retraction of base of penis. move buttocks aside and look for anterior/posterior shortening of the perineal structures.
** Bellows: lifting and dropping of pelvic floor. Look for deepening and flattening of buttock groove.

Source: Medtronic, Inc. Reprinted with permission of Medtronic, Inc. © 2008

Technique

The implantation of SNS is a two-stage procedure. The initial stage, or test, allows one to assess whether implantation of the device will be beneficial to the patient.

Many physicians perform the first stage or percutaneous nerve evaluation (PNE) in the office by introducing a unilateral or bilateral lead into the S3 foramen using local anesthesia. I have the luxury of utilizing fluoroscopy. Others have adopted placement of a permanent tined lead in the operating room in an attempt to minimize the number of false-negatives with the test and false-positive results with the second stage. PNE failures have the option of attempting the tined lead approach. The length of the test varies but generally is one week for OAB, and as long as three or four weeks for urinary retention.

Prior to insertion of the tined lead, patients receive prophylactic antibiotics and appropriate aseptic precautions. In the prone position the buttocks are held apart with tape retraction and draped to allow visualization of a bellows. The feet are left uncovered to assess for toe response.

The S3 foramen is generally located approximately 9 cm cephalad to the drop off of the sacrum and 1 to 2 cm lateral to the midline. Under fluoroscopy, the S3 foramina are located in the straight line visualized between the two lower aspects of the sacroiliac joint.

The foramen needle is introduced into the S3 foramen and stimulated. Plantarflexion of the great toe and bellows contraction of the perineal area confirm correct position. Simultaneous sensory responses help optimize lead placement (Table 14.1). The foramen needle is then removed and replaced with the white introducer sheath. The lead is introduced through the sheath exposing the four electrodes. Typically electrodes 2 and 3 straddle

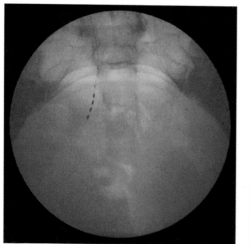 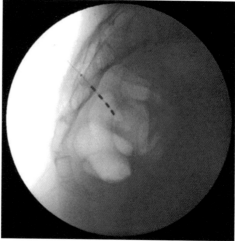

Figure 14.1 The lead is properly located in the S3 foramen noted in the anterior/posterior (a) and lateral (b) x-ray views.

the ventral surface of the sacrum (Figure 14.1a/1b).

A 3–4 cm incision is made in the upper buttock below the beltline and carried down through subcutaneous tissue for a few centimeters. The lead is passed from medial to lateral with the tunneling device where it is connected to the extension wire. The tunneling device is then used to transpose the extension wire from the medial aspect of the incision to an exit point on the contralateral side of the back. A sterile dressing is applied and the extension wire is connected to the external pulse generator. A greater than 50% improvement in lower urinary tract symptoms is considered a success and the patient is a good candidate for stage II.

During stage II the implantable pulse generator (IPG) is inserted. In the prone position the previously made buttock incision is opened and extended for a few centimeters. The subcutaneous pocket is enlarged to accommodate the IPG and to allow for a tension free closure. The extension wire is detached and removed, and the lead is

secured to the generator. Prior to closure electrode impedances are checked.

Some simple suggestions may make the test stimulation and subsequent implantation more successful:

1 Enter the S3 foramen as medial as possible, orienting the needle in a medial to lateral direction. This helps ensure that the lead and its four electrodes are parallel to the nerve achieving better contact with all four positions.

2 Be diligent when in S3 to get the best responses possible. Change the angle, axis, or depth of the foramen needle a number of times until you get preferably a good response in three or four electrodes. Responses at low amplitude (<3 amplitudes) are highly satisfactory.

3 Motor responses are adequate without sensory. When absent, raise the consciousness level of the patient and confirm S3 by utilizing sensory.

4 The more anterior the sensory responses the better – for instance, the vagina in women and the scrotum in men. Avoid

penile stimulation since it may limit subsequent amplitude increases by being too irritating.

5 Avoid injection of local anesthesia into the foramen as it may attenuate responses to stimulation.

6 It's not the battery! Changing the external generator battery in the hope of correcting a non-response is rarely the solution. Reposition the foramen needle.

7 Do not be overly concerned if the side used for the tined lead is different from that of the PNE. Use the side that intraoperatively provides the best responses.

8 Work with a great Medtronic representative. I have the luxury of working with a fabulous representative. He is superb in the operating room and his assistance in trouble-shooting and patient care is outstanding. Hats off to Glen.

KEY POINT

- Be diligent in locating the best S3 response and work with a great manufacturer representative.

Troubleshooting sacral nerve stimulation

A number of adverse events have been reported with SNS. It is important to be able to troubleshoot a patient who presents with a decreased or absent SNS response who was doing well previously or one complaining of another problem. Testing impedances of the electrodes is paramount to the process.

KEY POINT

- Effective troubleshooting helps to maximize the success of sacral nerve stimulation.

Impedance describes the resistance to the flow of electrons through a circuit. Typically normal SNS impedance measures between 400–1500 ohms. An open circuit is one in which there is no flow as a result of too much resistance. This occurs with a broken lead and the impedance generally exceeds 4000 ohms. A short circuit is one with too little resistance resulting in excessive current flow, diminishing battery life. Short circuits typically have measured impedances of <50 ohms. The circuit begins in the IPG, traveling through the lead wires and electrodes to the patient's tissue, and back through either another electrode tracing the same path (bipolar), or directly to the IPG case (unipolar).

The most common causes of open circuits include a fractured lead or extension wire and loose connections. Patients generally feel no stimulation since there is no current flow. Unipolar measurements are most useful in diagnosing open circuits because they isolate each individual electrode. Crushed wires touching each other or fluid intrusion into connectors may cause short circuits. Patients often experience stimulation over the IPG or no stimulation.

Bipolar measurements are best for identifying shorts between two wires.

Impedance measurements are recommended at the time of implantation, at the first programming visit, and any time there is a problem. Each electrode is interrogated for its intactness allowing a skilled programmer to program around the problem, maintaining the device's function.

Patients presenting with discomfort over the IPG either are experiencing a pocket related problem or an output related one. Pocket related events include infection, a device too close to a bony prominence or beltline, and a pocket too tight or too loose. Pain and tenderness with redness or incisional drainage is typical of infection. Antibiotics may temporarily improve symptoms but the recommended management is explantation of the entire device. Output related problems resulting in IPG pain include increased patient sensitivity to unipolar stimulation or current leaks.

Switching the IPG on and off helps differentiate between device and pocket related problems. Persistent discomfort while off rules out an output related one. Some patients are sensitive to the unipolar mode since the IPG is the positive pole and switching to bipolar eliminates pain in some cases. When short circuits are located the device can often be reprogrammed to use different electrodes, alleviating the problem. If reprogramming fails, revision may be necessary.

Commonly, patients present with recurrent symptoms associated with either perceived stimulation in the wrong location or absent stimulation. Unipolar interrogation allows one to map out where the patient feels the stimulation. Programming bipolar combinations and increasing the pulse width can also be beneficial. When reprogramming fails, revision for lead repositioning or relocation to the other side may be necessary. In those experiencing no sensation, remaining battery life and inadvertent on–off is assessed. Impedances are next checked for the presence of open and short circuits. Similarly, when programming around the malfunctioning lead cannot be achieved revision is recommended.

Maximizing therapy with a treatment algorithm

In order to maximize efficacy and to help millions of OAB patients we need to embrace and liberally offer all three neuromodulation therapies to them. In order to do so I recommend the adoption of an OAB treatment algorithm in order to drive efficacy. Let me present mine to you (Figure 14.2).

My patients are initially treated with a combination of antimuscarinics and behavioral therapy. Nearly all patients are started on behavioral treatments including fluid modifications, bladder retraining, and pelvic floor rehabilitation. Many patients

KEY POINT

• A treatment algorithm for OAB helps drive efficacy.

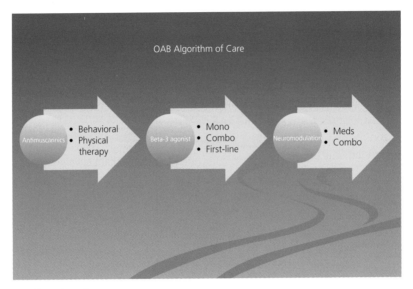

Figure 14.2 OAB algorithm of care.

are offered appointments with our in-house physical therapy team who are experts in treating patients with voiding dysfunction.

When patients fail two (and perhaps three) antimuscarinics, they are offered myrbetriq. We have had tremendous success treating ROAB with myrbetriq either as monotherapy or in combination with antimusarinics. In milder cases I tend to switch to myrbetriq and in the more severe partial responding population I often add the Beta-3 agent. The efficacy and tolerability of myrbetriq has been such that I would not be surprised if it becomes first-line therapy for many urologists prior to starting antimuscarinics.

When medical and behavioral therapy does not reach the patient's treatment goal, I offer nearly all ROAB patients neuro-modulation. Each of the three treatments have their inherent advantages and disadvantages and in my opinion it should be the patient's choice of which one best suits them, not mine. Utilizing a common sense

approach, many elderly patients with multiple co-morbidities are only offered PTNS.

Of course ROAB patients who have not exhausted all of the available antimuscarinics have the option of trying a fourth or fifth medication and in rare cases this may be beneficial.

Patients declining neuromodulation and who have exhausted all pharmaceuticals unfortunately have reached the end of my treatment algorithm. Those who fail a neuromodulation therapy are usually re-offered the other two options, depending on patient factors. In addition, partial responders to neuromodulation may be restarted on an OAB agent that has helped in the past to help augment their therapy.

The algorithm is simple and in my opinion helps maximize efficacy. The moment the pen or keypad orders an OAB agent the patient is on a path to be offered neuromodulation unless they reach their treatment goal with conservative therapies. Patients are educated about the process and that the treatment options are their choice, not mine. I find it equally rewarding to help patients with medication, behavioral therapy, neuro-modulation, or with a combination of treatments. I strongly encourage my colleagues to adopt such an algorithm and no longer accept the limited care many of our patients are currently receiving.

References

1 International Neurododulation Society. www.neuromodulation.com. Accessed Jan. 22, 2013.

2 Mekhail NA, Cheng J, Narouze S, et al. Clinical applications of neurostimulation: forty years later. *Pain Pract.* 2010;**10**(2):103–112.

3 Stewart WF, Van Rooyen JB, Cundiff GW, et al. Prevalence and burden of overactive bladder in the United States. *World J Urol.* 1999;**44**:56–66.

4 Coyne KS, Sexton CC, Kopp ZS, et al. The impact of overactive bladder on mental health, work productivity and health-related quality of life in the UK and Sweden: results from EpiLUTS. *BJU Int.* 2011;**108**:1459–1471.

5 Abrams P, Kelleher CJ, Kerr LA, Rogers RG: Overactive bladder significantly affects quality of life. *Am J Manag Care* **6**: S580–S590, 2000.

6 Liberman JN, Hunt TL, Stewart WF, et al. Health-related quality of life among adults with symptoms of overactive bladder: results from a U.S. community-based survey. *Urology* 2001;**57**:1044–1050.

7 Brown JS, McGhan WF, Chokroverty S. Comorbidities associated with overactive bladder. *Am J Manag Care* 2000;**6**:S574–S579.

8 Brown JS, Vittinghoff E, Wyman JF, et al. Urinary incontinence: does it increase risk for falls and fractures? Study of Osteoporotic Fractures Research Group. *J Am Geriatr Soc.* 2000; **48**:721–725.

9 Wagner TH, Hu TW. Economic costs of urinary incontinence in 1995. *Urology* 1998;**51**: 355–361

10 Ganz ML, Smalarz AM, Krupski TL, et al. Economic costs of overactive bladder in the United States. *Urology* 2010; **75**(3):526–532.

11 Burgio KL. Influence of behavior modification on overactive bladder. *Urology* 2002; **60**(5suppl.1); 72–76.

12 Gormley EA, Lightner DJ, Burgio KL, et al. Diagnosis and treatment of overactive bladder (non-neurogenic) in adults: AUA/SUFU guideline. *J Urol.* 2012;**188**:2455–2463.

13 Brostrom S, Hallas J. Persistence of antimuscarinic drug use. *Eur J Clin Pharm.* 2009;**65**(3): 309–314.

14 Leng WW, Chancellor MB. How sacral nerve stimulation neuromodulation works. *Urol Clin North Am.* 2005;**32**:11–18.

15 Van der Pal F, Heesakkers JP, Bemelmans BL. Current opinion on the working mechanisms of neuromodulation in the treatment of lower urinary tract dysfunction. *Curr Opin Urol.* 2006;**16**(4):261–267.

16 Schmidt RA, Jonas U, Oleson KA, et al. Sacral nerve stimulation for treatment of refractory urinary urge incontinence. *Sacral Nerve Stimulation Study Group. J Urol.* 1999;**162**(2): 352–357.

17 Hassouna MM, Siegel SW, Lycklama AAB, et al. Sacral neuromodulation in the treatment of urgency-frequency symptoms: a multicenter study on efficacy and safety. *J Urol.* 2000;**163**: 1849–1854.

18 van Kerrebroeck PE, van Voskuilen AC, Heesakkers JP, et al. Results of sacral neuromodulation therapy for urinary voiding dysfunction: outcomes of a prospective, worldwide clinical study. *J Urol.* 2007:**178**(5):2029–2034.

19 Groen J, Bertil F, Blok M, et al. Sacral neuromodulation as treatment for refractory idiopathic urge urinary incontinence: 5-year results of a longitudinal study in 60 women. *J Urol.* 2011;**186**:954–959.

20 Leong RK, Marcelissen TA, Nieman FH, et al. Satisfaction and patient experience with sacral neuromodulation: results of a single center sample survey. *J Urol.* 2011;**185**:588–592.

21 http://manuals.medtronic.com/manuals/mri [accessed Sep. 2014]

22 Chartier-Kastler EJ, Ruud Bosch JLH, Perrigot M, et al. Long-term results of sacral nerve stimulation (S3) for the treatment of neurogenic refractory urge incontinence related to detrusor hyperrflexia. *J Urol.* 2000;**164**: 1476–1480.

23 Comiter CV. Sacral neuromodulaton for the symptomatic treatment of refractory interstitial cystitis: a prospective study. *J Urol.* 2003; **169**:1369–1373.

24 Peters KM, Konstandt D. Sacral neuromodulation decreases narcotic requirements in refractory interstitial cystitis. *BJU Int.* 2001;**93**:777–779.

25 Sherman ND, Jamison MG, Webster GD, et al. Sacral neuromodulation for the treatment of refractory urge incontinence after stress incontinence surgery. *Amer J Obstet Gynecol.* 2005; **193**:2083–2087.

26 Humphreys MR, Vandersteen DR, Slezak JM, et al. Preliminary results of sacral neuromodulation in 23 children. *J Urol.* 2006;**176**:2227–2231.

27 Lenis AT, Gill BC, Carmel ME, et al. Patterns of hardware related electrode failures in sacral nerve stimulation devices. *J Urol.* 2013; **190**:175–179.

28 Firoozi F, Gill B, Ingber MS, et al. Increasing patient preparedness for sacral neuromodulation improves patient reported outcomes despite leaving objective measures of success unchanged. *J Urol.* 2013;**190**:594–597.

29 Siegel S, Bennett J, Mangel J, et al. Results of a prospective, randomized, multicenter study evaluating the safety and efficacy of InterStim therapy at 6-month follow-up in subjects with symptoms of overactive bladder [abstract]. *Female Pelvic Med Reconstr Surg.* 2012;**18**(5S):S114.

30 Borawski KM, Foster RT, Webster GD, et al. Predicting implantation with a neuromodulator using two different test stimulation techniques: a prospective randomized study in urge incontinent women. *Neurourol and Urodyn.* 2007;**26**(1):14–18.

31 Marcelissen T, Leong R, Serroyen J, et al. Is the screening method of sacral neuromodulation a prognostic factor for long-term success? *J Urol.* 2011;**185**(2):583–587.

CHAPTER 15

Posterior tibial nerve stimulation

John Heesakkers

Department of Urology, Radboud University Medical Center, Nijmegen, The Netherlands

---

KEY POINTS

- Overactive Bladder Syndrome (OAB) is an innervation issue.
- Correction of the innervation system may correct OAB complaints.
- The posterior tibial nerve originates in the pelvis.
- Stimulating the posterior tibial nerve can correct OAB symptoms.
- Good quality studies show the positive and clinical relevant effect in OAB.

Introduction

Neuromodulation of the lower urinary tract is extensively applied in patients with Overactive Bladder (OAB) complaints. The best known and best documented technique is sacral nerve stimulation. Posterior Tibial Nerve Stimulation (PTNS) is the second most extensively documented way of nerve stimulation. The exploration of the best technique of electrical stimulation of the lower urinary, including sex organs is guided by three principles:

1 Stimulation should be done via the least invasive way.

   For this reason transcutaneous stimulation with surface electrodes or stimulation probes would suit best.

2 Stimulation should be in an area that is acceptable and not embarrassing for patients.

   This makes sacral dermatomes or legs appropriate areas for stimulation.

3 Stimulation should be practical to apply. Continuous stimulation is therefore less ideal and discontinuous stimulation is easier than continuous stimulation.

Ways of peripheral neuromodulation

The nerves that innervate the lower urinary tract originate from the lumbar, sacral, and coccygeal segmental nerves from L2 to S4 (Figure 15.1). Afferent and

---

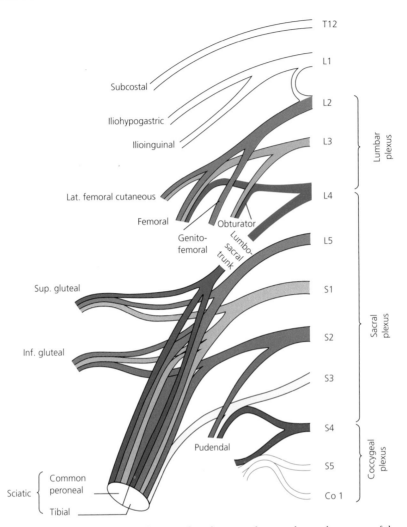

Figure 15.1 Organization of the lower lumbar, sacral, and coccygeal nerve plexus, the merger of the various roots and the most important nerves that branch from the merged nerve plexus. The tibial nerve has it's offspring in the sacral roots of mainly S2 and S3. Source: Basic Human Anatomy: A Regional Study of Human Structure. Source: http://www.dartmouth.edu/~humananatomy/figures/chapter_30/30-6.HTM#top. Reproduced with permission of Ronan O'Rahilly, MD. (For color detail, please see color plate section).

efferent fibers from these segmental sacral roots merge in the periphery outside the spinal cord. After merging, the nerve fibers continue as combined nerves that have lost their segmental innervation pattern. The sciatic nerve is composed of fibers from L4 to S3. The posterior tibial nerve is a part of the sciatic nerve. Peripheral neuromodula-tion of the lower urinary tract has been attempted via stimulation of one of the involved nerves, such as the dorsal genital nerve or the posterior tibial nerve. It can also be done by the overlying skin or by stimulating the dermatomes that are inner-vated by the same nerve as the ones that innervate the lower urinary tract.

History

It is an ancient Chinese custom to perform acupuncture on the lower leg. With this technique, developed in China over 5000 years ago, the "energetic harmony" of the urogenital tract might be restored by way of stimulation of specific points. Wilhelmus ten Rhyne (1647–1700) was a Dutch physician who was employed by the Dutch East India Company in 1673, where he encountered eastern traditional medicine (Figure 15.2). In 1683, he published a book entitled *Dissertatio de Arthritide: Mantissa Schematica: De Acupunctura: Et Orationes Tres*. He wrote about the art of needling for treating diseases, including those of the lower urinary tract. He called this technique "*Acupunctura*" and it was the first Western detailed study on that matter.

One of the most commonly used acupuncture points used for gynecological, fertility, digestive, urinary, sexual, and emotional disorders is the SanYinJiao point, or Spleen 6. It can be translated as "Three Yin Intersection," because it is the meeting point of the three yin channels of the leg: Spleen, Liver, and Kidney. SanYinJiao, SP-6 or Spleen 6 is located on the medial side of the lower leg, about 6–8 cm cephalad to the prominence of the medial malleolus. It lies close to the medial crest of the tibia. The location of the SP-6 acupuncture point and the organs affected by this kind of acupuncture has remarkable similarities with posterior tibial nerve stimulation. When electrical current is applied to the acupuncture needle the technique is called electrical acupuncture. Especially when electroacupuncture is performed with similar stimulation parameters (2–15 Hz, 10–20 mA), it is likely that nerve stimulation is the effective treatment. Similar effects as with tibial nerve stimulation therefore might be expected on the pelvic organs, as well as on the spleen and on the liver.

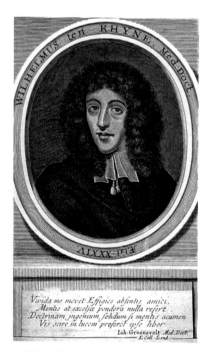

Figure 15.2 Wilhelmus ten Rhyne, the first Western physician to describe the ancient Chinese technique of acupuncture. Source: http://en.wikipedia.org/wiki/Willem_ten_Rhijne#.

Posterior tibial nerve stimulation

The fundamental feature of neuromodulation is that nerves are stimulated and not energy pathways or other routes that do not have any anatomical substrate. Nerve stimulation ideally has an efferent motor effect and an afferent sensory effect. Stimulation of the posterior tibial nerve results in great toe flexion or fanning of the toes. The sensory effect is a radiation tickling sensation of the foot sole. McGuire was the first to explore tibial nerve stimulation in 1983. [2] He performed transcutaneous posterior tibial nerve stimulation in 15 patients with detrusor overactivity because of a neurological disease.

Inspired by this previous work by McGuire, Marshall Stoller started research on percutaneous tibial nerve stimulation (PTNS) as neuromodulative treatment in lower urinary tract dysfunction. After initial testing in pig-tailed monkeys, [3] PTNS was later investigated in humans with promising results. This new initiative was the start of the worldwide development and exploration of PTNS.

Historic overview	
5000 BC	Acupuncture of lower leg in China
1683	Wilhelmus ten Rhyne writes *Dissertatio de Arthritide: Mantissa Schematica: De Acupunctura: Et Orationes Tres*
1983	Ed McGuire performs transcutaneous posterior tibial nerve stimulation
1987	Percutaneous tibial nerve stimulation by Marshall Stoller
1999	Clinical introduction of PTNS
2006	First publication on tibial nerve implant by van der Pal
2009	First randomized controlled trial by Peters

Technique

PTNS is performed in patients placed in the supine position with the medial malleolus pointing upwards. A 34 gauge stainless steel needle is inserted approximately 3 to 4 cm, about 3 fingerbreadths, cephalad to the medial malleolus between the posterior margin of the tibia and soleus muscle. A stick-on electrode is placed on the same leg near the arch of the foot. The needle and electrode are connected to a low voltage (9 volts) stimulator (Urgent PC®, Uroplasty Inc, Minnetonka, MN) with an adjustable pulse intensity of 0 to 10 mA, a fixed pulse width of 200 microseconds, and a frequency of 20 Hz. The amplitude is slowly increased until the large toe starts to curl or toes start to fan. If the large toe does not curl or pain occurs near the insertion site, the stimulation device is switched off and the procedure is repeated. If the large toe curls or toes start to fan, stimulation is applied at an intensity well tolerated by the patient. If necessary the amplitude can be increased during the session. In general, patients undergo 12 outpatient treatment sessions, each lasting 30 minutes, one to three times per week. If a good response occurs the patient is offered chronic treatment. [4]

Working mechanism

At the moment the working mechanism of neuromodulation, including PTNS, is still not completely understood. However, it is postulated that symptoms of OAB including incontinence may represent an alteration of the pelvic neuromuscular environment via changes in the inhibitory and excitatory signals of the voiding reflex. It is thought that electrical stimulation of the sacral nerve roots modulates the afferent neural reflex pathways between the spinal cord or pons and pelvic organs. As the ascending sensory pathway inputs and guarding reflex pathway are modulated, storage may be facilitated.

Blok et al. looked at the effects of acute and chronic sacral neurostimulation on PET images of the brain. [5] In the acute phase, brain areas are involved that have to do with sensorimotor learning. These are the areas located in the right post-central gyrus, the left parietal cortex, the medial prefrontal cortex, and the right insula. Furthermore, there was activation in the ventromedial orbitofrontal cortex, and decreased activation in the left medial cerebellum.

However, chronic sacral neurostimulation decreased activity in the cerebellum, midbrain, and adjacent midline thalamus and limbic cortical areas previously implicated in the control of micturition and urinary storage. They postulated that neuromodulation modulates predominantly areas involved in sensorimotor learning, which might become less active during the course of chronic SN.

In analogy to sacral neuromodulation, central effects have been studied in PTNS. Finazzi Agro et al. studied the effect of PTNS and sham stimulation on Short Latency somatosensory evoked potentials (SL-SEP) and long latency somatosensory evoked potentials (LL-SEP). [6] Somatosensory evoked potentials (SEP) reflect information processing in the brain after stimulation of the peripheral somatosensory system. In particular, LL-SEP seems to provide information on the function of somatosensory associative cortical structures. LL-SEP changes imply that a long time after stimulation (one day after treatment) changes in SEP occur. They showed that the amplitude of LL-SEP changes of P80 and P100 waves in the active PTNS group was significantly higher as compared to the placebo group.

The recorded P80 and P100 amplitude increase might reflect long-term modifications in synaptic efficiency through the somatosensory pathway induced by repetitive peripheral nerve stimulation. Long-term potentiation (LTP) and depression (LTD) of excitatory synaptic transmission can contribute to experience-dependent modifications of brain function, including learning and memory. Thus, a plastic reorganization of the cortical network triggered by peripheral neuromodulation can be hypothesized as a mechanism of action of PTNS. They concluded that PTNS effects are mediated by suprasacral centers of stimulus elaboration involving finally cortical associative areas. This is in line with the theories about the working mechanism of sacral nerve stimulation.

If one considers applying PTNS for improvement of clinical conditions one has to accept that:

- It is possible to positively influence the innervation system of the lower urinary tract by stimulation of the tibial nerve at the ankle.
- There is no direct sensation in the bladder area nor motor action of muscles in or adjacent to the pelvic floor during tibial nerve stimulation.
- Discontinuous stimulation during a limited period of time once to thrice a week is sufficient to have a beneficial effect.

Clinical results

Since the introduction of PTNS in 1999, several studies have been performed evaluating its effectiveness in especially patients with OAB dry and OAB wet and non-obstructive urinary retention.

Almost all studies on overactive bladder used micturition diaries and general and/or disease specific quality of life questionnaires to measure the effects of PTNS. [7,8] Subjective success was found in 59–64% of patients. [7, 8] Objective success, defined most of the time as more than 50% decrease in incontinence episodes and/or micturition frequency, was found in 47–56% of patients. [8, 9]

Urodynamic studies especially measured by cystometry may provide more objective data on the efficacy of percutaneous tibial nerve stimulation. When acute PTNS is performed as soon as detrusor overactivity is observed during cystometry, the suppressive effects in neurological patients are contradicting. [10, 11]

Frequency/volume chart data and quality of life scores improved significantly. Of the participants with pre- and post-treatment urodynamic data, only a few showed complete abolishment of detrusor overactivity. [12] Nevertheless, increments in cystometric bladder capacity and in volume at DI were significant. Subjects without detrusor overactivity at baseline appeared 1.7 times more prone to respond to PTNS. The more the bladder overactivity was pronounced, the less these patients were found to respond to PTNS.

Once a positive treatment outcome has been obtained with PTNS, a maintenance program is needed to avoid recurrence of complaints. One study evaluated the necessity of maintenance therapy by means of a six-week pause of therapy in successfully treated PTNS patients, leading to over 50% worsening of main symptoms in almost all patients. Restarting PTNS afterwards improved complaints to the level present before the break in treatment. [13]

One of the most important studies on PTNS was performed by Peters et al. [14] The so-called Study of UrgentPC versus Sham Effectiveness in Treatment of Overactive Bladder Symptoms (SUmiT) was a multicenter, double-blind, randomized, controlled trial comparing the efficacy of percutaneous tibial nerve stimulation to

sham through 12 weeks of therapy. The breakthrough was that a validated sham arm was developed and used as a comparator. This was the first time that the net effect apart from the placebo effect could be measured. In two groups of 110 patients the improvement in global response assessment (GRA), voiding diary parameters, and overactive bladder and quality of life questionnaires was evaluated. The GRA is a self-reported seven-point scale that shows whether an individual perceives a change due to the treatment. Individuals who noted a moderate or marked improvement were regarded as successfully treated patients. Voiding diary parameters after 12 weeks of therapy showed percutaneous tibial nerve stimulation subjects had statistically significant improvements in frequency, nighttime voids, voids with moderate to severe urgency, and urinary urge incontinence episodes compared to sham. The GRA in the PTNS subjects showed 55% reporting moderately or markedly improved responses compared to 21% in the sham group.

Another sham controlled study was performed by Finazzi et al. with similar results. [[15]]

PTNS implies that patients have to have repeat treatments. The tapering studies show that once every two or three weeks is sufficient in those patients that benefit from PTNS. Another major question is what the long-term success of PTNS is. Peters et al. followed 50 participants from the SUmiT Trial who met the primary effectiveness endpoint after 12-weekly PTNS. [16] These patients were prescribed a fixed-schedule 14-week tapering protocol followed by a personal treatment plan aimed at sustaining OAB symptom improvement. Of this group, 29 patients completed the 36-month protocol and received a median of 1.1 treatments per month. At three years, 77% maintained moderate or marked improvement in OAB symptoms. Compared to baseline, median voids per day decreased from 12.0 to 8.7, and urge incontinence episodes per day decreased from 3.3 to 0.3. All quality of life parameters remained markedly improved from baseline through three years.

- PTNS improves OAB symptoms based on voiding diary parameters in 47–56% of patients.
- Subjective improvement is obtained in 60% of patients.
- PTNS increases cystometric capacity and delays the onset of, but does not abolish, detrusor overactivity.
- Maintenance therapy is necessary to sustain the effect of therapy.
- PTNS improved bladder symptoms measured with GRA in 55% of patients as compared to 21% in a sham treated group.
- After 3 years, 77% of patients responding to initial therapy experienced moderate to marked improvement of OAB symptoms.
- A pilot study implies that the Urgent SQ implant appears to be a safe and effective treatment for OAB.

Prognostic factors for PTNS

Little data are available about prognostic factors for success or failure of PTNS. Studies on urodynamic changes by PTNS suggest that in the case of overactive bladder without detrusor overactivity, patients are more prone to a successful treatment

outcome. [12] Clinical parameters for predicting SNS outcome were also tested in 132 patients treated with PTNS, but showed no significance. [17] Also, a history of sexual and/or physical abuse did not alter PTNS treatment outcome. However, a low total score at baseline in the SF-36 general quality of life questionnaire proved to be predictive for not obtaining objective nor subjective success. Especially patients with a low SF-36 Mental Component Summary were prone to fail. These patients also scored worse on disease-specific quality of life questionnaires, although they had no different disease severity compared to patients with good mental health.

- Subjects with mental problems don't seem to be ideal candidates for PTNS.

Urgent-SQ; the PTNS implant

Rather quickly after the modern clinical development of PTNS, it was recognized that the repeated return to the clinic, once weekly or once bi- or triweekly, would finally lead to a logistic problem, with patients returning to the clinic approximately one to two times per month. If all successfully treated patients returned every week, this would lead to a jammed outpatient clinic. More importantly, the travel burden for patients would be high and PTNS treatment on-demand would not be possible. Therefore an implant was developed that was placed at the tibial nerve at the ankle that could be operated via radiofrequency activation with an external stimulator: the Urgent-SQ (Figures 15.3 and 15.4).

The pioneering work was done by van der Pal et al. [18] They looked at

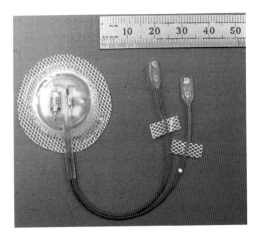

Figure 15.3 The Urgent-SQ implant consisting of an internal electromagnetic pulse receiver, the body with two leads, and monopolar platinum electrodes. (For color detail, please see color plate section).

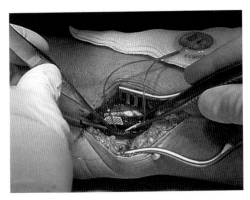

Figure 15.4 Site of implantation during surgery. The two electrodes are placed on two opposite sides of the tibial nerve just proximal to the medial malleolus. (For color detail, please see color plate section).

eight patients with refractory overactive bladder who were treated with the Urgent-SQ. After implanting the device, the patients could operate the implant by means of an external stimulator. Patients were evaluated at 3, 6, and 12 months follow-up. The primary objective was >=50% reduction in the number of incontinence

episodes and/or voids on bladder diary. At 3, 6, and 12 months, respectively five, six, and four patients met the primary objective. At 3- and 6-month follow-up, voiding and quality of life parameters had significantly improved. Urinary tract infection, temporary walking difficulties, and spontaneous radiating sensations were reported as adverse

events and no local infection, erosion, or dislocation.

Janssen et al. reported about the long-term efficacy and safety of these patients in an open-label study. [19] The seven patients who still had the implant were contacted after nine years and evaluated with an interview, physical examination, ankle x-ray, voiding diaries, and completed questionnaires about adverse events, performance, efficacy, safety, and quality of life with the validated I-QoL. Results showed that six of the seven patients still had sensory and loco-motor responses on stimulation at nine-year follow-up. Four patients who had a successful treatment response at one year still used the device. The implants were intact with no migration and/or displacement. Two patients experienced minor discomfort. The conclusion was that after nine years the Urgent-SQ implant was a safe therapy for OAB.

Future perspectives

Percutaneous tibial nerve stimulation is a minimally invasive, easily accessible neuromodulation technique and has proven its benefit in overactive bladder and non-obstructive urinary retention. Regretfully, in chronic pelvic pain the effects seem to be only modest. At this moment quite some "circumstantial" evidence exists for its efficacy based on animal studies and clinical studies including urodynamic parameters. In the case that PTNS becomes a more established treatment modality, no doubt other indications will be explored. Subjects for further investigation of areas that have already some clinical efficacy data are children, neurologic patients, and patients with fecal incontinence.

Almost all research done on PTNS used the same stimulation protocol: PTNS was performed in 10 to 12 weekly sessions, each lasting for 30 minutes. Stimulation parameters were preset and rather fixed and every time only one needle was inserted. It may be well anticipated that changes in treatment scheme and/or stimulation parameters could lead to a different, possibly even better, outcome. The same goes for bilateral instead of unilateral therapy. It is evident that an accelerated stimulation scheme has the advantage of achieving clinical results faster. [20] Regarding stimulation parameters, it is rather widely agreed that pulse intensity in neuromodulation should be set at a well tolerable level. As it is suggested that frequency is optimal at more unpleasantly low levels (5–6 Hz), [21] studies on PTNS with pulse frequencies below 20 Hz may produce interesting results. The same goes for changes in pulse duration, in PTNS the standard setting is 0.2 ms.

The recent revitalization of the Urgent-SQ gives other possibilities. Efforts should be undertaken to refine the pre-implant testing phase in order to decrease the amount of unnecessarily treated patients. Hopefully this will eventually lead to the ideal implant: an effective and safe, easily controllable device that is operated by patients themselves in flexible, individualized treatment schemes.

References

1 Ten Rhyne W. Dissertatio de arthritide mantissa schematica, de acupunctura: Et Orationes tres, I. De chymiae et botaniae antiquitate et dignitate, II. De hysionomia, III. De monstris. 1683.

2 McGuire EJ, Zhang SC, Horwinski ER, Lytton B. Treatment of motor and sensory detrusor instability by electrical stimulation. *J Urol.* 1983 Jan;**129**(1):78–79.

3 Stoller ML, Copeland S, Millard AR et al. The efficacy of acupuncture in reversing unstable bladder in pig-tailed monkeys. [abstract 2]. J Urol 1987;(suppl 137): 104A.

4 Govier FE, Litwiller S, Nitti V et al. Percutaneous afferent neuromodulation for the refractory overactive bladder: results of a multicenter study. *J Urol.* 2001;**165**:1193–1198.

5 Blok BF, Groen J, Bosch JL, et al. Different brain effects during chronic and acute sacral neuromodulation in urge incontinent patients with implanted neurostimulators. *BJU Int.* 2006 Dec;**98**(6):1238–1243.

6 Finazzi-Agrò E, Rocchi C, Pachatz C, et al. Percutaneous tibial nerve stimulation produces effects on brain activity: study on the modifications of the long latency somatosensory evoked potentials. *Neurourol Urodyn.* 2009;**28**(4): 320–324.

7 van Balken MR, Vandoninck V, Gisolf KW, et al. Posterior tibial nerve stimulation as neuromodulative treatment of lower urinary tract dysfunction. *J Urol.* 2001;**166**:914–918.

8 Vandoninck V, Van Balken MR, Finazzi Agró E, et al. Posterior tibial nerve stimulation in the treatment of urge incontinence. *Neurourol Urodyn.* 2003;**22**:17–23.

9 Klingler HC, Pycha A, Schmidbauer J Marberger M. Use of peripheral neuromodulation of the S3 region for treatment of detrusor overactivity: a urodynamic-based study. *Urology* 2000; **56**:766–771.

10 Kabay SC, Yucel M, Kabay S. Acute effect of posterior tibial nerve stimulation on neurogenic detrusor overactivity in patients with multiple sclerosis: urodynamic study. *Urology* 2008;**71**:641–645.

11 Fjorback MV, van Rey FS, van der Pal F, et al. Acute urodynamic effects of posterior tibial nerve stimulation on neurogenic detrusor overactivity in patients with MS. *Eur Urol.* 2007 Feb;**51**(2):464–470.

12 Vandoninck V, van Balken MR, Finazzi Agrò E, et al. Percutaneous tibial nerve stimulation in the treatment of overactive bladder: urodynamic data. *Neurourol Urodyn.* 2003;**22**(3):227–232.

13 Van der Pal F, van Balken MR, Heesakkers JP, et al. Percutaneous tibial nerve stimulation (PTNS) in the treatment of refractory overactive bladder syndrome: is maintenance treatment a necessity? *BJU Int.* 2006;**97**:547–550.

14 Peters KM, Carrico DJ, Perez-Marrero RA, et al. Randomized trial of percutaneous tibial nerve stimulation versus Sham efficacy in the treatment of overactive bladder syndrome: results from the SUmiT trial. *J Urol.* 2010 Apr;**183**(4):1438-43. doi: 10.1016/j.juro.2009.12.036. Epub 2010 Feb 20. PubMed PMID: 20171677.

15 Finazzi-Agrò E, Petta F, Sciobica F, et al. Percutaneous tibial nerve stimulation effects on detrusor overactivity incontinence are not due to a placebo effect: a randomized, double-blind, placebo controlled trial. *J Urol.* 2010 Nov; **184**(5):2001–2006.

16 Peters KM, Carrico DJ, Wooldridge LS, et al. Percutaneous tibial nerve stimulation for the long-term treatment of overactive bladder:3-year results of the STEP Study. *J Urol.* 2013 Jun; **189**(6):2194–2201.

17 van Balken MR, Vergunst H, Bemelmans BL. Prognostic factors for successful percutaneous tibial nerve stimulation. *Eur Urol.* 2006;**49**: 360–365.

18 Van der Pal F, van Balken MR, Heesakkers JP, et al. Implant driven tibial nerve stimulation in the treatment of refractory overactive bladder syndrome: 12-month follow up. *Neuromodulation* 2006;**9**:163–171.

19 Janssen DA, Farag F, Heesakkers JP. Urgent-SQ implant in treatment of overactive bladder syndrome: 9-year follow-up study. *Neurourol Urodyn.* 2013 Jun;**32**(5):472–475.

20 20.Finazzi Agro E, Campagna A, Sciobica F et al. Posterior tibial nerve stimulation: is the once-a-week protocol the best option? *Minerva Urol Nefrol.* 2005;**57**:119–123.

21 Fall M, Lindstrom S. Electrical stimulation. A physiologic approach to the treatment of urinary incontinence. *Urol Clin North Am.* 1991; **18**:393–407.

CHAPTER 16

Botulinum toxin for the overactive bladder

Apostolos Apostolidis

Aristotle University of Thessaloniki, Thessaloniki, Greece

KEY POINTS

- Botulinum neurotoxin type A (BoNT/A), delivered via intradetrusor injections, is now an approved second-line treatment for incontinence associated with Neurogenic Detrusor Overactivity (NDO) and for OAB symptoms in adults.

- Its mechanism of action when injected in the bladder is still incompletely understood, but it appears to affect multiple target molecules in both the afferent and efferent bladder pathways, while central effects are under investigation.

- Its efficacy in refractory incontinence and other symptoms associated with either neurogenic or idiopathic detrusor overactivity is supported by a large body of high level evidence. These results come mostly from single-injection studies.

- Further to medical parameters of clinical efficacy, BoNT/A significantly improves patients' quality of life.

- The vast majority of high level data concern onabotulinumtoxinA, which has been more comprehensively studied than abobotulinumtoxinA.

- Sustained efficacy seems to be achieved with repeat injections in those choosing to be retreated, at least in the neurogenic patient population, but the level of evidence remains low. Data on duration of efficacy, treatment persistence/discontinuation, and predictors of response to treatment are very limited.

- There is great heterogeneity in the literature on injection techniques, doses, and dilutions used for either of the two most used formulations. Efforts are being directed to standardization of the injection technique following the registration trials.

- The treatment is considered to be safe overall with predictable and reversible side-effects. Urinary tract infections are the most common adverse event in the IDO/OAB population. Reduction of the "predictable" side-effect of incomplete bladder emptying and need for post-treatment self-catheterizations was considered when the approved dose of 100 U onabotulinuimtoxinA was chosen for the IDO/OAB population.

- Results on the cost-effectiveness of BoNT/A when compared to other second-line OAB treatments have so far been inconclusive.

Overactive Bladder: Practical Management, First Edition. Edited by Jacques Corcos, Scott MacDiarmid and John Heesakkers.
© 2015 John Wiley & Sons, Ltd. Published 2015 by John Wiley & Sons, Ltd.

Introduction: A new second-line treatment for incontinence

Botulinum neurotoxin type A (BoNT/A), delivered via intradetrusor injections, is now an approved second-line treatment for incontinence associated with Neurogenic Detrusor Overactivity (NDO) and for OAB symptoms in adults. In 2011, the US FDA granted approval for the use of the onabotulinumtoxinA (BOTOX™) format for urinary incontinence associated with NDO in adult neurological patients with inadequate response to or reduced tolerance of an anticholinergic medication. As the registration trials had included only adult patients with stable spinal cord injury (SCI) below the cervical level or with multiple sclerosis, the license currently stands mainly for these groups of neurological patients. The approval expanded in January 2013 to include treatment of adults with OAB who cannot use or do not adequately respond to anticholinergics. Similar approvals have been granted or awaited in a number of European countries.

Practical facts about BoNT/A

Botulinum neurotoxin (BoNT), a neurotoxin produced by *Clostridium botulinum*, is found in seven serotypes (A–G), of which BoNT-A (Figure 16.1) has the longest duration of action and is the most commonly used in clinical practice, having been licensed for a number of indications (strabismus, blepharospasm, cervical dystonia, hyperhidrosis, NDO-incontinence, OAB). BoNT/A is available in various commercial forms, namely Botox® (Allergan Pharmaceuticals, Irvine, CA, USA), Dysport® (Ipsen Biopharm Ltd, Slough, UK), Xeomin®, (Merz Pharma GmbH & Co. KGaA, Frankfurt, Germany),

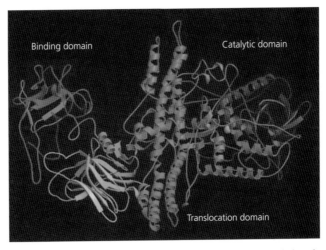

Figure 16.1 BoNT/A consists of a heavy and a light chain linked by a disulphide bond. Source: Lacy, D.B., Tepp, W., Cohen, A.C., DasGupta, B.R., Stevens, R.C. (PDB-Bild 3BTA) [CC-BY-SA-2.0-de (http://creativecommons.org/licenses/by-sa/2.0/de/deed.en)], via Wikimedia Commons. (For color detail, please see color plate section).

Prosigne (Lanzhou Biological Products, Lanzhou, China), and PurTox (Mentor Corporation, Madison, WI, USA). Although all products are derivatives of the same serotype, differences in isolation, extraction, purification, and formulation protocols used by the various companies result in a variance in the clinical characteristics of the brands. As a consequence the doses are not inter-changeable between brands and to under-line this, non-proprietary names have been recently introduced (onabotulinum-toxinA for Botox®, abobotulinumtoxinA for Dysport®, and incobotulinumtoxinA for Xeomin®). In addition, clinical dose conversion studies for the lower urinary tract do not exist and the proposed dose equivalences (1U Botox® equivalent to 1U Xeomin® and 3U Dysport®) do not neces-sarily apply in the LUT.

How does BoNT/A act when injected in the bladder?

BoNT/A consists of a heavy and a light chain linked by a disulphide bond (Figure 16.1). Its action is exerted via binding to its receptor synaptic vesicle protein 2 (SV2), [1] and cleavage of the substrate for its action, the Synaptosomal Associated Protein with a molecular weight of 25kD (SNAP25). [2] The latter is part of the SNARE (soluble N-ethylmaleimidesen-sitive fusion attachment protein receptor) complex which also includes the proteins synaptobrevin (vesicle associated mem-brane protein -VAMP) and syntaxin. Both SV2 and SNAP25 have been identi-fied in abundance in nerve fibers in the detrusor and the suburothelium. The high-est density of the two proteins was found in parasympathetic nerves, but sympathetic and sensory fibers also express SV2 and SNAP25. [3]

BoNT/A was originally applied in the human bladder aiming for an ultrapo-tent anticholinergic effect and a transient detrusor muscle paralysis, since its acknowledged mechanism of action in skeletal muscles involved blocking acetyl-choline release from synaptic vesicles in the synaptic cleft. The toxin is known to bind to SV2 by the heavy chain before being internalized by the nerve terminal. The light chain then passes into the cytosol where it inactivates the SNARE complex via cleavage of SNAP25. This dis-rupts the mechanism of fusion of synaptic vesicles to the cytoplasmic membrane which is necessary for neurotrans-mitter release. The effect is reversible, as the parental nerve terminal gradually develops lateral axonal sprouts, which eventually regress as the terminal regains functionality. [4]

Current evidence, however, points towards an alternative mechanism of action in the bladder, heavily involving the afferent bladder pathways [5] (Figure 16.2). By con-trast, a reversible reduction of the release of ACh from the detrusor muscle has, to date, been demonstrated only in animal *in vitro* conditions simulating parasympathetic overactivity. [6] The reduction in voiding detrusor pressures and/or detrusor under-activity shown in several clinical trials sug-gests an anticholinergic effect on the human detrusor which may be associated with the decrease in post-treatment density of mus-carinic receptors found in a recent human study. [7] This study also identified a decrease in purinergic detrusor receptors.

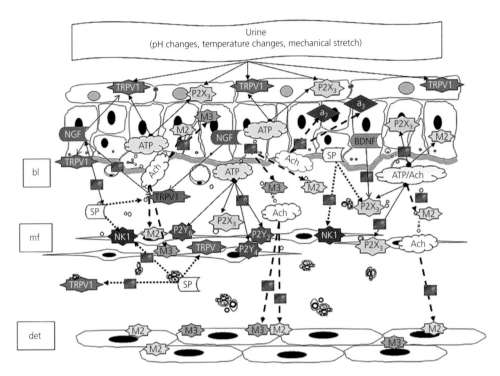

Figure 16.2 BoNT/A has been proposed to affect at multiple levels the complex system of interactions between the release of neurotransmitters and actions on receptors located on the bladder pathways which are thought to be involved in mechanosensation. This cartoon representation of the human bladder wall with known or proposed location of receptors and sites of release of neuropeptides and growth factors has been updated from the relevant Figure in reference [5]. Abbreviations: bl=basal lamina of urothelium, mf=myofibroblast layer, det= detrusor muscle. All connections identified by arrows (see reference [5] for arrow identification) are thought to be upregulated in detrusor overactivity. Apostolidis 2006 [5]. Source: Reproduced with permission of Elsevier. (For color detail, please see color plate section).

Abbreviations:

TRPV1:	Transient Receptor Potential Vanilloid 1
$P2X_3$:	ionotropic purinergic receptor type 3
$P2Y_2/P2Y_4/P2Y_6$:	metabotropic purinergic receptors types 2, 4 and 6
M2/M3:	muscarinic acetylcholine receptors types 2 and 3
α_3, α_7:	nicotinic acetylcholine receptors types 3 and 7
NK1:	Neurokinin receptor type 1 (SP receptor)
SP:	Substance P
NGF:	Nerve Growth Factor
BDNF:	Brain Derived Neurotrophic Factor
ACh:	Acetylcholine, ATP - Adenosine Triphosphate

Together with the reduction in suburothelial purinergic receptors, [8] it appears that BoNT/A may exert a potent effect on the purinergic component of human bladder pathways, which is enhanced in conditions of bladder overactivity. In this respect, it was shown that the urothelially released ATP is also blocked by BoNT/A in spinalized animals. [9] By contrast, a similar effect on the urothelial relase of ACh has been questioned, as the Vesicular Acetylcholine Transporter could not be detected by various methods in the human bladder urothelium. [10] A neuronal cholinergic effect, on the other hand, is supported by a study in normal and SCI animals, where BoNT/A treatment decreased the bladder contractions evoked by electrical stimulation of spinal nerves without altering intrinsic contractions. [11] However, this neuronal effect differs from the one in skeletal muscles, since a single BoNT/A injection in the human detrusor was not found to induce significant nerve sprouting. [12]

It has been proposed that lack of neuronal sprouting is associated with the prolonged bladder effect compared to the effect on skeletal muscles. It may be partly due to the post-BoNT/A reduction of bladder nerve growth factor (NGF) levels. [13] Decreased NGF may also contribute to the reduction in suburothelial levels of the transient receptor potential TRPV1 (vanilloid or capsaicin receptor), which is involved in mechanosensation and pain mechanims. This, however, could be also via a direct effect of BoNT/A on receptor trafficking. [5] As urine NGF and Brain-Derived Neurotrophic Factor (BDNF) levels were also decreased after BoNT/A bladder injections, an effect on urothelially released neurotrophins was proposed. [14, 15] Despite, however, the speculated urothelial effect of the toxin, neither SV2 nor SNAP-25 could be detected by immunohistochemistry in human urothelial cells, contrary to their abundance in the suburothelium. [3]

Further to the apparent lack of neuronal sprouting in the detrusor and suburothe-lium, [8, 12] other mechanisms to explain the long duration of effect of the toxin when injected in the bladder include the persistence of the cleaved SNAP25 product at the neuromuscular junction, [16] an effect on both preganglionic and postganglionic parasympathetic fibers, [17, 18] a central desensitization effect [8] and neural plasticity. [19] A spinal desensitization effect of BoNT/A was seen in animal models of inflammation-induced bladder overactivity, where intravesical administration of BoNT/A resulted in reduced c-fos cell counts at the L6-S1 spinal cord segments. [20] Further, neural plasticity has been proposed as the main factor regulating the partial restoration to normal levels of urothelial and suburothelial muscarinic receptors following successful BoNT/A treatment of detrusor overactivity symptoms. [19]

Neurogenic detrusor overactivity and BoNT/A
Efficacy

The level of evidence (LOE) for the use of BoNT/A in NDO is the highest. It is built upon two meta-analyses, a recent one in SCI-associated NDO [21] and an older one comprising both NDO and OAB studies up to early 2010, [22] several systematic reviews, [22–26] eight (8) randomized trials of which six (6) are placebo-controlled, [27–32] and two (2) are active comparator-controlled trials [33, 34] (Table 16.1), four LOE2 studies, [35–38] and a wealth of LOE3 publications from increasing number of centers worldwide.

All LOE1 studies to date have reported on the onabotulinumtoxinA (BOTOX®) preparation, apart from a single study using abobotulinumtoxinA (Dysport®) in

Table 16.1 Results from LOE1 studies on the use of BoNT/A in patients with refractory NDO (authors in alphabetical order).

Study	Pts No	F/U	Preparation/Dose	%Δ leaks	%Δ MCC	%Δ MDP
Apostolidis et al. [33]	16	6 wk	Placebo	−35	62	−5
	19		Botox/50 U	−29	64	−38
	21		Botox/100 U	−37	136	−54
	17		Botox/200 U	−55	86	−52
Chen and Kuo [35]	38	6 mo	Botox/200 U		77	−42
	34		Botox/300 U		43	−64
Cruz et al. [30]	92	6 wk	Placebo	−36	2.6	15
	92		Botox/200	−67	63	−55
	91		Botox/300	−62	64	−64
Ehren et al. [29]	17	26 wk	Dysport /500		60	−74
	10		Placebo		0	−22
Giannantoni et al. [34]	12	6 mo	Botox/300	−71	75	−40
Ginsberg et al. [32]	149	6 wk	Placebo	−31	6	−4.7
	135		Botox/200	−65	60	−68
	132		Botox/300	−73	66	29
Hershorn et al. [31]	25	6 wk	Placebo	13	−11	18
	27		Botox/300	−57	75	46
Schurch et al. [28]	21	6 wk	Placebo	−7	18	
	19		Botox/200	−52	72	
	19		Botox/300	−54	58	

Source: Adapted with permisson from [26].

comparison to placebo [28] (Table 16.1). Overall, onabotulinumtoxinA has been more comprehensively studied than abobotulinumtoxinA. [25] A single LOE3 study has reported on the Prosigne® BoNT/A preparation. [39]

Despite the variability in study designs, results consistently confirm the efficacy of BoNT/A in the treatment of refractory NDO-associated incontinence (Tables 16.1 and 16.2). A systematic review recorded mean post-treatment continence rates of 71% with onabotulinumtoxinA and 66% with abobotulinumtoxinA in all LOE studies. [25] Respective complete continence rates, however, were only as high as 40–41% with onabotulinumtoxinA compared to 7.6–10% with placebo in the FDA registration trials [29, 31] (LOE1). A trend for better clinical outcomes in LOE3 studies was also noted in an update of the latter review (Table 16.2), as the decrease in the mean number of incontinence episodes was 80% in LOE3 studies compared to 68% ($p=0.07$) in LOE1–2 studies. [26] Nevertheless, further to the clinical improvement, significant ameliorations have been also demonstrated in urodynamic parameters usually evaluated in NDO patients, such as maximum cystometric capacity (MCC, 68 and 86% mean increase in LOE1–2 and LOE3 studies, respectively), maximum detrusor pressure (MDP, 42% mean decrease in all studies) and reflex volume (RV, 61 and 74% mean increase in LOE1–2 and LOE3 studies, respectively) [23–26] (Tables 16.1 and 16.2). BoNT/A is also able to minimize involuntary detrusor

Table 16.2 Mean and SEM of clinical and urodynamic outcomes of LOE1 and 2 versus LOE3 studies in patients receiving BoNT/A for NDO, also compared by preparation and dose where feasible. %Δ in all study endpoints refer to % change from baseline values.

All studies (SEM)	LOE	No studies/ No patients	%Δ daily leak	%Δ daily catheterization	%Δ MCC	%Δ RV	%Δ MDP	%UTI
Placebo	1	6/313	−19(10)	−2	13(10)	21	−2(6)	33
All BTX-A	1&2	12/ 874	−63(3)	−18(4)	68(6)	61(11)	−42(9)	39
All BTX-A	3	41/ 1840	−80(4)	−18(7)	86(9)	74(8)	−42(6)	10
P value Placebo Vs LOE1			0.006	0.01	0.002	<0.001	0.01	0.3
P value LOE1 Vs LO2&3			0.01	0.94	0.1	0.36	0.98	<0.001
onabotulinumtoxinA all	1&2	10/752	−63(5)	−18(4)	72(5)	48(13)	−40(9)	39
onabotulinumtoxinA all	3	33/1400	−77(4)	−20(5)	91(12)	71(8)	−41(8)	13
P value			0.03	0.77	0.22	0.19	0.94	<0.001
onabotulinumtoxinA 300iu	1&2	8/383	−71(5)	−17(6)	70(5)	49(23)	−31(15)	38
onabotulinumtoxinA 300iu	3	25/1156	−82(4)	−24(4)	77(10)	108(47)	−40(10)	14
P value			0.09	0.4	0.49	0.3	0.66	0.006
abobotulinumtoxinA all	1&2	3/122			27 (3)	56(19)		
abobotulinumtoxinA all	3	8/433			74 (7)	91(5)		
P value					0.006	0.34		

Source: Adapted with permisson from [26].

contractions (IDC); these were abolished in 60–69% of the patients treated with onabotulinumtoxinA in the two registration trials as opposed to 17.4–19% of those who received placebo. [29, 31]

Although both the onabotulinumtoxinA and abobotulinumtoxinA preparations appear to be efficacious in NDO, [25] there are no direct comparisons for dose, efficacy, and safety in patients with NDO or OAB. Results of a single, non-randomized study on 42 patients suggest that the BOTOX® (onabotulinumtoxinA) formulation may be more efficacious than the Prosigne® formulation in improving MCC and incontinence in patients with refractory NDO. [39]

Onset and duration of effect

While the earliest documented clinical benefits in most LOE1 studies have been recorded at two weeks post-treatment when the first follow-up visit was designed to take place, open-label studies reported significant improvements in urgency, daytime frequency, and nocturia recorded in bladder diaries as early as 48 hours and in associated incontinence as early as 72 hours in NDO patients still experiencing bladder sensation. [40]

A long duration of efficacy has been established in the literature: the beneficial effects of a single onabotulinumtoxinA injection may last 6–16 months compared to 5–12 months for a single abobotulinumtoxinA injection. [25] Such extraordinary results were confirmed in the FDA regulatory approval trials which covered a total 691 patients; the median time to retreatment was 37–42 weeks for onabotulinumtoxinA compared to 13–14 weeks for placebo. [29, 31] Results of the three-year extension study on the efficacy of repeat treatments are awaited. The level of evidence for efficacy and safety of the toxin when used in repeat treatment sessions remains low, but the number of LOE3 studies reporting on the sustained efficacy of either of the two formulations with results from various centers is steadily growing. [41–49] A single randomized study compared two doses of onabotulinumtoxinA (200 U vs. 300 U) administered every six months for up to two injections (LOE1–2). [34] The two doses were found to be comparable for improvements in incontinence and urodynamic parameters, with the exception of IDC, which responded better to the higher dose ($p=0.01$).

Antimuscarinics and BoNT/A: A measure of efficacy or a BoNT/A efficacy enhancer?

A large proportion of patients injected with a BoNT/A formulation are still using antimuscarinics at the time of injection, despite what is deemed as an inadequate response to the oral medication. In earlier studies, patients were asked to regulate on demand the antimuscarinic dose and overall use following a BoNT/A injection. Significant reductions in both the use and dose of anti-incontinence medication became apparent during maximum efficacy of the

toxin in open-label studies, [41, 50, 51] but also in two RCTs which allowed titration of the antimuscarinics dose on demand. [28, 30] Specifically designed studies to examine possible additional benefits from the concomitant use of antimuscarinics are still lacking, but a *post hoc* analysis of the phase 3 regulatory trials suggested that patients on antimuscarinics had similar improvements in incontinence rates, urodynamic parameters, and quality of life as those not using medication. [52]

Predictors of response to treatment

While the use of antimuscarinics may be a measure but cannot be used as a predictor of clinical efficacy, research has not identified any robust determinants of treatment efficacy in NDO. With reported overall failure rates of 5–25% for onabotulinumtoxinA and 10–32% for abobotulinumtoxinA, [25] only longer duration of MS has been proposed to be a predicting factor of treatment failure in a single LOE3 study. [53] Speculation that treatment failure may be associated with the formation of neutralizing BoNT/A antibodies has been perplexed by the wide range of reported antibody formation rates following treatment (0–35%). [54–57] Further, a controlled study in children found no association between antibody formation and treatment failure, despite an initial increased rate of antibody formation in patients receiving repeat versus single injections (71 versus 38%). [58]

Do all neurogenic patient populations respond the same to the toxin?

Although direct comparisons of efficacy between patient populations are lacking, BoNT/A appears to be highly efficacious in both MS and SCI patients, [29, 31] who comprise the vast majority of study participants to date, mostly in mixed studies, with only small case series reporting on patients with Parkinson's disease or cerebrovascular accident (CVA). [59–62] Two studies coming from a single center discuss efficacy and safety of the treatment in MS patients only. They found significant, long-lasting improvements in clinical, urodynamic, and quality of life parameters with repeat injections using the highest dose of onabotulinumtoxinA (300 U). [48, 63] A third report involved the MS subpopulation of one of the FDA registration trials ($n = 154$ patients) who were randomized to receive placebo, 200 U, or 300 U onabotulinumtoxinA. The 200 U dose achieved similar efficacy in incontinence as the 300 U dose, but with lower rates of post-treatment CIC (24.3 vs. 37.5%) and UTI (58.5 vs. 70%). Finally, in a small study SCI patients achieved better continence rates and lower detrusor pressures compared to CVA patients. [62]

BoNT/A bladder injections have a dramatic effect on quality of life (QOL)

This has been demonstrated in RCTs with either of the two most commonly used preparations. It was the primary outcome in the single published RCT with abobotulinumtoxinA. NDO patients injected with 500 U Dysport® had a more significant change in QOL parameters and intake of anticholinergics compared to placebo-treated patients up to 26 weeks post-treatment. [28] Subanalyses of the RCTs using onabotulinumtoxinA also revealed that QOL scores, usually assessed with the I-QOL questionnaire, had improved significantly more than in the placebo groups for up to 36 weeks post-treatment.

[29, 30, 64] It has been proposed that changes in troublesome clinical symptoms may be a more representative reflection of the QOL improvements than the equally significant changes in urodynamic parameters. [50]

Doses: The higher the better?

The majority of published studies have used 300 U onabotulinumtoxinA in NDO patients, but a breakthrough in changing the most commonly used dose could be identified with the first randomized, placebo-controlled trial in 2005. [27] Although not an objective of this small-sized study, it was evident in reported results that 200 U onabotulinumtoxinA could achieve similar, if not more sustainable, effects as the 300 U dose. The suggested plateau in the efficacy of the toxin was later confirmed in the large registration trials, which demonstrated similar efficacy and a more favorable adverse event profile for the 200 U compared to the 300 U onabotulinumtoxinA dose. [29, 31] At the same time, a dose-response study using lower doses of onabotulinumtoxinA provided some evidence for a more significant clinical benefit of the 200 U dose compared to the 50 U and 100 U doses in SCI patients with NDO. [32] Based on such findings, the 200 U onabotulinumtoxinA dose was licensed for the treatment of refractory NDO incontinence.

As the recommended 200 U dose is associated with a 22–25% incidence of *de novo* post-treatment clean intermittent catheterizations, which rises to 35% with the previously used 300 U dose, [29, 31] the efficacy and safety of a lower dose was tested in a pilot study using 100 U onabotulinumtoxinA in MS patients, who may opt for preservation of voiding function as opposed to SCI patients with commonly absent or severely impaired bladder sensation. Interestingly, the dose produced significant decreases in daytime frequency, nocturia, urgency, and associated incontinence for a mean 8 months in the 12 patients studied. At the same time, despite the increase in PVR, the need for CIC was minimized. [65]

The few studies comparing different doses of abobotulinumtoxinA are inconclusive due to either inadequate sample size or lack of randomization. [35, 47, 66] A randomized, double-blind study comparing 500 U to 750 U abobotulinumtoxinA could identify a trend for better clinical and urodynamic improvements with the 750 U dose. [36] No clear dose-response could be found in a case-control study, although higher doses of abobotulinumtoxinA (750 U and 1000 U) appeared to achieve longer lasting effects than the 500 U dose. [66]

Injection technique and dilutions: does volume matter?

There is a widespread notion that the toxin is efficacious independent of dilution volume, number of injection sites, or site of injection. Thus, few studies have examined correlations between those variables and the toxin's efficacy and safety. Nevertheless, as in the majority of published studies onabotulinumtoxinA was delivered at 30 injection sites and in the regulatory trials the same number of injection sites was used when administering either 300 U or 200 U BOTOX®, the licensed formulation advises such a dilution that would allow injection at 30 injection sites. A high dilution volume and number of injection sites is supported by experimental data, where activity of

the toxin was assessed via distribution of the cleaved SNAP25 product [18] although a clinical study comparing 10 to 30 injection sites (300 U Botox®) could find no difference in the changes of incontinence episodes and cystometric capacity between the two injection techniques. [67] Dilution in 30 ml delivered at 30 sites appears to be most common when injecting abobotulinumtoxinA too, despite a large variance in the number of injection sites and dilution volumes (10–30 injection sites, dilution volumes 5–30 ml). [25]

The proposed site of injection also remains unchanged from the technique originally described by Schurch et al. where injections were delivered into the detrusor muscle sparing the trigone [68] (Figure 16.3). This technique has been applied in the majority of published studies [24] although a comparative study suggested that trigonal injections may produce better continence rates and more significant improvements in reflex volume than detrusor injections alone. [37] There is no robust data on the use of a rigid versus flexible cystoscopes and on the type of injection needles. The tendency is, however to use finer injection needles, [24, 69, 70] and a typified needle is now marketed for bladder BoNT/A injections (http://www.porges.com/en-uk/otherurologyproducts/lower-urinary-tract/bonee).

As, however, delivery of BoNT/A via bladder wall injections may be associated with some complications, including a degree of discomfort in patients with reminiscent or unaltered bladder sensation, alternative delivery techniques are being investigated. Preclinical studies examined intravesical instillations of BoNT/A encapsulated in liposomes [71] or via electromotive drug

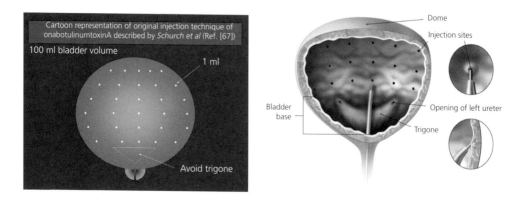

Figure 16.3 2D (left) and 3D (right) cartoon representation of the onabotulinumtoxinA bladder injection technique in NDO/OAB patients. According to the original description by Schurch et al. [68], each 100 U toxin vial was diluted in 10 ml normal saline, and 1 ml of the dilute was delivered at each injection site. The bladder wall is virtually mapped by the surgeon and injection sites should be at a distance of ≥ 1 cm from each other and exclude the trigone in a half-full bladder. The injection needle should be adequately inserted (up to 4 mm) to achieve a detrusor muscle delivery, minimizing at the same time the risk of injecting outside a thinned bladder wall by overdistension. Schurch 2000 [68]. Source: Reproduced with permission of Elsevier. (For color detail, please see color plate section).

administration (EMDA), [72] with interesting results. A pilot study of EMDA-administered BoNT/A in children with myelomeningocele reported significant improvements in urodynamic and clinical parameters. [73]

Is BoNT/A injected in the bladder safe?

The most common "adverse event" (AE) is the significant increase in post-void residual in patients not using CIC prior to treatment and the subsequent need to start CIC. As this is clearly related to the mechanism of action of the toxin, it is debated as a proper AE since it is to be anticipated. Interestingly, in the large placebo-controlled trials, 12–22% of the placebo-treated patients were also started on CIC post-treatment, suggesting patient management issues even before study entry. Nevertheless, an additional 20–25% and 27–30% of the patients

needed to initiate CIC post-treatment with 200 U and 300 U onabotulinumtoxinA, respectively.

The increased rate of *de novo* CIC in the BoNT/A-treated patients accounts for a higher incidence of urinary tract infections (UTIs) in those treated with onabotulinumtoxinA as opposed to placebo-treated patients [29, 31] (Table 16.2). This RCT finding may appear to contradict earlier prospective studies that had reported significant reductions in the incidence of UTIs for up to six months to six years post-treatment with BoNT/A. [46, 74, 75] The most likely explanation for this apparent discrepancy, however, must be that RCTs also report cases of asymptomatic bacteriuria as UTIs, whereas open-label studies reported only symptomatic UTIs. Asymptomatic bacteriuria/UTIs are associated with CIC. [31]

Muscle weakness might potentially be a serious adverse event; still, it is not clearly defined in clinical studies and has been described also by terms such as hypoasthenia or fatigue. The overall incidence from combined literature data is 0.005% in patients receiving onabotulinumtoxinA and 0.026% in patients receiving abobotulinumtoxinA, [25] but considerably higher rates were reported in certain studies. In two of the most recent RCTs, 8.8–11% of BOTOX-treated participants reported fatigue as opposed to 0–1% of the placebo-treated, [29, 30] while a much lower incidence was recorded in the third RCT. [31] The effect resolves spontaneously after 2–8 weeks and appears to be dose-related for abobotulinumtoxinA, with most cases reported in patients injected with 750–1000 U, but not for onabotulinumtoxinA. [29, 31, 44, 76]

Other reported clinical AEs include haematuria, constipation, and flu-like symptoms. [25, 29, 31] Quantitative and qualitative, mostly positive, changes of semen have been described in SCI patients. [77] Despite initial reservations of injecting the trigone in order to avoid possible vesicoureteral reflux, this was not proven to be an issue in small trials. [37, 78, 79]

Concerns about autonomic and histological secondary effects have been raised. [80, 81] Preclinical evidence supports a post-treatment reduction in autonomic dysreflexia incidence, [82] but clinical studies report somewhat higher rates of autonomic dysfunction incidents in toxin-treated patients compared to placebo. [30, 31] Findings of neuromuscular jitter in single-fiber EMG recordings post-treatment in one-third of the patients cannot be considered as definitive since the study was neither comparative or controlled. [83] Based on sparse human studies, it appears that BoNT/A does not cause bladder wall fibrosis or apoptosis, [84–87] while evidence points even towards a reduction of the fibrotic elements. [84] However, a possible increase in inflammation and eosinophilic infiltration of the bladder wall with repeat injections warrants further investigation. [85]

OAB/Idiopathic Detrusor Overactivity (IDO) and BoNT/A

Efficacy

A total of 56 studies with a minimum patient sample of 10 patients each have reported on the use of BoNT/A in OAB/IDO, of which 16 are randomized studies [64, 88–99] (Table 16.3). In the vast majority of studies onabotlulinumtoxinA was used, and the treatment was again found to be highly efficacious. A mean 57% complete continence rate was estimated in an earlier systematic review, [25] but this did not include the most recent large RCTs, which reported disappointingly low continence rates (22.9, 27, and 31%) [93, 95, 97] (Table 16.4). Indeed, there is a wide variance in reported outcomes of a single treatment cycle, particularly between the largest RCT and the largest open-label study to date (22.9 vs. 86% incontinence-free patients). [97, 100] Improvements above the placebo effect were seen in all OAB symptoms (daily frequency, urgency, urgency incontinence, and nocturia) and in urodynamic parameters such as MCC and MDP.

Most improvements were again better in lower LOE studies, with MCC and daily frequency achieving or trending for significance when compared to LOE1-2 studies (Frequency: 29 vs. 40%, $p=0.08$ – MCC: 32 vs. 58%, $p=0.003$). [26] Treatment efficacy

Table 16.3 Results from LOE1 studies on the use of BoNT/A in patients with refractory non-neurogenic OAB symptoms.

Study	No pts	F/U	Preparation /Dose	%Δ daily frequency	% Δ daily urgency	% Δ daily leak	% Δ MCC	% Δ MDP	% Δ QOL
Altaweel et al. [101]	11	3 mo	Botox/100	−47	−60	−45	24	−28	UDI6=−50 IIQ-7=−42
	11		Botox/200	−49	−59	−32	51	−27	UDI6=−41 IIQ-7=−44
Brubaker et al. [89]	15	3 mo	Placebo			−5			
	28		Botox/200			−85			
Chapple et al. [96]	271	6 wk	Placebo	−7	−12	−25			IQOL =19
	277		Botox/100	−18	−45	−62			IQOL =73
Denys et al. [94]	29		Placebo	−9	−31	−31	10	49	IQOL =30
	21		Botox/50	−11	−16	−51	8	51	IQOL =38
	22		Botox/100	−30	−34	−54	8	37	IQOL =96
	27		Botox/150	−32	−53	−56	17	50	IQOL =110
Dmochowski et al. [91]	43	12 wk	Placebo				19	5	KHQ=−7
	56		Botox/50				19	16	KHQ =−11
	55		Botox/100				28	−4	KHQ =−19
	50		Botox/150				39	−22	KHQ =−21
	52		Botox/200				33	−21	KHQ =−20
	55		botox/300				48	−4	KHQ =−19
Flynn et al. [90]	7	6 wk	Placebo	−7		9			UDI6=7.4 IIQ–7=0
	15		Botox 200/300	−12		−58			UDI6=−38 IIQ-7=−67
Gousse et al. [102]	30	6 wk	Botox/100						
	30		Botox/150						
Jabs et al. [103]	10	6 mo	Placebo	6		8	−21		UDI6=−18 IIQ-7=−7
	11		Botox/100	−26		−67	13		UDI6=−49 IIQ-7=−50
Kuo [104]	37	3 mo	Botox/100	−15	0.8	−57	21	−16	
	35			−17	−6	−59	17	−7	
	33			−20	−7	−28	27	−15	
Nitti et al. [97]	280	6 wk	Placebo	−1.1	−13	−24			
	277		Botox/100	−15	−35	−64			
Sahai et al. [88]	18	4 wk	Placebo	−7	−18	−19	−15	−4	UDI6=−5 IIQ-7=−28
	16		Botox/ 200	−49	−79	−62	72	−55	UDI6=−48 IIQ-7=−67
Tincello et al. [93]	98	6 wk	Placebo	−10	−20	−14			IQOL=32

Source: Adapted with permisson from [26].

Table 16.4 Mean and SEM of clinical and urodynamic outcomes of LOE1 and 2 versus LOE3 studies in patients receiving BoNT/A for OAB, also compared by preparation and dose where feasible. %Δ in all study endpoints refer to % change from baseline values.

All studies (SEM)	LOE	No studies/ No patients	%Δ daily frequency	%Δ daily urgency	%Δ daily leak	%Δ MCC	%Δ MDP	%ISC	%UTI
Placebo	1	9/772	−5(2)	−19(3)	−13(5)	−2(10)	17(17)	0	7
All BTX-A	1 & 2	16/ 1380	−29(3)	−38(6)	−59(4)	32(5)	−31(6)	12	21
All BTX-A	3	40/2673	−40(4)	−49(8)	−69(6)	58(7)	−29(6)	16	14
P value Placebo Vs LOE1			<0.001	0.02	<0.001	0.01	0.04	<0.001	<0.001
P value LOE1 Vs LO2&3			0.08	0.3	0.15	0.003	0.88	<0.001	0.01
onabotulinumtoxinA all	1&2	15/1358	−29(3)	−38(6)	−59(4)	28(4)	−23(5)	12	21
onabotulinumtoxinA all	3	34/2302	−38(5)	−51(9)	−70(6)	59(7)	−29(7)	13	14
P value			0.12	0.27	0.14	<0.001	0.49	0.4	0.01
onabotulinumtoxinA 200iu	1&2	5/195	−40(9)	−69(6)	−68(14)	52(11)	−34(10)	24	34
onabotulinumtoxinA 200iu	3	15/847	−34(4)	−49(15)	−79(10)	59(18)	−19(12)	31	10
P value			0.53	0.3	0.53	0.79	0.38	0.08	<0.001
onabotulinumtoxinA 100iu	1&2	10/886	−28	−30(6)	−55(4)	23(4)		7	18
onabotulinumtoxinA 100iu	3	8/744	−38	−51(33)	−63(9)	56(6)		10	16
P value			0.23	0.28	0.41	<0.001		0.09	0.4

Source: Adapted with permisson from [26].

appears to be dose-dependent as the continence rates in a dose-response study were 15.9, 29.8, 37.0, 40.8, 50.9, and 57.1% in the placebo, and 50, 100, 150, 200, and 300 U onabotulinmtoxinA groups, respectively. [91]

Interestingly, failure rates appear to be higher in idiopathic OAB studies than in NDO studies. Treatment benefit was reported by only 60.8 and 62.8% in the two largest RCTs [96, 97] with a placebo effect approaching 30%. Similarly, a landmark earlier study which had raised awareness on the high post-treatment rates of increased post-void residuals and UTIs had

also reported a clinical response in approximately 60% of treated women. [89] This may be partly associated with patients' expectations from the treatment. In a cohort of women with OAB/IDO, the majority of women (>75%) would expect to become fully continent, to have a minimization of their urgency, and a voiding frequency of <8 times/day, and would be happy with a beneficial effect lasting ≥9 months if injected with BoNT/A. Preferences were no different between treatment-naïve and women already on antimuscarinics. [105] Other, open-label studies, reported better outcomes. In the largest study of repeat injections in IDO patients ($n=100$), 24% discontinued the treatment, but only 13% because of poor efficacy, with the dislike for CIC accounting for the remaining 11% of the drop-outs. Comparative, open-label studies found no differences in efficacy between IDO/OAB and NDO populations treated with either the same [106, 107] or different doses of BoNT/A. [108] Elderly patients may also benefit from the treatment as demonstrated in a small series of 21 patients with a mean age of 81 years who received 200 U onabotulinumtoxinA. A mean duration of symptomatic improvement of seven months was reported, with no treatment-related AEs. [109]

Efficacy seems to be maintained with repeat injections, but the LOE is low and few published large series exist. [110, 111]

Onset and duration of effect

Similar to the NDO populations, in OAB RCTs the earliest time-point where a positive effect was recorded was two weeks post-injection as per study design. Another RCT reported an improvement in OAB symptoms at day 8, but this became significant one month post-treatment. Open-label studies identified an earlier response within the first week of treatment. In a small study of eight patients examining the daily changes in OAB symptoms after injection of 200 U onabotulinumtoxinA, Kalsi et al. found significant reductions in urgency, frequency, and urgency incontinence as of day 4. [40] In a large study of 100 patients treated with 100 U, the mean time to loss of urgency was five days. [100] A similar result was reported in a study of 35 OAB patients treated with 200 U Botox®. [112]

By contrast to the NDO literature, little data exists on duration of effect in OAB.

The majority of LOE1 studies had outcomes reported at 3–6 months, with a single RCT estimating a mean 373 days of treatment benefit for the women who responded to treatment. [89] A long-lasting effect with inter-injection intervals of at least 300 days was also found in a cohort of patients who received up to eight repeat injections (mean time to re-injection 322 days), [110] and an even longer duration of effect (min. 12 – max.15 months) in another large series who received up to five injections. [111] All studies which reported durable mid-term effects had used 200 U onabotulinumtoxinA in the vast majority of their patients. [89, 110, 111]

Doses

In a dose-ranging study using doses between 50 and 300 U onabotulinumtoxinA , even the lower dose of 50 U was found to improve OAB symptoms compared to placebo, although not consistently. Similar to the NDO population, analysis of clinical and urodynamic data suggested a plateau in efficacy at doses of 100–150 U onabotulinumtoxinA. When the rates of AEs (CIC and UTI) were also considered it was decided that the 100 U dose combined the best clinical and AE profile, [91] later receiving approval for refractory OAB treatment. Still, there appears to be a large gap in efficacy concerning complete continence between the approved 100 U and the 200 U dose which was most commonly investigated in the earlier RCTs (37 vs. 51%). These findings complemented open-label studies also estimating that 51% of the patients had achieved complete continence with a single 200 U Botox® injection. [113] Results remain difficult to interpret as another RCT – though underpowered – reported 55 and 50% continence rates with 100 and 150 U onabotulinumtoxinA, respectively. [94]

Studies comparing different doses are sparse and inadequately powered. In a randomized trial, patients receiving 150 U Botox® seemed to achieve better continence rates if incontinent (58 vs. 25%) and restoration of micturition frequency if dry (90 vs. 60%) when compared to those who received 100 U, but differences were not statistically significant, possibly due to the small sample size. [114] No differences were seen in AE profile between the two doses. These findings are contradicted by another randomized and a non-randomized study, which found no clinically relevant differences between 100 U and 200 U and 100 U and 150 U onabotulinumtoxinA, respectively. [101, 115]

Antimuscarinics and BoNT/A in OAB/IDO

Going a step further from the question of the additive role of antimuscarinics arising from the NDO studies, an alternative double-blind, double-placebo-controlled study directly compared 100 U onabotulinumtoxinA to oral antimuscarinics (solifenacin or tropsium), but in a mixed patient population in terms of previous use of antimuscarinics for urgency incontinence. Interestingly, results showed no difference between the two groups in reduction of incontinence episodes and QOL improvement, but BOTOX® was more effective in achieving complete continence (27 vs. 13%). [95] Following discontinuation of oral medication, a more durable effect could be seen for patients in the onabotulinumtoxinA group. No significant interactions were found between treatment group and prior use of antimuscarinics. Between

those who were treated with Botox®, patients who had failed antimuscarinics due to inadequate efficacy showed a lesser treatment benefit compared to those who had discontinued due to an unfavorable AE profile (60 vs. 86%, $p = 0.02$). [116]

Quality of life: much better after BoNT/A treatment in OAB/IDO

Improved QOL is a consistent finding in all RCTs as well as in open-label studies, independent of questionnaire used (usually I-QOL or UDI6 & IIQ7). [64, 90, 94, 96–99] The improvement in QOL seems to be sustained with repeat treatments. [111] Importantly, despite the fact that fear of increased PVR and need for CIC may prevent patients from having the treatment or discontinue it, [105, 110] a retrospective study claimed that QOL was not affected by the use of CIC. [117]

Predictors of response to treatment

In the first effort to identify poor responders to treatment, Schmid et al. in their cohort of 100 IDO/OAB patients suggested that poor bladder compliance, low MCC (<100 ml), and bladder wall fibrosis may be associated with lower efficacy. Younger age (55 vs. 68 years, $p = 0.03$) and OAB-associated incontinence (as opposed to OAB-dry) were related to a better clinical response in another – univariate – analysis. [118] In the same analysis, higher maximal detrusor pressures showed a tendency to correlate with better efficacy (49 vs. 29 cm H_2O, $p = 0.06$). This finding may appear to partly contradict earlier data by Sahai et al. who found that high max. P_{det} (>110 cm H_2O) may predict poor response to treatment with a high specificity and sensitivity. [119] Neither of the two studies clarified whether max. P_{det} referred to an involuntary detrusor contraction upon filling. Finally, the presence of DO upon baseline urodynamic investigation does not appear to predict treatment outcomes, [92] but post-treatment UTIs or incidents of hematuria were found to be associated with poorer outcomes. [122]

Injection technique

A great variance exists again concerning dilution volumes, site of injections (detrusor vs. suburothelium, trigonal vs. nontrigonal) and number of injection sites. Consistent with the notion that "volume matters," the original 20 ml dilution used for the 200 U onabotulinumtoxinA (1 ml per injection site) was preserved throughout the regulatory trials using 100 U (0.5 ml per injection site). [91, 96, 97] Trigone-including injections of abobotulinumtoxinA were found to be superior to trigone-sparing injections in terms of OAB symptomatic improvement, [121] but another randomized, actively-controlled study using 100 U onabotulinumtoxinA found no differences in efficacy between trigone-including and trigone-sparing injections. [104] Risk of vesicoureteric reflux does not increase with trigonal injections. [104, 121, 122]

Adverse events: A clearer profile in OAB/IDO

There is a unanimous agreement and high LOE in the literature that BoNT/A bladder injections for OAB/IDO are associated with increased post-void residuals, an increased need for post-treatment self-catherizations as well as an increased rate of UTIs. OnabotulinumtoxinA was also found to be associated with a higher rate of UTIs and need for post-treatment CIC in a direct comparison with antimuscarinics, although with a less common dry mouth effect. [95]

Both major side-effects appear to be largely dose-dependent, but a plateau may come after a certain dose, and 300 U onabotulinumtoxinA seem to have similar or even lower rates of CIC and UTIs as the 200 U dose. The proportion of patients requiring CIC were 0, 3.6, 9.1, 12.7, 18.2, and 16.4% for placebo, and 50, 100, 150, 200, and 300 U groups, respectively. Indeed, the 200 U which appeared to be favored in the earlier RCTs and in large open-label studies has been linked to CIC rates ranging between 21 and 43%. [88, 89, 91, 111] By contrast, significantly lower CIC rates have been reported for the 100 U dose: 0%–9% of patients in large multicenter RCTs were started on CIC, [91, 94–97] which complemented results of the largest open-label study using 100U (4%). [100] However, these results are always subject to the definition and management differences of a large PVR. For example, only 41% of patients with a post-treatment PVR of >200 ml initiated CIC in the phase 3 pivotal trial. [96] The loss in efficacy is counterbalanced by the higher AE rate of the higher dose (increased PVR, post-treatment catheterizations, and UTIs).

Urinary tract infections appear to be the most common adverse event in IDO/OAB patients, with a wide range of reported incidence. In RCTs using 200 U onabotulinumtoxinA, the incidence ranged between 7 and 44% compared to 0–22% for placebo. [88, 89, 93] The dose-finding study recorded UTI in 16.3, 33.9, 44, 48.1, and 34.5% of patients randomized to receive placebo, 50, 100, 150, 200, and 300 U onabotulinumtoxinA respectively. This adverse event seems to be associated with the increase in post-void residuals.

Efforts have been made to predict some of the most common side-effects. In a urodynamic analysis, Sahai et al. proposed poor pre-treatment detrusor contractility as a predictor of incomplete bladder emptying and need for CIC. A projected isovolumetric pressure (PIP1) in women < 50 and a bladder contractility index (BCI) in men < 120 combined good sensitivity and specificity for prediction of poor bladder emptying post-BoNT/A injections. [123] Male gender and incomplete bladder emptying even before treatment (PVR ≥ 100 ml) increased the likelihood of post-treatment retention, while the presence of medical comorbidity was associated with a high PVR. Urinary tract infections were found to occur more commonly in women and in men with retaining prostate. [122]

The economics of BoNT/A: Is it cost-effective to inject the overactive bladder with BoNT/A?

A UK study based on data from patients who had been injected with either 300 U (NDO) or 200 U (IDO/OAB) and had a > 50% symptomatic improvement used projected quality-of-life improvements and concluded that bladder BoNT/A injections are cost-effective for either NDO or IDO/OAB, on an estimated cost of £6000 per quality adjusted life year (QALY). [124] This analysis, however, was performed on an estimated inter-injection interval of 19.5 months. A European study in NDO patients found that intradetrusor BoNT-A may halve the treatment costs of incontinence, possibly via a decrease in the incidence of UTIs and in the use of pro-continence medication and incontinence protection. [125] BoNT/A

costs were found to be comparable to augmentation cystoplasty at five years in the NDO patients, but with a rather unrealistic mean duration of effect of five months per treatment session and with a ≤40% incidence of augmentation cystoplasty associated complications. [126] A USA study comparing BoNT/A to sacral neuromodulation (SNM) and augmentation cystoplasty for IDO/OAB patients for up to three years identified BoNT/A to be the least costly intervention. Further analysis found that SNM persisted as the most costly intervention in all scenarios of outcomes and risks. [128] Somewhat conflicting results were published for another two studies comparing BoNT/A to SNM. Both found SNM to be cost-effective compared to BoNT/A at five and ten years, respectively. [128, 129]

Concluding remarks

A large body of evidence supports the efficacy and overall safety of BoNT/A for bladder use in both the NDO and OAB/IDO populations, but they were produced mostly by tertiary referral centers in either open-label studies or RCTs. Following approval for use in both indications, the widespread use of the toxin in refractory overactive bladder patients will produce real-life data which are awaited with great interest. Standardization of peri- and post-treatment patient care as well as of injection techniques (if possible) could be a way towards more homogeneous analyzable results, and could help maximize treatment benefits for the patient but also protect this valuable second-line treatment. More research is needed on the mechanism of action, safety, long-term use of the toxin, and the development of alternative delivery techniques.

References

1 Dong M, Yeh F, Tepp WH et al., SV2 is the protein receptor for botulinum neurotoxin A. *Science*, 2006. **312**(5773):592–6.

2 Dolly O, Synaptic transmission: inhibition of neurotransmitter release by botulinum toxins. *Headache* 2003;**43** Suppl 1:S16–24.

3 Coelho A, Dinis P, Pinto R, et al., Distribution of the high–affinity binding site and intracellular target of botulinum toxin type a in the human bladder. *Eur Urol.* 2010;**57**(5):884–890.

4 de Paiva A, Meunier FA, Molgo J et al. Functional repair of motor endplates after botulinum neurotoxin type A poisoning: biphasic switch of synaptic activity between nerve sprouts and their parent terminals. *Proc Natl Acad Sci USA* 1999;**96**:3200–3205.

5 Apostolidis A, Dasgupta P, Fowler CJ, Proposed mechanism for the efficacy of injected botulinum toxin in the treatment of human detrusor overactivity. *Eur Urol.* 2006;**49**(4):644–650.

6 Smith CP, Franks ME, McNeil BK, et al., Effect of botulinum toxin A on the autonomic nervous system of the rat lower urinary tract. *J Urol.* 2003;**169**:1896–900.

7 Schulte-Baukloh H, Priefert J, Knispel HH, et al. Botulinum toxin a detrusor injections reduce postsynaptic muscular m2, m3, p2x2, and p2x3 receptors in children and adolescents who have neurogenic detrusor overactivity: A single-blind study. *Urology* 2013;**81**(5):1052–1057.

8 Apostolidis A, Popat R, Yiangou Y, et al., Decreased sensory receptors p2x3 and trpv1 in suburothelial nerve fibers following intradetrusor injections of botulinum toxin for human detrusor overactivity. *J Urol.* 2005;**174**(3):977–983.

9 Khera M, Somogyi GT, Kiss S, et al. Botulinum toxin A inhibits ATP release from bladder urothelium after chronic spinal cord injury. *Neurochem Int.* 2004;**45**(7):987–993.

10 Yoshida M, Masunaga K, Satoji Y, et al. Basic and clinical aspects of non–neuronal acetylcholine: expression of non–neuronal acetylcholine in urothelium and its clinical significance. *J Pharmacol Sci.* 2008;**106**(2):193–198.

11 Ikeda Y, Zabbarova IV, Birder LA, et al. Botulinum neurotoxin serotype A suppresses neurotransmitter release from afferent as well as efferent nerves in the urinary bladder. *Eur Urol.* 2012;**62**(6):1157–1164.

12 Haferkamp A, Schurch B, Reitz A, et al. Lack of ultrastructural detrusor changes following endoscopic injection of Botulinum toxin type A in overactive neurogenic bladder. *Eur Urol.* 2004;**46**:784–791.

13 Giannantoni A, Di Stasi SM, Nardicchi V, et al., Botulinum–A toxin injections into the detrusor muscle decrease nerve growth factor bladder tissue levels in patients with neurogenic detrusor overactivity. *J Urol.* 2006;**175**(6):2341–2344.

14 Liu HT, Chancellor MB, Kuo HC. Urinary nerve growth factor levels are elevated in patients with detrusor overactivity and decreased in responders to detrusor botulinum toxin–a injection. *Eur Urol.* 2009 Oct;**56**(4):700–706.

15 Pinto R, Lopes T, Frias B, et al., Trigonal injection of botulinum toxin A in patients with refractory bladder pain syndrome/interstitial cystitis. *Eur Urol.* 2010;**58**(3):360–365.

16 Schulte-Baukloh H, Zurawski TH, Knispel HH, et al. Persistence of the synaptosomal–associated protein–25 cleavage product after intradetrusor botulinum toxin A injections in patients with myelomeningocele showing an inadequate response to treatment. *BJU Int.* 2007;**100**(5):1075–1080.

17 Coelho A, Cruz F, Cruz CD, Avelino A. Effect of onabotulinumtoxinA on intramural parasympathetic ganglia: an experimental study in the guinea pig bladder. *J Urol.* 2012;**187**(3):1121–1126.

18 Coelho A, Cruz F, Cruz CD, Avelino A. Spread of onabotulinumtoxinA after bladder injection. Experimental study using the distribution of cleaved SNAP–25 as the marker of the toxin action. *Eur Urol.* 2012;**61**(6):1178–1184.

19 Datta SN, Roosen A, Pullen A, et al., Immunohistochemical expression of muscarinic receptors in the urothelium and suburothelium of neurogenic and idiopathic overactive human bladders, and changes with botulinum neurotoxin administration. *J Urol.* 2010;**184**(6):2578–2585.

20 Vemulakonda VM, Somogyi GT, Kiss S, et al. Inhibitory effect of intravesically applied botulinum toxin A in chronic bladder inflammation. *J Urol.* 2005;**173**(2):621–624.

21 Mehta S, Hill D, McIntyre A, et al., Meta-analysis of botulinum toxin A detrusor injections in the treatment of neurogenic detrusor overactivity after spinal cord injury. *Arch Phys Med Rehabil.* 2013 Aug; **94**(8):1473–1481.

22 Duthie JB, Vincent M, Herbison GP, et al. Botulinum toxin injections for adults with overactive bladder syndrome. *Cochrane Database Syst Rev.* 2011;**12**:CD005493.

23 Karsenty G, Denys P, Amarenco G, et al., Botulinum toxin A (Botox) intradetrusor injections in adults with neurogenic detrusor overactivity/neurogenic overactive bladder: a systematic literature review. *Eur Urol.* 2008;**53**(2):275–287.

24 Apostolidis A, Dasgupta P, Denys P, et al., Recommendations on the use of botulinum toxin in the treatment of lower urinary tract disorders and pelvic floor dysfunctions: a european consensus panel report. *Eur Urol.* 2009;**55**:100–120.

25 Mangera A, Andersson KE, Apostolidis A, et al. Contemporary management of lower urinary tract disease with botulinum toxin A: a systematic review of botox (onabotulinumtoxinA) and dysport (abobotulinumtoxinA). *Eur Urol.* 2011;**60**(4):784–795.

26 Mangera A, Apostolidis A, Andersson KE, et al., An updated systematic review and statistical comparison of standardised mean outcomes for the use of botulinum toxin in the management of lower urinary tract disorders. *Eur Urol.* 2014;**65**(5):981–990.

27 Schurch B, de Seze M, Denys P, et al. Botulinum toxin type A is a safe and effective treatment for neurogenic urinary incontinence: results of a single treatment, randomized, placebo controlled 6–month study. *J Urol.* 2005;**174**(1):196–200.

28 Ehren I, Volz D, Farrelly E, et al. Efficacy and impact of botulinum toxin A on quality of life in patients with neurogenic detrusor overactivity: a randomised, placebo–controlled, double–blind study. *Scand J Urol Nephrol.* 2007;**41**(4):335–340.

29 Cruz F, Herschorn S, Aliotta P, et al., Efficacy and safety of onabotulinumtoxinA in patients with urinary incontinence due to neurogenic detrusor overactivity: a randomised, double–blind, placebo–controlled trial. *Eur Urol.* 2011;**60**(4):742–750.

30 Herschorn S, Gajewski J, Ethans K, et al. Efficacy of botulinum toxin A injection for neurogenic detrusor overactivity and urinary incontinence: a randomized, double–blind trial. *J Urol.* 2011;**185**(6):2229–2235.

31 Ginsberg D, Gousse A, Keppenne V, et al., Phase 3 efficacy and tolerability study of onabotulinumtoxinA for urinary incontinence from neurogenic detrusor overactivity. *J Urol.* 2012;**187**(6):2131–2139.

32 Apostolidis A, Thompson C, Yan X, Mourad S. An exploratory, placebo–controlled, dose–response study of the efficacy and safety of onabotulinumtoxinA in spinal cord injury patients with urinary incontinence due to neurogenic detrusor overactivity. *World J Urol.* 2013 Dec;**31**(6):1469–1474.

33 Giannantoni A, Di Stasi SM, Stephen RL, et al. Intravesical resiniferatoxin versus botulinum–A toxin injections for neurogenic detrusor overactivity: a prospective randomized study. *J Urol.* 2004;**172**(1):240–243.

34 Chen YC, Kuo HC. The therapeutic effects of repeated detrusor injections between 200 or 300 units of onabotulinumtoxina in chronic spinal cord injured patients. *Neurourol Urodyn.* 2014 Jan;**33**(1):129–134.

35 Grosse J, Kramer G, Jakse G. Comparing two types of botulinum-A toxin detrusor injections in patients with severe neurogenic detrusor overactivity: a case-control study. *BJU Int.* 2009;**104**(5):651–656.

36 Grise P, Ruffion A, Denys P, et al. Efficacy and tolerability of botulinum toxin type A in patients with neurogenic detrusor overactivity and without concomitant anticholinergic therapy: comparison of two doses. *Eur Urol.* 2010;**58**(5):759–766.

37 Abdel-Meguid TA. Botulinum toxin–A injections into neurogenic overactive bladder—to include or exclude the trigone? A prospective, randomized, controlled trial. *J Urol.* 2010; **184**(6):2423–2428.

38 Krhut J, Samal V, Nemec D, Zvara P. Intradetrusor versus suburothelial onabotulinumtoxinA injections for neurogenic

detrusor overactivity: a pilot study. *Spinal Cord* 2012;**50**(12):904–907.

39 Gomes CM, de Castro Filho JE, Rejowski RF, et al. Experience with different botulinum toxins for the treatment of refractory neurogenic detrusor overactivity. *Int Braz J Urol.* 2010;**36**(1):66–74.

40 Kalsi V, Apostolidis A, Gonzales G, et al. Early effect on the overactive bladder symptoms following botulinum neurotoxin type A injections for detrusor overactivity. *Eur Urol.* 2008;**54**: 181–187.

41 Grosse J, Kramer G, Stohrer M. Success of repeat detrusor injections of botulinum A toxin in patients with severe neurogenic detrusor overactivity and incontinence. *Eur Urol.* 2005;**47**(5):653–659.

42 Karsenty G, Reitz A, Lindemann G. Persistence of therapeutic effect after repeated injections of botulinum toxin type A to treat incontinence due to neurogenic detrusor overactivity. *Urology* 2006;**68**(6):1193–1197.

43 Reitz A, Denys P, Fermanian C, et al. Do repeat intradetrusor botulinum toxin type A injections yield valuable results? Clinical and urodynamic results after five injections in patients with neurogenic detrusor overactivity. *Eur Urol.* 2007;**52**(6):1729–1735.

44 Del Popolo G, Filocamo MT, Li Marzi V, et al., Neurogenic detrusor overactivity treated with english botulinum toxin A: 8-year experience of one single centre. *Eur Urol.* 2008;**53**(5): 1013–1020.

45 Stoehrer M, Wolff A, Kramer G, et al., Treatment of neurogenic detrusor overactivity with botulinum toxin A: the first seven years. *Urol Int.* 2009;**83**(4):379–385.

46 Giannantoni A, Mearini E, Del Zingaro M, Porena M. Six-year follow-up of botulinum toxin A intradetrusorial injections in patients with refractory neurogenic detrusor overactivity: clinical and urodynamic results. *Eur Urol.* 2009;**55**(3):705–711.

47 Ghalayini IF, Al-Ghazo MA, Elnasser ZA. Is efficacy of repeated intradetrusor botulinum toxin type A (Dysport((R))) injections dose dependent? Clinical and urodynamic results after four injections in patients with drug-resistant neurogenic detrusor overactivity. *Int Urol Nephrol.* 2009;**41**(4):805–813.

48 Khan S, Game X, Kalsi V, et al. Long–term effect on quality of life of repeat detrusor injections of botulinum neurotoxin A for detrusor overactivity in patients with multiple sclerosis. *J Urol.* 2011;**185**(4): 1344–1349.

49 Kuo HC, Liu SH. Effect of repeated detrusor onabotulinumtoxinA injections on bladder and renal function in patients with chronic spinal cord injuries. *Neurourol Urodyn.* 2011;**30**(8):1541–1545.

50 Kalsi V, Apostolidis A, Popat R et al. Quality of life changes in patients with neurogenic versus idiopathic detrusor overactivity after intradetrusor injections of botulinum neurotoxin type A and correlations with lower urinary tract symptoms and urodynamic changes. *Eur Urol.* 2006;**49**(3):528–535.

51 Reitz A, Stohrer M, Kramer G, et al. European experience of 200 cases treated with Botulinum–A toxin injections into the detrusor muscle for urinary incontinence due to neurogenic detrusor overactivity. *Eur Urol.* 2004;**45**:510–515.

52 Sievert KD, Heesakkers J, Ginsberg D. Efficacy of onabotulinumtoxinA in neurogenic detrusor overactivity is independent of concomitant anticholinergic use. *Eur Urol.* 2012; suppi: **11**:e461.

53 Deffontaines-Rufin S, Weil M, Verollet D, et al. Botulinum toxin A for the treatment of neurogenic detrusor overactivity in multiple sclerosis patients. *Int Braz J Urol.* 2011;**37** (5):642–648.

54 Schulte-Baukloh H, Bigalke H, Miller K. et al., Botulinum neurotoxin type A in urology: antibodies as a cause of therapy failure. *Int J Urol.* 2008;**15**(5):407–415; discussion 415.

55 Naumann M, Carruthers A, Carruthers J, et al., Meta-analysis of neutralizing antibody conversion with onabotulinumtoxinA (BOTOX(R)) across multiple indications. *Mov Disord.* 2010;**25**(13):2211–2218.

56 Hegele A, Frohme C, Varga Z, et al. Antibodies after botulinum toxin A injection into musculus detrusor vesicae: incidence and clinical relevance. *Urol Int.* 2011;**87**(4):439–444.

57 Schulte-Baukloh H, Herholz J, Bigalke H, et al. Results of a BoNT/A antibody study in children and adolescents after onabotulinumtoxin

A (Botox(R)) detrusor injection. *Urol Int.* 2011; **87**(4):434–438.

58 Kajbafzadeh AM, Nikfarjam L, Mahboubi AH, Dianat S. Antibody formation following botulinum toxin type A (dysport) injection in children with intractable bladder hyperreflexia. *Urology* 2010;**76**(1):233–237.

59 Giannantoni A, Rossi A, Mearini S, et al. Botulinum toxin A for overactive bladder and detrusor muscle overactivity in patients with Parkinson's disease and multiple system atrophy. *J Urol.* 2009;**182**(4):1453–1457.

60 Kulaksizoglu H, Parman Y. Use of botulinim toxin–A for the treatment of overactive bladder symptoms in patients with Parkinsons's disease. *Parkinsonism Relat Disord.* 2010;**16**(8):531–534.

61 Giannantoni A, Conte A, Proietti S, et al. Botulinum toxin type A in patients with Parkinson's disease and refractory overactive bladder. *J Urol.* 2011;**186**(3):960–964.

62 Kuo, HC. Therapeutic effects of suburothelial injection of botulinum A toxin for neurogenic detrusor overactivity due to chronic cerebrovascular accident and spinal cord lesions. *Urology* 2006;**67**(2):232–236.

63 Kalsi V, Gonzales G, Popat R, et al. Botulinum injections for the treatment of bladder symptoms of multiple sclerosis. *Ann Neurol.* 2007;**62**(5):452–457.

64 Schurch B, Denys P, Kozma CM, et al. Botulinum toxin A improves the quality of life of patients with neurogenic urinary incontinence. *Eur Urol.* 2007;**52**(3):850–858.

65 Mehnert U, Birzele J, Reuter K, Schurch B, The effect of botulinum toxin type A on overactive bladder symptoms in patients with multiple sclerosis: a pilot study. *J Urol.* 2011;**184**(3):1011–1016.

66 Ruffion A, Capelle O, Paparel P, et al. What is the optimum dose of type A botulinum toxin for treating neurogenic bladder overactivity? *BJU Int.* 2006;**97**(5):1030–1034.

67 Karsenty G, Carsenac A, Boy S, et al. Botulinum toxin– A (BTA) in the treatment of neurogenic detrudor overcativity (NDOI)– A prospective randomized study to compare 30 vs. 10 injection sites. *Eur Urol.* 2007;**2**:245.

68 Schurch B, Stohrer M, Kramer G, et al. Botulinum–A toxin for treating detrusor hyper-

reflexia in spinal cord injured patients: a new alternative to anticholinergic drugs? *Preliminary results. J Urol.* 2000;**164**(3 Pt 1):692–697.

69 Harper M, Popat R, DasGupta R, et al. A minimally invasive technique for outpatient local anaesthetic administration of intradetrusor botulinum toxin in intractable detrusor overactivity. *BJU Int.* 2003;**92**:325–326.

70 Schulte-Baukloh H, Knispel HH. A minimally invasive technique for outpatient local anaesthetic administration of intradetrusor botulinum toxin in intractable detrusor overactivity. *BJU Int.* 2005;**95**(3):454.

71 Chuang YC, Tyagi P, Huang CC, et al. Urodynamic and immunohistochemical evaluation of intravesical botulinum toxin A delivery using liposomes. *J Urol.* 2009;**182**(2):786–792.

72 Kajbafzadeh AM, Montaser-Kouhsari L, Ahmadi H, Sotoudeh M, Intravesical electromotive botulinum toxin type A administration: part I—Experimental study. *Urology* 2011;**77**(6):1460–1464.

73 Kajbafzadeh AM, Ahmadi H, Montaser–Kouhsari L, et al. Intravesical electromotive botulinum toxin type A administration–part ii: clinical application. *Urology* 2011;**77**(2):439–445.

74 Gamé X, Bentaleb Y, Thiry–Escudie I, et al. Detrusor injections of Botulinum toxin A in patients with neurogenic detrusor overactivity significantly decrease the incidence of symptomatic urinary tract infections. *Eur Urol.* 2006;**49**(4): suppl. 1 (A1107).

75 Wefer B, Ehlken B, Bremer J, et al. Treatment outcomes and resource use of patients with neurogenic detrusor overactivity receiving botulinum toxin A (BOTOX) therapy in Germany. *World J Urol.* 2010;**28**(3):385–390.

76 De Laet K, Wyndaele JJ. Adverse events after botulinum A toxin injection for neurogenic voiding disorders. *Spinal Cord* 2005;**43**(7):397–399.

77 Caremel R, Courtois F, Charvier K. Side effects of intradetrusor botulinum toxin injections on ejaculation and fertility in men with spinal cord injury: preliminary findings. *BJU Int.* 2012 Jun;**109**(11):1698–1702.

78 Mascarenhas F, Cocuzza M, Gomes CM, Leao N. Trigonal injection of botulinum toxin–A does not

cause vesicoureteral reflux in neurogenic patients. *Neurourol Urodyn.* 2008;**27**(4):311–314.

79 Alloussi SH, Lang C, Eichel R, et al. Videourodynamic changes of botulinum toxin A in patients with neurogenic bladder dysfunction (NBD) and idiopathic detrusor overactivity (IDO) refractory to drug treatment. *World J Urol.* 2012 Jun;**30**(3): 367–373.

80 Girlanda P, Vita G, Nicolosi C, et al. Botulinum toxin therapy: distant effects on neuromuscular transmission and autonomic nervous system. *J Neurol Neurosurg Psychiatry* 1992;**55**: 844–845.

81 Dutton JJ. Botulinum–A toxin in the treatment of craniocervical muscle spasms: short– and long–term, local and systemic effects. *Surv Ophthalmol.* 1996;**41**:51–65.

82 Elkelini MS, Bagli DJ, Fehlings M, Hassouna M. Effects of intravesical onabotulinumtoxinA on bladder dysfunction and autonomic dysreflexia after spinal cord injury: role of nerve growth factor. *BJU Int.* 2012;**109**(3):402–407.

83 Schnitzler A, Genet F, Durand MC, et al. Pilot study evaluating the safety of intradetrusor injections of botulinum toxin type A: investigation of generalized spread using single–fiber EMG. *Neurourol Urodyn.* 2011; **30**(8):1533–1537.

84 Comperat E, Reitz A, Delcourt A, et al. Histologic features in the urinary bladder wall affected from neurogenic overactivity – a comparison of inflammation, oedema and fibrosis with and without injection of botulinum toxin type A. *Eur Urol.* 2006;**50** (5):1058–1064.

85 Apostolidis A, Jacques TS, Freeman A, et al. Histological changes in the urothelium and suburothelium of human overactive bladder following intradetrusor injections of botulinum neurotoxin type A for the treatment of neurogenic or idiopathic detrusor overactivity. *Eur Urol.* 2008;**53**(6):1245–1253.

86 Pascali MP, Mosiello G, Boldrini R et al. Effects of botulinum toxin type A in the bladder wall of children with neurogenic bladder dysfunction: a comparison of histological features before and after injections. *J Urol.* 2011;**185**(6 Suppl):2552–2557.

87 Kessler TM, Khan S, Panicker JN, et al., In the human urothelium and suburothelium, intra-detrusor botulinum neurotoxin type A does not induce apoptosis: preliminary results. *Eur Urol.* 2010;**57**(5):879–883.

88 Sahai A, Khan MS, Dasgupta P. Efficacy of botulinum toxin–A for treating idiopathic detrusor overactivity: results from a single center, randomized, double–blind, placebo con-trolled trial. *J Urol.* 2007;**177**(6):2231–2236.

89 Brubaker L, Richter HE, Visco A, et al. Refractory idiopathic urge urinary inconti-nence and botulinum A injection. *J Urol.* 2008;**180**(1): 217–222.

90 Flynn MK, Amundsen CL, Perevich M, et al. Outcome of a randomized, double–blind, placebo controlled trial of botulinum A toxin for refractory overactive bladder. *J Urol.* 2009;**181**(6):2608–2615.

91 Dmochowski R, Chapple C, Nitti VW, et al. Efficacy and safety of onabotulinumtoxinA for idiopathic overactive bladder: a double–blind, placebo controlled, randomized, dose ranging trial. *J Urol.* 2010;**184**(6): 2416–2422.

92 Rovner E, Kennelly M, Schulte-Baukloh H, et al. Urodynamic results and clinical outcomes with intradetrusor injections of onabotu-linumtoxinA in a randomized, placebo–controlled dose–finding study in idiopathic overactive bladder. *Neurourol Urodyn.* 2011;**30** (4):556–562.

93 Tincello DG, Kenyon S, Abrams KR, et al., Botulinum toxin A versus placebo for refractory detrusor overactivity in women: a randomised blinded placebo-controlled trial of 240 women (the RELAX Study). *Eur Urol.* 2012;**62**: 507–514.

94 Denys P, Le Normand L, Ghout I, et al., Efficacy and safety of low doses of onabotu-linumtoxinA for the treatment of refractory idiopathic overactive bladder: a multicentre, double–blind, randomised, placebo-controlled dose-ranging study. *Eur Urol.* 2012;**61**(3): 520–529.

95 Visco AG, Brubaker L, Richter HE, et al., Anticholinergic therapy vs. onabotulinumtox-ina for urgency urinary incontinence. *N Engl J Med.* 2012;**367**(19):1803–1813.

96 Chapple C, Sievert KD, Macdiarmid S, et al. OnabotulinumtoxinA 100 U significantly improves all idiopathic overactive bladder

symptoms and quality of life in patients with overactive bladder and urinary incontinence: a randomised, double-blind, placebo-controlled trial. *Eur Urol*. 2013;**64**(2): 249–256.

97 Nitti VW, Dmochowski R, Herschorn S, et al. OnabotulinumtoxinA for the treatment of patients with overactive bladder and urinary incontinence: results of a phase 3, randomized, placebo controlled trial. *J Urol*. 2013;**189**(6): p. 2186–2193.

98 Sahai A, Dowson C, Khan MS, Dasgupta P. Improvement in quality of life after botulinum toxin–A injections for idiopathic detrusor overactivity: results from a randomized double-blind placebo-controlled trial. *BJU Int*. 2009;**103**(11):1509–1515.

99 Fowler CJ, Auerbach S, Ginsberg D, et al., OnabotulinumtoxinA improves health-related quality of life in patients with urinary incontinence due to idiopathic overactive bladder: a 36-week, double-blind, placebo-controlled, randomized, dose-ranging trial. *Eur Urol*. 2012;**62**(1):148–157.

100 Schmid DM, Sauermann P, Werner M et al., Experience with 100 cases treated with botulinum–A toxin injections in the detrusor muscle for idiopathic overactive bladder syndrome refractory to anticholinergics. *J Urol*. 2006;**176**(1):177–185.

101 Altaweel W, Mokhtar A, Rabah DM. Prospective randomized trial of 100u vs 200u Botox in the treatment of idiopathic overactive bladder. *Urol Ann*. 2011;**3**(2):66–70.

102 Gousse AE, Kanagarajah P, Ayyathurai R, et al. Repeat intradetrusor injections of onabotulinum toxin A for refractory idiopathic overactive bladder patients: a single–center experience. *Female Pelvic Med Reconstr Surg*, 2011;**17**(5): 253–257.

103 Jabs C, Carleton E. Efficacy of botulinum toxin A intradetrusor injections for non–neurogenic urinary urge incontinence: a randomized double–blind controlled trial. *J Obstet Gynaecol Can*. 2013;**35**(1):53–60.

104 Kuo HC, Bladder base/trigone injection is safe and as effective as bladder body injection of onabotulinumtoxinA for idiopathic detrusor overactivity refractory to antimuscarinics. *Neurourol Urodyn*. 2011;**30**(7): 1242–1248.

105 Digesu GA, Panayi D, Hendricken C, et al. Women's perspective of botulinum toxin treatment for overactive bladder symptoms. *Int Urogynecol J*. 2011;**22**(4): 425–431.

106 Kessler TM, Danuser H, Schumacher M, et al. Botulinum A toxin injections into the detrusor: an effective treatment in idiopathic and neurogenic detrusor overactivity? *Neurourol Urodyn*. 2005;**24**(3):231–236.

107 Ghalayini IF, Al-Ghazo MA, Intradetrusor injection of botulinum–A toxin in patients with idiopathic and neurogenic detrusor overactivity: urodynamic outcome and patient satisfaction. *Neurourol Urodyn*. 2007;**26**(4):531–536.

108 Popat R, Apostolidis A, Kalsi V, et al. A Comparison between the response of patients with idiopathic detrusor overactivity and neurogenic detrusor overactivity to the first intradetrusor injection of botulinum-A toxin. *J Urol*. 2005;**174**(3):984–988.

109 White WM, Pickens RB, Doggweiler R, Klein FA. Short-term efficacy of botulinum toxin A for refractory overactive bladder in the elderly population. *J Urol*. 2008;**180**(6):2522–2526.

110 Dowson C, Watkins J, Khan MS, et al. Repeated botulinum toxin type A injections for refractory overactive bladder: medium–term outcomes, safety profile, and discontinuation rates. *Eur Urol*. 2012;**61**(4):834–839.

111 Khan S, Kessler TM, Apostolidis A, et al. What a patient with refractory idiopathic detrusor overactivity should know about botulinum neurotoxin type A injection. *J Urol*. 2009;**181**(4):1773–1778.

112 Rapp DE, Lucioni A, Katz EE, et al. Use of botulinum-A toxin for the treatment of refractory overactive bladder symptoms: an initial experience. *Urology* 2004;**63**: 1071–1075.

113 Khan S, Panicker J, Roosen A, et al. Complete continence after botulinum neurotoxin type A injections for refractory idiopathic detrusor overactivity incontinence: patient–reported outcome at 4 weeks. *Eur Urol*. 2010;**57**(5): 891–896.

114 Cohen BL, Barboglio P, Rodriguez D, Gousse AE. Preliminary results of a dose–finding study for botulinum toxin–A in patients with idiopathic overactive bladder: 100 versus

150 units. *Neurourol Urodyn.* 2009;**28**(3): 205–208.

115 Kanagarajah P, Ayyathurai R, Caruso DJ, et al. Role of botulinum toxin–A in refractory idiopathic overactive bladder patients without detrusor overactivity. *Int Urol Nephrol.* 2011;**44**(1): 91–97.

116 Makovey I, Davis T, Guralnick ML, O'Connor RC. Botulinum toxin outcomes for idiopathic overactive bladder stratified by indication: lack of anticholinergic efficacy versus intolerability. *Neurourol Urodyn.* 2011;**30**(8):1538–1540.

117 Kessler TM, Khan S, Panicker J, et al. Clean intermittent self–catheterization after botulinum neurotoxin type A injections: short–term effect on quality of life. *Obstet Gynecol.* 2009;**113**(5):1046–1051.

118 Cohen BL, Caruso DJ, Kanagarajah P, Gousse AE. Predictors of response to intradetrusor botulinum toxin–A injections in patients with idiopathic overactive bladder. *Adv Urol.* 2009: 328364.

119 Sahai A, Khan MS, Le Gall N, Dasgupta P. Urodynamic assessment of poor responders after botulinum toxin–A treatment for over-active bladder. *Urology* 2008;**71**(3):455–459.

120 Kuo HC, Liao CH, Chung SD. Adverse events of intravesical botulinum toxin A injections for idiopathic detrusor overactivity: risk factors and influence on treatment outcome. *Eur Urol.* 2010;**58**(6): 919–926.

121 Manecksha RP, Cullen IM, Ahmad S, et al. Prospective randomised controlled trial comparing trigone-sparing versus trigone-including intradetrusor injection of abobotulinumtoxinA for refractory idiopathic detrusor overactivity. *Eur Urol.* 2012;**61**:928–935.

122 Karsenty G, Elzayat E, Delapparent T, et al. Botulinum toxin type A injections into the trigone to treat idiopathic overactive bladder do not induce vesicoureteral reflux. *J Urol,* 2007;**177**(3):1011–1014.

123 Sahai A, Sangster P, Kalsi V, et al. Assessment of urodynamic and detrusor contractility variables in patients with overactive bladder syndrome treated with botulinum toxin–A: is incomplete bladder emptying predictable? *BJU Int.* 2009;**103**(5):630–634.

124 Kalsi V, Popat RB, Apostolidis A, et al. Cost–consequence analysis evaluating the use of botulinum neurotoxin–A in patients with detrusor overactivity based on clinical outcomes observed at a single UK centre. *Eur Urol.* 2006;**49**(3):519–527.

125 Wefer B, Ehlken B, Bremer J, et al., Treatment outcomes and resource use of patients with neurogenic detrusor overactivity receiving botulinum toxin A (BOTOX((R))) therapy in Germany. *World J Urol.* 2010;**28**(3): 385–390.

126 Padmanabhan P, Scarpero HM, Milam DF, et al. Five–year cost analysis of intra–detrusor injection of botulinum toxin type A and augmentation cystoplasty for refractory neuro-genic detrusor overactivity. *World J Urol.* 2011;**29**(1): 51–57.

127 Watanabe, JH, Campbell JD, Ravelo A, et al. Cost analysis of interventions for anti-muscarinic refractory patients with overactive bladder. *Urology* 2010;**76**(4):835–840.

128 Leong RK, de Wachter SG, Joore MA, van Kerrebroeck PE. Cost–effectiveness analysis of sacral neuromodulation and botulinum toxin A treatment for patients with idiopathic overactive bladder. *BJU Int.* 2011;**108**(4): 558–564.

129 Arlandis S, Castro D, Errando C, et al. Cost–effectiveness of sacral neuromodulation compared to botulinum neurotoxin A or continued medical management in refractory overactive bladder. *Value Health* 2011;**14** (2):219–228.

SECTION 6
Surgery

CHAPTER 17

Surgical treatment for overactive bladder

Jerzy B. Gajewski and Fadi Sawaqed

Dalhousie University, Halifax, Canada

> **KEY POINTS**
>
> - Surgical treatment for OAB is reserved for refractory cases.
> - Careful consideration should be given to the patient's medical condition, needs, and expectations.
> - Bladder augmentation is the most commonly utilized technique.
> - Complications and consequences of surgery can be significant and should be discussed extensively with the patient before surgery.

Surgical treatment for OAB is reserved only for patients who fail all previous conservative managements. The surgical intervention should be tailored to the patient's bladder condition, overall medical status, physical abilities, and expectations. The patient should understand the consequences and possible complications of the procedure. This chapter will only discuss surgical treatment in adults.

Bladder augmentation

Several different surgical procedures have been utilized, however the most prevalent is bladder augmentation. The first ileocystoplasty was performed in dogs by Tizzoni in 1888. [1] Shortly after, it was followed by cystoplasty in humans, reported by Mikulicz in 1899. [2] It was not often used until the 1950s, when Couvelaire popularized it for the treatment of the small contracted tuberculous bladder. [3] Augmentation cystoplasty was introduced for idiopathic detrusor overactivity by Bramble et al. in 1982. [4] Fifteen adult patients with enuresis and/or severe urgency incontinence were treated by a modified form of enterocystoplasty, using sigmoid colon or ileum. Satisfactory results were obtained in 13 patients, who were dry both by day and by night.

Since then, many different surgeons have carried out augmentation for a variety of indications, using many different types of bowel segments like the stomach, the ileum, the caecum, and the ascending and sigmoid colon. [5] All have been used as

Overactive Bladder: Practical Management, First Edition. Edited by Jacques Corcos, Scott MacDiarmid and John Heesakkers.
© 2015 John Wiley & Sons, Ltd. Published 2015 by John Wiley & Sons, Ltd.

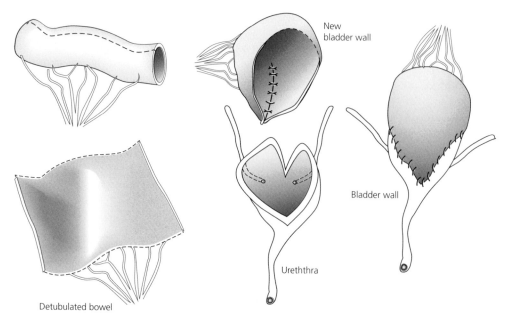

New bladder wall

Bladder wall

Ureththra

Detubulated bowel

Figure 17.1 "Clam" ileocystoplasty. Source: www.springerimages.com.

tubular or detubularized, simple or complex segments. Mundy et al. described "Clam" ileocystoplasty (Figure 17.1) for treatment of refractory urgency incontinence. [6] The success rate was 75%. Six patients were cured of their symptoms but needed clean intermittent catheterization (CIC) and four had their symptoms significantly improved by the operation. Authors also noticed that bladder compliance usually improved with the operation and detrusor overactivity was either abolished or reduced to an insignificant level. Voiding dysfunction, however, is a common postoperative problem and must be identified and treated.

Augmentation enterocystoplasty is usually done with the intraperitoneal approach. The "extraperitoneal" approach involves a small peritoneotomy to obtain the segment of bowel for augmentation. Reyblat et al. [7] compared operative and post-operative parameters and clinical outcomes of these two techniques. Patients in the extraperitoneal group had significantly shorter operative times (3.9 vs. 5.6 h); shorter hospital stays (8.0 vs. 10.5 days); and shorter waiting periods for the return of bowel function (3.5 vs. 4.9 days). There was no significant difference in complication rates. Post-operative continence was equally improved in both groups.

Ileocystoplasty is usually performed as an open surgical procedure. Recently however, with the advances in technology, laparoscopic [8] and robotic cystoplasty [9] have been introduced. Animal data indicate similar outcomes between open and robotic-assisted ileocystoplasty but incidences of complex adhesions post-surgery favor the robotic approach. [10]

Some series report mixed populations of idiopathic and neurogenic patients treated with clam cystoplasty. [11] After a clam enterocystoplasty, only half of the patients became dry and appliance-free.

The magnitude of the surgery and the voiding dysfunction associated with the relative lack of motivation of elderly patients made the operation less successful and more hazardous in those over the age of 65.

The Hasan et al. [12] study comprised 48 patients who underwent enterocystoplasty for idiopathic detrusor overactivity or neurogenic detrusor overactivity. Early symptomatic outcome was good in 83% of the patients. Nottingham Health Profile (NHP) scores revealed significant improvements in all domains. Long-term outcomes were less satisfactory, with recurrent urinary tract infections (UTI) in 37% of the patients, a need for long-term antibiotic therapy in 15%, and a change in bowel habits in 33%. Clean intermittent self catheterization (CISC) was performed in 85% of patients. The long-term outcome was better for neurogenic detrusor overactivity than idiopathic, 92 and 58% respectively.

Enterocystoplasty can also be used as a part of complex interventions. Lewis et al. [13] reviewed mixed-patient populations (78 patients) who underwent "clam" enterocystoplasty. Nearly half were non-neurogenic. Most patients were operated on for incontinence but 12 had upper tract damage, related either to urinary diversion or to poor bladder compliance in the early phase of filling. After surgery, most of the patients became dry (69). Some patients (30) voided spontaneously, (17) by activation of an artificial urinary sphincter or by self-intermittent catheterization (22). Four patients continued to have nocturnal enuresis, three diurnal enuresis, and two stress incontinence. One patient had a continent diversion.

In another report of mixed pathology, [14] 122 augmentation cystoplasties performed over an eight-year period were reviewed. The primary urodynamic diagnosis was reduced compliance in 92 (77%) patients and detrusor hyperreflexia/instability in the remainder. The clinical diagnostic groups were: spinal cord injury/disease in 32 (27%), myelodysplasia in 27 (22%), interstitial cystitis in 21 (17%), idiopathic detrusor instability in 13 (11%), radiation cystitis in 8 (7%), Hinman-Allen syndrome in 5 (4%), and miscellaneous in 11 (9%). A detubularized ileal or sigmoid augmentation was used in 82 (67%) patients. In 19 patients, augmentation accompanied undiversion. Sixteen patients had a simultaneous fascial sling for urethral incompetence. Bladder capacity was increased from a preoperative mean of 108 ml (range 15–500 ml) to 438 ml (200–1200 ml) post-operatively. Of the 106 assessable patients, 75% had excellent results.

A retrospective study on 32 patients with suprasacral spinal cord injury and neurogenic detrusor overactivity showed resolution of the incontinence in all patients with the follow-up of six years. An improvement in quality-of-life parameters was reported in 96.2%. Pre-operative vesico-ureteric reflux resolved completely in four out of five patients and improved from grade IV to grade II in one. [15]

The Goodwin "cup-patch technique" (Figure 17.2) uses an ileal segment, opened along its antimesenteric border and folded twice for bladder augmentation. [16] Nine patients with MS received surgical treatment using this technique. Outcomes included improvement in bladder capacity and resolution of vesico-ureteral reflux and improvement in renal function. [17] This technique is now widely used.

In the case of severe detrusor hypertrophy, supratrigonal cystectomy combined with cystoplasty can be considered.

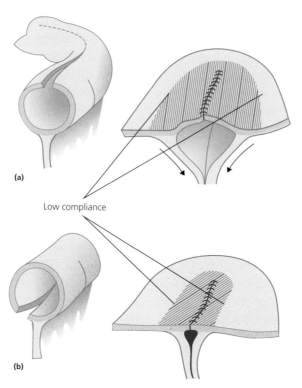

(a)

Low compliance

(b)

Figure 17.2 The low-compliance area is shown after antemesenteric (**a**) and perimesenteric (**b**) transection of the ileal segment. *BJU International*, Volume 88, Issue 6, pages 577–580, October 2001. Source: Reproduced with permission of John Wiley & Sons Ltd.

Ureteric reimplantation at the time of cystoplasty is mostly utilized in children, providing an 85% resolution of the reflux and acceptable morbidity. [18]

Long-term urodynamic outcome in 26 patients with neurogenic voiding dysfunction, who underwent augmentation enterocystoplasty alone or in conjunction with various continence or antireflux techniques showed good results. All but one patient (96%) in the series had near or complete resolution of urinary incontinence and mean total bladder capacity increased from 201 to 615 ml and mean maximum detrusor pressure decreased from 81 to 20 cm H_2O. [19]

Augmentation ileocystoplasty is a valuable alternative for patients with intrac-table urgency incontinence. However, these patients and their physicians should be aware of its limitations, specifically the possibility that incontinence may persist and the high probability of the need for self-catheterization, with potential subsequent urinary tract infection. [20] Contraindications to perform ileocystoplasty include significant inflammatory bowel disease or dysfunction and the inability to perform CIC.

Using an appropriate questionnaire in spinal cord injured patients, Khastgir et al. have found high patient-satisfaction rates in augmentation cystoplasty in addition to successful surgical outcomes. [15]

Different segments have been used by some centers; however, they have never

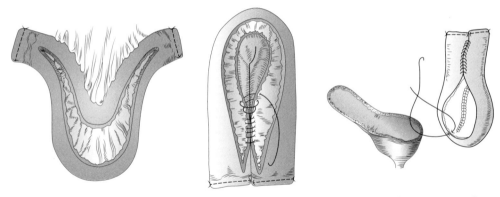

Figure 17.3 Sigmoid augmentation cystoplasty. http://emedicine.medscape.com/article/443916-overview. Source: Reproduced with permission of Medscape Reference (http://emedicine.medscape.com/).

reached the popularity of the ileal pouch. A sigmoid colon segment fashioned into a cup-patch and detubularized cecum was used for augmentation cystoplasty in neurogenic patients. Some patients had an additional artificial urinary sphincter implanted. There was a good clinical outcome in most patients after 15 months. [5]

Enterocystoplasty with ileum, cecum, and sigmoid (Fig 17.3) in combination with different surgical techniques has been used to prevent upper tract deterioration or urinary incontinence. In general, there was little difference in outcome with regard to which part of the bowel was used. [21] In a retrospective review, the sigmoid colon showed a trend towards a lower rate of small bowel obstruction with no difference in perforation or stone formation compared with ileum. [22] A good reservoir capacity can be achieved with both ileum and sigmoid post-operatively. However, ileum provided lower reservoir pressures and better compliance. Detubularized ileum seems to be better-suited than sigmoid for augmentation cystoplasty in patients with neurogenic bladder dysfunction. [23]

Biomaterials for cystoplasty have been used on an experimental basis. Only two pilot studies have been conducted with some promising results up to two years' follow-up. Clearly, more extensive trials must be conducted before this technique can be considered for routine surgical procedures. [24]

UDS evaluation post-augmentation

Urodynamic studies after augmentation enterocystoplasty, in comparison to patients without surgical intervention, showed larger maximal cystometry capacity, lower detrusor pressure, and improvement in bladder compliance. [19, 25] Detrusor overactivity may persist in some patients. [12]

Urinary incontinence may be secondary to poor sphincteric function in patients with and without prior augmentation. Strict follow-up of the patients after augmentation enterocystoplasty is necessary. [23] It was suggested that detrusor pressure <20 cm H_2O after augmentation surgery in myelodysplasia may predict better outcomes with regard to continence. [26] Long-term (6.3 yrs) follow-up in a single institution prospective study showed an 89% continence rate with clean intermittent catheterization (CIC), an increase in MCC, and a decrease in end filling pressure. [27]

A review of urodynamic findings in 23 "Clam" enterocystoplasty patients, [28] mostly with neurogenic detrusor overactivity and poor compliance, showed a significant improvement in bladder pressure in all but two patients. Overall, a long-term satisfactory outcome was achieved in 78% of patients.

Artificial urethral sphincter and augmentation

Successful outcomes could be improved by careful patient selection and by performing an anti-stress incontinence procedure, such as the implantation of an artificial urinary sphincter cuff or a cystourethropexy, where there is associated bladder outlet incompetence. Augmentation surgery can be combined with the insertion of an artificial urinary sphincter. Catto et al. reported a total of 108 sphincters failed due to infection (25%), tissue atrophy (5%), or mechanical reasons (25%). The overall infective failure rate was similar in patients who underwent simultaneous augmentation (30%), compared with the other patients (23%), although there was a statistically significant difference within the first three post-operative years. [29] Mor et al. implanted an artificial urinary sphincter cuff with augmentation cystoplasty in a mixed patient population and reported an 82% continence rate. [30] Venn and Mundy reported a 78% continence rate

with cystoplasty alone in patients with neuropathic bladders, increasing to 90% with the addition of an artificial urinary sphincter. The patients undergoing cystoplasty and AUS implantation for idiopathic detrusor overactivity had a 93% continence rate. [31] In another report, >90% continence was achieved in neurogenic patients after simultaneous cystoplasty and implantation of an AUS. [32]

Complications

Augmentation cystoplasty is associated with numerous possible complications and consequences. Post-surgery mortality has been calculated to be between 0% and 3.2%. [33, 34] Beyond obvious complications associated with anesthesia and open surgery, several specific problems involving ileocystoplasty have been reported. Small bowel obstruction, anastomotic leak, and wound-healing issues have been reported in between 2–6%. [35]

Voiding dysfunction is probably the most common complication, often by design. Bowel pouch and bladder wall division contribute to a decrease of detrusor contractility. Some patients can void spontaneously but the majority, especially patients with neurogenic bladder overactivity, need clean intermittent catheterization (CIC). [32]

Late complications (>30 days) include incisional hernia, anastomotic perforation, calculus formation, and urethral stricture. [20] Revision rate may be as high as 16%. Urinary incontinence may manifest in 13% of patients with half of these requiring surgical treatment. Pyelonephritis occurred in 11% patients. Reservoir rupture is rare, occurring in 4–13% of patients. [12, 36]

It is a serious and life-threatening complication. [37, 38]

Chronic bowel problems (20–50%) include diarrhea, fecal incontinence, and bowel movements at night. [30, 39] Irritable bowel syndrome is often associated with detrusor overactivity. Some of the bowel problems relate to the malabsorption of bile acid in the terminal ileum. Extended ileum resection to create the pouch may be a contributing factor. Giving cholestyramine sometimes improves bowel function. [40]

Vitamin B12 deficiency can develop due to resection of the terminal ileum. Therefore, it is imperative to leave 15–20 cm of the most distal terminal ileum to avoid this deficiency. Electrolyte abnormalities, more common in children, usually accompany ileal or cecum ileocystoplasty and manifest as a chloremic metabolic acidosis. Urea from the urine is metabolized into ammonium by bowel flora. The ammonium is then reabsorbed by the bowel pouch coupled with the loss of bicarbonates and metabolic acidosis. This leads to the net reabsorption of hydrogen ion, ammonium, and chloride. Renal potassium loss leads to hypokalemia, hypocalcemia, and hypomagnesemia. Good renal function and time (atrophy of bowel mucosa in the pouch) usually ameliorate electrolyte metabolisms.

Renal insufficiency may develop due to bacteriuria, chronic UTIs, vesicoureteral reflux, and unrecognized high-pressure bladder. [32, 41] It is independent from the bowel segment used for ileocystoplasty.

Stone formation in the bladder and upper urinary tract was reported in 9–15% of the patients after augmentation ileocystoplasty. [42] Patients on CIC, and those with incomplete emptying and UTIs with urease splitting bacteria, were at higher risk.

Mucus formation can be up to 40 gm [43] and contribute to voiding dysfunction, UTIs, stone formation, and even bladder perforations. Mucus production is more pronounced in colonic than ileal pouches. [44]

Asymptomatic bacteriuria is almost universal post ileocystoplasty because of strong adherence of the bacteria to bowel mucosa. It usually does not require treatment unless it is Proteus or Klebsiella bacteria. [45] Chronic bacteriuria has been considered as a risk factor for stone formation and voiding dysfunction. Prevalence of symptomatic UTIs requiring antibiotic range is from 5–40%. [32, 46]

Bladder cancer has been reported in patients with different cystoplasty procedures. [47] The incidence of bladder cancer, although higher than in the general population, is the same as in patients with neurogenic bladder. [48]

Detrusor myectomy autoaugmentation

Autoaugmentation (Fig 17.4) is achieved by removing the bladder muscle to allow the bladder mucosa to form a pseudo diverticulum. [49] This is a delicate procedure, requiring extensive removal of the detrusor. A large epithelial bulge is created, which functions to augment the storage properties of the bladder without using the bowel. It has been applied for both idiopathic and neurogenic OAB, although results are better in patients with idiopathic OAB. [49] Early reports were encouraging, and comparable to classical enterocystoplasty; [50, 51] however,

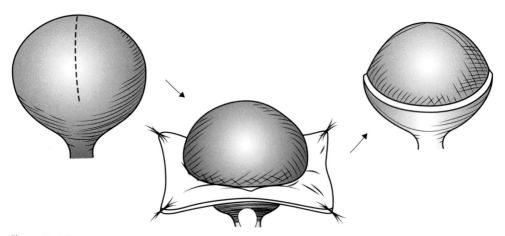

Figure 17.4 Detrusor myectomy. Ashraf Abou-Elela (2011). Source: Augmentation Cystoplasty: in Pretransplant Recepients, Understanding the Complexities of Kidney Transplantation, Prof. Jorge Ortiz (Ed.), ISBN: 978-953-307-819-9, InTech, Available from: http://www.intechopen.com/books/understanding-the-complexities-of-kidneytransplantation/augmentation-cystoplasty-in-pretransplant-recepients.

long-term outcomes were less satisfactory. [52–54] Almost half of the patients required clean intermittent self-catheterization afterward. [55]

Seromuscular enterocystoplasty (Fig 17.5) combines autoaugmentation with enterocystoplasty by covering the exposed mucosa-ony portion of the bladder with a detubularized segment of the bowel, devoid of mucosa. [56] The short-term outcomes are encouraging but the procedure is limited to specialized centers. [20] Overall, there is limited data to recommend autoaugmentation for adults.

Denervation procedures

Denervation procedures have been applied to idiopathic OAB, in general. Usually, bladder denervation can be accomplished with injection of anesthetic or ablative chemicals. Dilute phenol (6%) has been used for injection into the trigone. [57] Outcomes have been very

disappointing, sometimes resulting in horrific complications involving vesico-vaginal fistula. [58]

Another approach utilizes surgical dissection of the peripheral nerves (pelvic nerve). Ingelman-Sundberg denervation, which was initially described in 1959, [59] was performed during radical hysterectomy for motor urgency. In later years, it was modified to use a vaginal or combined vaginal and abdominal approach. [60] Although success rates were reported to be as high as 70%, there is a lack of long-term data. The denervation procedures have never achieved widespread popularity.

Sacral rhizotomy (S2-5), through an extra or intradural approach, has also been used for bladder deafferentation. The consequence of this procedure, however, is denervation of sphincteric and erectile function. It has been utilized with a Finetech-Brindley stimulator to overcome sphincteric activity during bladder contraction. [61] The complexity of the procedure

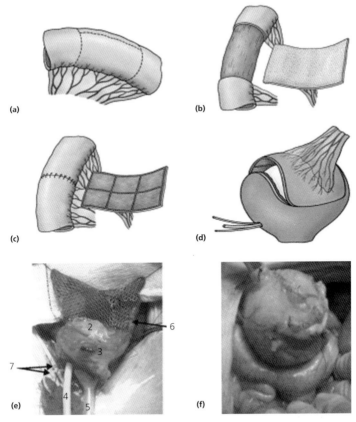

Figure 17.5 The different stages of composite cystoplasty. (a) To develop a vascularized, de-epithelialized seromuscular segement, a Foley catheter was inserted rectally and the balloon filled with sterile water within the portion of sigmoid bowel to be dissected. The dissection limits of the bowel and mesentery were defined. (b) Using the balloon as a support, the seromuscular layer of the bowel was incized and separated from the lamina propria deep to the mucosa. (c) The vascularized, deepithelialized patch was isolated and received the autologous tissue-engineered urothelial cell sheet in complex with the Vicryl mesh. The mesenteric fenestration was closed to prevent internal hernia. (d) The bladder was opened widely and augmented with the composite bowel segment. Gentle distension of the augmented bladder was maintained with a silicone vesical conformer. Urine was diverted post-operatively with ureteric stents and a Malecot suprapubic catheter. Stages (c) and (d), respectively, are illustrated in (e) and (f) during an actual composite cystoplasty operation. (e1) Patches of Vicryl mesh supporting urothelial cell sheets against de-epithelialized colon; (e2) vesical conformer (collapsed); (e3) opened native bladder; (e4) Malecot suprapubic catheter; (e5) filling tube for vesical conformer; (e6) detubularized colon; (e7) ureteric catheters. Turner A, Subramanian R, Thomas DF, Hinley J, Abbas SK, Stahlschmidt J, Southgate J. Transplantation of Autologous Differentiated Urothelium in an Experimental Model of Composite Cystoplasty, *J. Eur Urol*. 2011 Mar; 59(3):447–54. Source: Reproduced with permission of Elsevier. (For color detail, please see color plate section).

and technical challenges preclude this technique from gaining wide acceptance.

Cystolysis, described by Mundy, includes a transection of the posterior and postero-lateral aspects of the bladder wall with a successful outcome reported in 74% of cases. Because of late-stage bladder muscle atrophy the procedure has been abandoned. [62]

Urinary diversion

Urinary diversion is an ultimate and last-resort treatment for patients with detrusor overactivity. Cases that require this form of treatment are often related to neurogenic detrusor overactivity. It should be reserved for patients with significant upper urinary tract changes, refractory to other treatment modalities. It may also be suggested in cases involving significantly disabled quadriplegics. In some cases of detrusor overactivity, a continent diversion may be considered in those who are able to catheterize a continent stoma. Concomitant cystectomy should be contemplated at the same time as diversion surgery because of the high (20%) risk of pyocystis. [63]

Summary

Surgical intervention in patients with idiopathic or neurogenic detrusor overactivity is a valid therapeutic option and should be considered for refractory detrusor overactivity. Ileocystoplasty is considered to be the most effective, with minimal complications, although any segment of the bowel can be considered. It is difficult to provide recommendations for adults regarding gastrocystoplasty and ureterocystoplasty as data is insufficient. Denervation procedures have only historical value.

Careful consideration should be given to patients' overall medical condition, as well as to their family health caretakers' expectations. Discussion should include a detailed description of the surgical procedure and its possible complications and consequences. The cognitive status, dexterity, and mobility of patients should also be evaluated. The final decision regarding the type of procedure must be tailored to patients' needs and expectations as well as to the surgeon's familiarity and expertise.

References

1. Tizzoni G, Foggi A. Die wiederhestellung der harnblase. *Centralbl F Chir.* 1888; **15**:921–932.
2. Von Mikulicz J. Zur operation der angebarenen blaßen-Spalte. *Zentralbl Chir.* 1889; **20**:641–643.
3. Couvelaire R. La petite vessie des tuberculeux genito-urinaires: essai de classification, places et variantes des cysto-intestinoplasties. *J Urol. (Paris).* 1950;**56**:381–434.
4. Bramble FJ. The treatment of adult enuresis and urge incontinence by enterocystoplasty. *Br J Urol.* 1982;**54**:693–696.
5. Sidi AA, Becher EF, Reddy PK et al. Augmentation enterocystoplasty for the management of voiding dysfunction in spinal cord injury patients. *J Urol.* 1990;**143**: 83–85.
6. Mundy AR, Stephenson TP. 'Clam' ileocystoplasty for the treatment of refractory urge incontinence. *Br J Urol.* 1985;**57**:641–646.
7. Reyblat P, Chan KG, Josephson DY, et al. Comparison of extraperitoneal and intraperitoneal augmentation enterocystoplasty for neurogenic bladder in spinal cord injury patients. *World J Urol.* 2009 Feb;**27**(1):63–68.
8. Meng MV, Anwar HP, Elliott SP, Stoller ML. Pure laparoscopic enterocystoplasty. *J Urol.* 2002;**167**:1386.
9. Il-Sang K, Jaw-Whan L, Ill-Young S. Robot-assisted laparoscopic augmentation ileocystoplasty: a case report. *Int Neurourol J.* 2010 April;**14**(1):61–64.
10. Razmaria AA, Marchetti PE, Prasad SM, et al. Does robotic-assisted laparoscopic ileocystoplasty (rali) reduce peritoneal adhesions compared to open surgery? BJU Int. 2013;Jun 13:doi: 10.1111/bju.12284. [Epub ahead of print]
11. Mark SD, McRae CU, Arnold EP, Gowland SP. Clam cystoplasty for the overactive bladder: a review of 23 cases. *Aust N Z J Surg.* 1994 Feb;**64**(2):88–90.
12. Hasan ST, Marshall C, Robson WA, Neal DE. Clinical outcome and quality of life following enterocystoplasty for idiopathic detrusor

instability and neurogenic bladder dysfunction. *Br J Urol.* 1995 Nov;**76**(5):551–557.

13. Lewis DK, Morgan JR, Weston PM, Stephenson TP. The "clam": indications and complications. *Br J Urol.* 1990 May;**65**(5):488–491.

14. Flood HD, Malhotra SJ, O'Connell HE, et al. Long-term results and complications using augmentation cystoplasty in reconstructive urology. *Neurourol Urodyn.* 1995;**14**(4):297–309.

15. Khastgir J, Hamid R, Arya M, et al. Surgical and patient reported outcomes of 'clam' augmentation ileocystoplasty in spinal cord injured patients. *Eur Urol.* 2003 Mar;**43**(3):263–269.

16. Goodwin WE, Winter CC, Barker WF. discussion 671. "Cup-patch" technique of ileocystoplasty for bladder enlargement or partial substitution. *J Urol.* 2002 Aug;**168**(2):667–670.

17. Zachoval R, Pitha J, Medova E, et al. Augmentation cystoplasty in patients with multiple sclerosis. *Urol Int.* 2003;**70**(1):21–6.

18. Hayashi Y, Kato Y, Okazaki T, et al. The effectiveness of ureteric reimplantation during bladder augmentation for high grade vesicoureteric reflux in patients with neurogenic bladder; long-term outcome. *J Pediatr Surg.* 2007;**42**:1998–2001.

19. Quek ML, Ginsberg DA. Long-term urodynamics followup of bladder augmentation for neurogenic bladder. *J Urol.* 2003 Jan;**169**(1):195–198.

20. Awad SA, Al-Zahrani HM, Gajewski JB, Bourque-Kehoe AA. Long-term results and complications of augmentation ileocystoplasty for idiopathic urge incontinence in women. *BJU.* 1998;**81**:569–573.

21. Lockhart JL, Bejany D, Politano VA. Augmentation cystoplasty in the management of neurogenic bladder disease and urinary incontinence. *J Urol.* 1986;**135**:969–971.

22. Shekarriz B, Uphadhyay J, Demirbilek S, et al. Surgical complications of bladder augmentation: comparison between various enterocystoplasties in 133 patients. *Urology* 2000; **55**:123–128.

23. Radomski SB, Herschorn S, Stone AR. Urodynamic comparison of ileum vs. sigmoid in augmentation cystoplasty for neurogenic bladder dysfunction. *Neurourol Urodyn.* 1995; **14**(3):231–237.

24. Yoo JJ, Olson J, Atala A, Kim B. Regenerative medicine strategies for treating neurogenic bladder. *Int Neurourol J.* 2011 Sep;**15**:109–119.

25. Vainrib M, Reyblat P, Ginsberg DA. Differences in urodynamic study variables in adult patients with neurogenic bladder and myelomeningocele before and after augmentation enterocystoplasty. *Neurourol Urodyn.* 2013;**32**:250–253.

26. Medel R, Ruarte AC, Herrera M, et al. Urinary continence outcome after augmentation ileocystoplasty as a single surgical procedure in patients with myelodysplasia. *J Urol.* 2002 Oct;**168**(4 Pt 2):1849–1852.

27. Chartier-Kastler EJ, Mongiat-Artus P, Bitker MO, et al. Long-term results of augmentation cystoplasty in spinal cord injury patients. *Spinal Cord.* 2000 Aug;**38**(8):490–494.

28. Beier-Holgersen R, Kirkeby LT, Nordling J. 'Clam' ileocystoplasty. *Scand J Urol Nephrol.* 1994 Mar;**28**(1):55–58

29. Catto JW, Natarajan V, Tophill PR. Simultaneous augmentation cystoplasty is associated with earlier rather than increased artificial urinary sphincter infection. *J Urol.* 2005 Apr;**173**(4):1237–1241.

30. Mor Y, Leibovitch I, Golomb J, et al. Lower urinary tract reconstruction by augmentation cystoplasty and insertion of artificial urinary sphincter cuff only: long term follow-up. *Prog Urol.* 2004 Jun;**14**(3):310–314.

31. Venn SN, Mundy AR. Long-term results of augmentation cystoplasty. *Eur Urol.* 1998;**34** Suppl 1:40–42.

32. Singh G, Thomas DG. Artificial urinary sphincter in patients with neurogenic bladder dysfunction. *B J Urol.*1996; **77**(2): 252–255.

33. Herschom S, Hewitt RJ. Patient perspective of long term outcome of augmentation cystoplasty for neurogenic bladder. *Urology* 1998; **52**: 672.

34. Cheng C, Hendry WF, Kirby RS, Whitfield HN. Detubularisation in cystoplasty: clinical review. *BJU* 1991;**67**(3):303–307.

35. Greenwell TJ, Venn SN, Mundy AR. Augmentation cystoplasty. *BJU Int.* 2001; **88**: 511.

36. Metcalfe PD, Casale AJ, Kaefer MA et al. Spontaneous bladder perforations: a report of SOD augmentations in children and analysis of risk. *J Urol.* 2006;**175**: 1466.

37. DeFoor W, Tackett L, Minevich E et al. Risk factors for spontaneous bladder perforation

after augmentation cystoplasty. *Urology* 2003; **62**:737.

38. Couillard D, Vapne k J, Rentzepis M. et al. Fatal perforation of augmemation cystoplasty in an adult. *Urology* 1993;**42**:585.

39. N'Dow J, Leung H, Marshall C et al. Bowel dysfunction after bladder reconstruction. *J Urol.* 1998;**159**:1470.

40. Pattni S, Walters JRF. Recent advances in the understanding of bile acid malabsorption. *Br Med Bull.* 2009;**92**:79.

41. Fontaine E, Leaver R, Woodhouse C. The effect of intestinal urinary reservoirs on renal function: a 10-year follow-up. *BJU Int.* 2000;**86**:195.

42. Nurse D, McInerney P, Thomas PJ, Mundy MS. Stones in enterocystoplasties. *Br J Urol.* 1996;**77**:684.

43. Murray K, Nurse D, Mundy A. Secreto-motor function of intestinal segments used in lower urinary tract reconstruction. *Br J Urol.* 1987;**60**:532.

44. Hamid R, Robertson WG, Woodhouse CRJ. Comparison of biochemistry and diet in patients with enterocystoplasty who do and do not form stones. *BJU lnt.* 2008;**101**: 1427.

45. Akerlund S, Campanello M, Kaijser B and Jonsson O. Bacteriuria in patients with a continent ileal reservoir for urinary diversion does not regularly require antibiotic treatment. *Br J Urol.* 1994;**74**:177–181.

46. Khoury JM, Timmons SL, Corbel L, Webster GD. Complications of enterocystoplasty. *Urology* 1992;**40**:9–14.

47. Veenboer PW, de Kort LM. Bladder carcinoma in a 31-year-old female spina bifida patient with an auto-augmented bladder. *Int Urol Nephrol.* 2012 Aug;**44**(4):1027–1030.

48. Higuchi IT, Granberg CF, Fox JA, Husmann DA. Augmentation cystoplasty and risk of neoplasia: fact, fiction and controversy. *J Urol.* 2010;**184**:2492–2496.

49. Swami KS, Feneley RCL, Hammonds JC, Abrams P. Detrusor myectomy for detrusor overactivity: a minimum 1 year follow-up. *Brit J Urol.* 1998;**81**:68–72.

50. Leng WW, Blalock HJ, Fredriksson WH, et al. Enterocystoplasty or detrusor myectomy? Comparison of indications and outcomes for bladder augmentation. *J Urol.* 1999 Mar;**161**(3): 758–763.

51. Veenboer PW, Nadorp S, de Jong TP, et al. Enterocystoplasty vs detrusorectomy: outcome in the adult with spina bifida. *J Urol.* 2013 Mar;**189**(3):1066–1070.

52. Cartwright PC, Snow BW. Bladder autoaugmentation: early clinical experience. *J Urol.* 1989 Aug;**142**(2 Pt 2):505–508; discussion 520–521.

53. Lindley RM, Mackinnon AE, Shipstone D, Tophill PR. Long-term outcome in bladder detrusorectomy augmentation. *Eur J Pediatr Surg.* 2003 Dec;**13** Suppl 1:S7–12.

54. Aslam MZ, Agarwal M. Detrusor myectomy: long-term functional outcomes. *Int J Urol.* 2012 Dec;**19**(12):1099–1102.

55. Kumar SP, Abrams PH. Detrusor myectomy: long-term results with a minimum follow-up of 2 years. *BJU Int.* 2005 Aug;**96**(3):341–344.

56. Bunson H, Manivel JC, Dayanc M, et al. Seromuscular colocystoplasty lined with urothelium: Experimental study. *Urology* 1994;**44**:773–748.

57. Blackford NN, Murray K, Stephenson TP, et al. Transvesical infiltration of the pelvic plexuses with phenol. *Br J Urol.* 1984; **56**: 647–649.

58. Chapple CR, Hampson SJ, Turner-Warwick RT, Worth PH. Subtrigonal phenol injection: how safe and effective is it? *Br J Urol.* 1991;**68**: 483–486.

59. Ingelman-Sundberg A. Partial denervation of the bladder. A new operation for the treatment of urge incontinence and similar conditions in women. *Acta Obstet Gynecol Scand.* 1959;**38**:487.

60. Cespedes DR, Cross CA, McGuire EJ. Modified Ingelman-Sundberg bladder denervation procedure for intractable urge incontinence. *J Urol.* 1996;**156**:1744–1747.

61. Brindley GS, Polkey CE, Rushton DN. Sacral anterior root stimulation for bladder control in paraplegia. *Paraplegia* 1982;**20**:363–381.

62. Mundy AR. Long-term results of bladder transection for urge incontinence. *Br J Urol.* 1983;**5**:642–644.

63. Koziol I, Hackler RH. Cutaneous ureteroileostomy in spinal cord injured patients: a 15-year experience. *J Urol.* 1975;**114**:709–711.

Special Populations and Synthesis

CHAPTER 18

Overactive bladder in older people

Adrian Wagg

Department of Medicine, University of Alberta, Edmonton, AB, Canada

---

KEY POINTS

- Overactive bladder (OAB) can have a considerable negative impact on quality of life, typically resulting in embarrassment, loss of dignity, and a withdrawal from social activities and interactions.

- Treatment of OAB in older people often requires multi-component interventions in the manner of a typical geriatric syndrome.

- Consideration should be given to those conditions and medications that might be amenable to treatment or alteration which might have a beneficial effect on the continence status of an older person.

- Although there continues to be a paucity of clinical intervention evidence relating to the frail elderly, there is no reason to assume that interventions which are proven to be effective in community dwelling older people might not be effective for them.

Introduction

Overactive bladder (OAB) can have a considerable negative impact on quality of life, typically resulting in embarrassment, loss of dignity, and a withdrawal from social activities and interactions, [1] perhaps increasing the likelihood of social isolation, a significant factor associated with functional decline in the elderly. [2] Population-based surveys have shown that OAB is a common disorder across adult life but its prevalence increases in association with age. For example, in a cross-sectional survey of 19 165 adults in Canada, Germany, Italy, Sweden, and the United Kingdom (the

EPIC study) the overall prevalence of OAB was 11.8%. The overall rates were similar between men and women, and increased with age; urgency was reported in 19.1% of men and 18.3% of women aged 60 years or over. In a population-based survey of 5204 adults in the United States (the NOBLE study), the overall prevalence of OAB was 16% in men and 16.9% in women; the increase in prevalence was age-related. [3–5] Available evidence from longitudinal studies suggests that OAB symptoms appear to progress in association with age, in terms of prevalence and severity, in both men and women. In men interviewed in 1992 and again in 2003, the proportion of men with

---

Overactive Bladder: Practical Management, First Edition. Edited by Jacques Corcos, Scott MacDiarmid and John Heesakkers.
© 2015 John Wiley & Sons, Ltd. Published 2015 by John Wiley & Sons, Ltd.

OAB increased from 15.6 to 44.4% and the proportion with urgency incontinence increased from 1.9 to 7.4%.[6] A similar pattern was observed in women over a 16-year period with a marked overall increase in the prevalence of urgency incontinence, from 17 to 26%. [7]

OAB has a proven negative impact on health related quality of life (HRQL) and affected people score significantly worse than their age matched counterparts without OAB in domains of physical and social functioning. [8, 9] Apart from the impact attributable to its lower urinary tract symptoms, OAB is associated with a number of health-related problems in older people. Published data show an increased risk of falls and fractures, sleep disturbance, depression, urinary tract infection, and risk of institutionalization associated with urinary incontinence. [10, 11] Older people affected by OAB also constitute a difficult to treat group that receives less optimal management than their younger counterparts. Finding a well-tolerated treatment in these patients who often have concomitant co-morbidities and take multiple medications is difficult. Treatment of this condition in older people often requires multi-component interventions in the manner of a typical geriatric syndrome.

Who are the elderly?

Whereas aging for many is characterized as "a progressive, generalized impairment of function resulting in a loss of adaptive response to stress (loss of biological reserve) and in a growing risk of age-associated disease," [12] there has been a change in the physical wellness of older people in the "baby boomer" generation which has led to reductions in late life disability. [13] Chronological age is not a useful marker with which to label such a heterogeneous group; some people at age 60 may be afflicted with multiple chronic diseases, whereas one may often encounter people aged 90 at a high level of physical and mental functioning without co-morbidity. A simple distinction might be drawn between the robust and frail elderly. Frailty as a concept has a number of definitions which center on the concept of biological reserve. The "frailty phenotype" combines impaired physical activity, mobility, balance, muscle strength, motor processing, cognition, nutrition, and endurance. [14–16] It is not identical to disability and the presence of co-existing disease (co-morbidity). In a study of older people meeting strict "phenotypic" criteria for frailty, 22% of the sample also had both co-morbidity and disability; 46% had co-morbidity without disability; 6% disability without co-morbidity, and 27% had neither. [15] Frailty may also be defined in a more mechanistic fashion, by summing the total number of pre-existing biomedical and social co-morbidities existing in each person; this frailty index predicts death, disability, and hospitalization. Frail people, however defined, have a higher risk of intercurrent disease, increased disability, hospitalization, and death than those without frailty. [17]

Overactive bladder – pathophysiology in older people

Urgency incontinence, or overactive bladder, is the commonest cause of urinary incontinence in older people. Urinary urgency becomes increasingly prevalent in late life and is probably the result of an interaction between bladder and lower urinary tract dysfunction and a diminution of central control of urgency as much as the phenomenon being related to bladder disease. When considering the evidence for age-related changes in lower urinary tract function in older people, data are often limited to either cross-sectional studies or studies in older people with lower urinary tract symptoms without either age matched cases or controls. Normal aging changes are difficult to study, because data including large numbers of individuals spanning decades are necessary to definitively separate "normal aging" from confounding factors and co-morbidity. Cross-sectional studies are subject to confounding by co-morbidity and time-dependent cohort effects. Thus, many studies actually describe "age related" associations rather than changes which occur with normal aging. Our state of knowledge of normal function is often similarly limited, but where they exist, cystometric data reveal an increased prevalence of detrusor overactivity in older people, coupled with a reduced bladder capacity, smaller voided volume, reduced sensation of filling, and increased prevalence of ineffective voiding. [18–21] In many older people, detrusor overactivity and impaired emptying often co-exist; a condition termed detrusor hyperactivity with impaired contractility (DHIC). [22–24] In these cases, the bladder does not empty efficiently in the absence of any outlet obstruction; as much as this is a true entity it is likely that it is simply a reflection of two common conditions which occur together frequently.

Ultrastructural studies of the bladder demonstrate cellular changes associated with age-related changes in detrusor function. One series involved comparisons of the symptomatic and asymptomatic aged 65 to 96, using urodynamic testing and electron microscopy of bladder biopsy specimens. [25–30] A consistent correlation between specific urodynamic findings and bladder ultrastructure was observed, although there has been considerable debate about the veracity of these findings and they have been disputed by the findings of a later study which found the ultrastructural changes described evenly distributed between specimens from those with normal bladders and those showing detrusor overactivity. [31]

There is increasing evidence for urgency incontinence in older people being a reflection of alteration of central control as much as an end organ disease. Functional PET scanning in young, healthy volunteers shows that the periaqueductal gray matter (PAG), pons, and ventral and dorsal portions of the pontine tegmentum are active during bladder filling. [32] Functional MRI studies in older people suggest that failure of activation in areas of the brain relating to continence, such as the orbitofrontal regions and the insula, may lessen the ability to suppress urgency, [33] and patients with multiple sclerosis who have lesions in the PAG are more likely to have urinary symptoms than those without. [34] There is a known association between vascular risk factors and LUTS, [35] and the presence of white matter hyperintensities within periventricular and subcortical regions of the brain is associated with functional and cognitive impairment, an increased incidence of urinary urgency and detrusor overactivity, and a difficulty in maintaining continence on cystometry. [36, 37] Damage to the anterior thalamic radiation appears to be significantly associated with incontinence and does not need to be bilateral to cause the problem. Response to bladder filling in the dorsal anterior cingulate gyrus and adjacent supplementary motor area is abnormally pronounced in patients with urgency incontinence. [33, 38] Whether the incidence of incontinence can be altered through aggressive vascular risk factor control is not known, but there is a suggestion that, in those with the highest white matter hyperintensity load, high dose statins and control of hypertension may be associated with lesion regression. [39]

Multi-morbidity

Multi-morbidity in older people is the norm. The number of people with more than one life altering chronic medical condition increases in association with age and in the seventh decade of life, only 20% of people will be without co-morbid conditions. Co-existing medical conditions have the potential to have an adverse impact on an older person's experience of urinary incontinence and OAB. In studies, the presence of incontinence as defined by the use of continence pads was positively associated with one or more geriatric syndromes such as falls, impaired mobility, or cognitive impairment. [40] Clearly those conditions which affect mobility will render urgency more difficult to deal with; conditions which have an impact on fluid handling, such as heart failure or other salt and water retaining conditions, will also place additional stress on "the system" and may make OAB symptoms "worse." Consideration should be given to those conditions which might be amenable to treatment and which might

Table 18.1 Co-morbid conditions affecting continence status

• peripheral vascular disease	• Stroke
	• Dementia
• diabetes mellitus	• Diffuse Lewy body
• congestive heart failure	(DLB) disease
• venous insufficiency	• Parkinson's disease
• chronic lung disease	• Normal Pressure
• falls and contractures	Hydrocephalus
• obesity	• Recurrent infection
• impaired mobility	• Constipation

Source: Ouslander, J.G. and J.F. Schnelle, *Incontinence in the nursing home.* Ann Intern Med, 1995. **122**(6): p. 438–49. McGrother C, Donaldson M. Continence in Health Care Needs Assessment http://www.hcna.bham. ac.uk/documents/02_HCNA3_D3.pdf.

have a beneficial effect on the continence status of an older person (Table 18.1). Needless to say, there is little evidence of beneficial impact in the literature and much is a result of custom and practice. However, there is increasing evidence for the benefits of exercise in older people, ranging from the community dwelling to institutionalized elderly. [41, 42] Clearly, improving gait speed and stamina alone may be enough to allow an older person to deal with urinary urgency and make it to the bathroom on time, as much as altering the underlying pathophysiology of OAB.

Polypharmacy

The other key feature that perhaps characterizes older people is the number of medications they take. Those over 65 years of age comprise between 12–16% of the population in the USA, UK, and Canada but consume 32, 50, and 45% of prescribed medications respectively. [43–46] This is of importance in dealing with urgency incontinence in the elderly for two reasons;

firstly, a number of medications may themselves exacerbate either lower urinary tract symptoms or incontinence and secondly, a reduction in the number of medications with anticholinergic properties taken by a cognitively at risk older person may be desirable if an antimuscarinic needs to be prescribed to manage OAB. The possibility that UI could be caused by a medication should be taken into account before prescribing drug treatment for UI in older persons. In one study, the risk of difficulty in controlling urination in community dwelling older women taking medications with LUT effects was about 30% higher compared to those who did not take such medications (OR 1.31 (95% CI 1.05–1.21)).

Overall, 20.5% of these women reported incident incontinence at Year 4 (three years from baseline). In a report from the Health, Aging and Body Composition Study, which examined 959 elderly community dwelling women, multi-variate logistic regression analyses revealed that current users of alpha blockers (adjusted odds ratio (AOR) =4.98, 95% confidence interval (CI) =1.96–12.64) and estrogen (AOR=1.60, 95% CI=1.08–2.36) had a greater risk of urinary incontinence than non-users. There was no greater risk of UI associated with current use of anticholinergics, central nervous system medications, or diuretics. [47] Medications that potentially increase the likelihood of continent toileting are shown in Table 18.2.

Table 18.2 Medications with potential to worsen urinary incontinence

Medication	Potential or actual effect
α adrenoreceptor antagonists	Decrease smooth muscle tone in the urethra and may precipitate stress urinary incontinence in women
Angiotensin converting enzyme (ACE) inhibitors	Cause cough that can exacerbate stress urinary incontinence
Agents with antimuscarinic properties	May cause ineffective voiding and constipation that can contribute to incontinence. May cause cognitive impairment and reduce effective toileting ability (high dose, cognitively at risk)
Calcium channel blockers	May cause constipation (verapamil) that can contribute to incontinence. May cause dependent oedema (amlodipine, nifedipine) which can contribute to nocturnal polyuria
Cholinesterase inhibitors	Can precipitate urgency incontinence through cholinergic action
Diuretics	Cause diuresis and precipitate incontinence
Lithium	Polyuria due to diabetes insipidus like state
Opioid analgesics	May cause constipation, confusion, and immobility – all of which can contribute to incontinence
Tramadol	Associated with constipation and impaired emptying
Psychotropic drugs	May cause confusion and impaired mobility and precipitate incontinence
Sedatives, Hypnotics, Antipsychotics	
Histamine$_1$ receptor antagonists	Most have anticholinergic effects
Selective serotonin re-uptake inhibitors (sertraline identified)	Increase cholinergic transmission and may lead to urgency urinary incontinence
Gabapentin	Can cause oedema, leads to polyuria while supine and exacerbate nocturia and nighttime incontinence
Glitazones	
Non-steroidal anti-inflammatory agents	

Cholinesterase inhibitors

Of particular interest is the use of cholinesterase inhibitors (CEI) for Alzheimer's disease. These drugs are associated with an increased risk of urinary urgency and urgency incontinence; evidence comes from individual case reports and then a case series of 216 consecutive patients with probable Alzheimer's disease. [48–50] Cholinesterase inhibitor treatment was associated with a 7% risk of new incontinence: the highest risk was seen in those with the most behavioral problems, with a lower risk in those who responded to treatment. Further evidence for an interaction between anticholinergics and CEIs comes from a database study of nursing home residents. [51] Residents with dementia, newly treated with cholinesterase inhibitors, were more likely to be prescribed a bladder anticholinergic than those residents with dementia not given a cholinesterase inhibitor. Intuitively, one might think that the use of a bladder antimuscarinic with a cholinesterase inhibitor might not only fail to improve OAB (taking that the CEI is producing benefit and cannot be stopped) but also cancel out any improvement in cognitive status. Things are not so clear cut, however, and there is some moderate quality evidence which might guide concomitant treatment. In one study, use of antimuscarinics (extended-release oxybutynin and tolterodine) and cholinesterase inhibitors in nursing home residents was associated with a decline in ADL function in the most functionally able residents but there was no detected worsening of cognition, this may however have been because the cognitive measure (MDS-COG) was inadequately sensitive. More importantly, there was no case of delirium observed. [52] In a study of 46 subjects with UI and dementia to assess the cognitive impact of trospium chloride in older people treated with galantamine over a six-month period, no effect on cognition or ADL was detected over the duration of the study. A within group analysis demonstrated an improvement in nocturia and reduction in pad use in this combination group. [53] Finally, a small study reported some positive effect of the treatment of UI with propiverine in subjects with probable Alzheimer's disease taking cholinesterase inhibitors. [54] The current weight of evidence appears to be that a positive outcome in terms of bladder control can be achieved without a significant detriment in either cognition or ADL, but a prospective trial has yet to be done. An early review of the effect of the drug on continence and cognitive status should be performed to ensure safe and effective prescribing.

Lifestyle, behavioral, and conservative therapies for OAB in older people

Alterations in lifestyle, behavioral techniques, and conservative management are recommended prior to more invasive therapies in most national and international guidelines for the management of incontinence and OAB. Such recommendations are, needless to say, made in the light of a paucity of data from older and frail older people. However, for the robust elderly, there is no reason to suspect that interventions which work in the middle aged and community dwelling elderly should not be effective in the less robust. Attention should be paid, however, to the nature of the intervention, the wishes and expectations of the patient, and – where relevant – those of the caregiver. Several lifestyle interventions for OAB have been evaluated in healthier older and younger women, including dietary modification, fluid selection and management, and constipation management. [55–57] Some of these interventions may be inappropriate or impractical to use in frail older people, yet advanced age alone should not preclude their use if assessment warrants this. Inadequate fluid intake and dehydration are common in older people, more so in those who limit their fluid intake for fear of leakage or urgency, and the dangers of dehydration and orthostatic hypotension probably outweigh those of OAB. Three studies in older people that examined increasing or normalizing fluid intake in older people suggested that this might improve general UI. [58–60] For example, caffeine reduction, recommended in some guidelines and based upon evidence of only moderate quality, is often difficult to achieve in practice and the benefits of so doing often limited. Behavioral techniques for UI in older people have not been specifically targeted at OAB, other than those utilizing bladder retraining, for which data are few and often combined with other interventions. A Cochrane review recommends bladder retraining as an appropriate first-line conservative intervention, but notes the relatively low quality of data and the wide variation in regimens employed. [61] Behavioral techniques, requiring learning, aim at increasing spontaneous toileting and improving continence in frail older people. The "gold standard," prompted voiding, often combined with functional exercise training to improve gait speed and stamina, has proved to be effective in frail older adults and is recommended for those capable of learning. A three-day trial should ideally lead to a 30% reduction in the need for wet checks and an increase in spontaneous toileting, but if this is not achieved then a return to "check and change" is recommended. [62, 63] Behavioral techniques in residential long-term care are difficult to maintain, given current staff to resident ratios and the intensity of intervention required to sustain the associated benefits. All of the available techniques – prompted voiding, [64] habit retraining, [65] and timed voiding [66] – require active participation of a caregiver, limiting their applicability to all older people.

Pharmacological interventions for older people

Older people appear to experience more severe disease than younger people. [67, 68] The oldest old, those over 75 years of age, also appear – from at least two pooled analyses of drug treatment for OAB – to require higher doses of medication to achieve maximal benefits of drug therapy. [69, 70] The reason for this may be due to pathophysiology at the more severe end of the spectrum; that older people are less able to perform or persist at behavioral and other conservative measures, or that higher serum levels of drug are required for symptom control despite a reduction in the density of bladder muscarinic receptors. Whatever the reason, the need for anticholinergic drug therapy in older people is often under-recognized and OAB under-treated. There is an understandable concern about adverse effects from medication, from which older people are more likely to suffer, leading to higher withdrawal rates from treatment but also concerns regarding falls, adverse cognitive effects, and the precipitation of delirium. Bladder antimuscarinics are included in the most recent Beer's criteria for potentially inappropriate medication use in older adults; for those with chronic constipation, dementia, or at risk of delirium. [71] There is, however, an increasing amount of data concerning the absence of effect on falls and precipitation of delirium in older people when treated for OAB, which should help to reassure those who are perhaps over cautious in their approach to treatment. [72, 73]

Specific age-related changes in pharmacokinetics, alteration in drug absorption, distribution, metabolism, and clearance, and their potential effect on UI drugs, include alterations in volumes of distribution depending upon changes in lean body mass and the relative lipophilicity of compounds, alterations in hepatic metabolism reductions in renal clearance, and an increase in the permeability of the blood–brain barrier. Whereas medication pharmacokinetics studies in older adults are in limited numbers, there are few, if any, studies involving the oldest old or those with significant co-morbidity. Older people are therefore at higher risk of ADEs from antimuscarinics because of age and co-morbidity-related changes in muscarinic receptor number and distribution, blood–brain barrier transport, and drug metabolism. The majority of data on the efficacy of antimuscarinics in older people comes from pooled analyses of trials involving community dwelling older adults. Only relatively recently have we seen trials prospectively planned to recruit and

retain older people and report on efficacy and safety of agents. Even so, the majority of these trials are short lasting, usually 12-week randomized placebo-controlled trials, with only two open-label extensions. Data on more complex older people come from two trials of oxybutynin immediate- [74] and extended-release, [75] and, more recently, from a study of fesoterodine. [76]

Oxybutynin

In long-term care residents who had failed prompted voiding alone, the addition of titrated oxybutynin-IR resulted in a significant but modest reduction in incontinence versus placebo. [74] The need for wet-checks did not differ between treatment arms, leading the authors to conclude that the improvement was not clinically significant. One or fewer episodes of daytime UI was achieved by 40% on drug but only 18% on placebo ($p < 0.05$). In a randomized two-month trial in frail community dwelling older people, oxybutynin-IR plus bladder training was superior to bladder training alone in improving urinary frequency but not UI. [77] A study in 416 community dwelling older persons found 68% reported a partial or complete symptomatic cure with 2.5 mg three times daily; 30% of subjects experienced ADEs, but only 10% withdrew because of them. [78] Only one RCT in frailer older people examined the efficacy of oxybutynin-ER but was underpowered. [75] In agreement with other meta-analyses, [79] oxybutynin was associated with a higher incidence of adverse effects than the other, newer, antimuscarinics.

Tolterodine

Older patients in tolterodine ER studies were all community dwelling, although several trials include elderly persons in their ninth and tenth decades, the mean age of participants was much lower (64 years) and results were not stratified by age. Overall, studies showed efficacy of tolterodine when compared with placebo over the typical 12 weeks of the study. [80–82] In a secondary analysis of a large, open-label German trial of tolterodine- IR 2 mg twice daily, higher age was significantly associated with "less favorable efficacy." [83] However, the absolute difference in odds was only 0.019, there was no association of tolerability with age, only mean age is described, and UI frequency was based on patient report – not bladder diaries, all of which fail to add up to a clinically meaningful difference. A trial of one-year duration of the addition of tolterodine ER 4 mg to alpha blocker or 5 ARA therapy in older men (mean age 74.9 years) resulted in a between group, statistically significant, decrease in the storage symptom score on the IPSS. [84]

Darifenacin

The first large pre-planned study of newer antimuscarinics in older people was of darifenacin for OAB in persons aged ≥ 65 (mean 72), in which there was no statistically significant difference between drug and placebo for the primary endpoint, UI frequency. There were statistically significant improvements with the drug for frequency of micturition and quality of life. [85] A two-year extension study in subjects > 65 was reported, showing maintenance of

OAB symptom improvement, with 44.4% patients achieving > or = 90% reduction in incontinence episodes for the 64% (137/214) subjects remaining in the study. [86] The potential for cognitive adverse effects has been prospectively studied. In a three-period crossover RCT in 129 older subjects, mean age 71 – of whom 88% had co-morbid medical conditions and 93% were on other medications – cognition was assessed using a standardized computerized test battery. Darifenacin did not adversely affect cognition compared to placebo. [87] A subsequent study in cognitively intact older people ($n = 49$, mean age 66) compared titrated darifenacin and oxybutynin-ER with placebo over threeweeks. Oxybutynin-ER but not darifenacin or placebo adversely affected delayed recall on the Name-Face Association test. [88]

Fesoterodine

Fesoterodine is a pro-drug which is rapidly and completely metabolized to 5-hydroxymethyl tolterodine, the main active metabolite of tolterodine. A pharmacokinetic study which included older people found no clinically meaningful effect on 5-HMT pharmacokinetics or pharmacodynamics after single dose administration of fesoterodine 8 mg. [89] The efficacy of fesoterodine has also been studied in a European trial (SOFIA) in 794 elderly men and women with OAB: [90] 46% of subjects reported urgency incontinence episodes at baseline, and 64% had prior treatment with antimuscarinics. At week 12, the improvement from baseline in urgency episodes, micturition frequency, nocturnal micturition, treatment benefit scales, and incontinence pad use all were statistically significantly greater with fesoterodine than with placebo. A 12-week open-label follow-up study revealed a maintained efficacy amongst those on fesoterodine and an achievement of similar effect on those switched from placebo to fesoterodine, with no unexpected safety concerns. [91] Fesoterodine has also been tested in medically complex older people as assessed by the Vulnerable Elders Survey-13, [92] which identifies those at risk of death in the following two years. This 12-week double-blind, placebo-controlled study including 562 people of mean age 75 years resulted in mean reductions in UUI episodes and 24-h micturition frequency at week 12 versus placebo. [76] The commonest treatment-related adverse events across all of these studies were dry mouth reaching – at maxima – 33% in the SOFIA study, and constipation at 11.1% in the vulnerable elders study. The cognitive safety of fesoterodine has been assessed in a single study of cognitively intact older subjects, using alprazolam as an active control, and placebo. There were no statistically significant changes in performance on a computer assisted battery of cognitive tests at either dose of fesoterodine versus placebo.[93]

Solifenacin

A secondary analysis of pooled Phase III data in patients aged 65 and older (all community dwelling, mean age 72) found similar efficacy to that reported for younger and middle aged persons. However, direct comparison with subjects < 65 yrs from the same pooled trials was not done. [69] Data from an open-label, 12-week trial in patients treated by community urologists

found that overall treatment-emergent adverse events were more likely in patients aged > 80 years and taking concomitant medications. A *post hoc* subgroup analysis on tolerability of solifenacin versus oxybutynin in older subjects reported that the incidence and severity of adverse events with solifenacin were similar between younger and older patients. Solifenacin 5 mg/day was associated with fewer episodes and lower severity of dry mouth, and a lower discontinuation rate. [94] Solifenacin showed no evidence of impaired cognition or self-ratings of mood and alertness versus placebo in an exploratory study in 12 cognitively intact older subjects, and in a three-way crossover design the cognitive effects of chronic dosing of 5 mg solifenacin, placebo, and 5 mg bid of oxybutynin were compared in 23 older subjects with mild cognitive impairment. There was no statistically significant effect on cognition of solifenacin versus placebo. Oxybutynin 5 mg bid was associated with impairment in power and speed of attention in a *post hoc* analysis of pooled time points at 1 + 2 h post dose. [95]

Trospium chloride

Although promoted for use in the elderly because of the reduced likelihood that the drug crosses the blood–brain barrier, trospium has only systematically been evaluated in "younger elderly," and results have not been stratified by age. [96] The effect of 60 mg trospium chloride once daily over 10 days on either learning or memory was assessed in 12 cognitively intact older people with no observable change in standardized testing. Additionally, no trospium was detectable in the CSF of the subjects at day 10. [97] As part of a larger study of trospuim chloride 20 mg bid, 26 patients with UUI and dementia, were treated with galantamine and trospium. There was no observable decrement in either cognition, measured by MMSE, or ability in terms of activities of daily living in the dually treated group and some improvement in continence outcomes. [53]

Propiverine hydrochloride

In 46 patients with dementia (mean age 81), there was a 40% decrease in urgency UI with propiverine 20 mg/day for 2 weeks, similar to two small Japanese trials and a German trial in 98 patients. [58, 98–100] A further study on cognition, only published in abstract form, revealed no observable change in MMSE over 12 weeks treatment in men and women > 70 years of age, including those with lower MMSE scores. There was neither formal diagnosis of MCI, nor formal reporting of adverse events. [101].

Mirabegron

There are data on the comparative pharmacokinetics of mirabegron, a beta adrenoreceptor 3 agonist. In this study, there were no statistically significant differences in mirabegron exposure between older volunteers aged 55 years and above and younger volunteers (18–45 years). Similar results were obtained for those aged 65 years and above. AUC was predicted to be 11% higher in a subject aged 90 years of age. Data on efficacy in patients over 65 years of age come from pooled analyses of registration trials and additional safety data

from longer term extension studies. Primary efficacy outcomes were change from baseline to final visit in mean number of incontinence episodes/24 hours and mean number of micturitions/24 hours. Tolerability was assessed by the incidence of treatment-emergent adverse events. Mirabegron at 25 mg (US/Canada) and 50 mg (elsewhere) once-daily reduced the mean numbers of incontinence episodes and micturitions/24 hours from baseline to final visit. Mirabegron was well tolerated: in both age groups, hypertension and urinary tract infection were among the most common adverse events over 12 weeks and 1 year. [102]

Botulinum toxin

There is one open-label uncontrolled study which has examined the short-term use of botulinum toxin in 21 patients over the age of 75 years. [103] There was no report of co-morbidity and subjects described as refractory to or intolerant of anticholinergic medications without detail were included, suggesting considerable selection. After 1 month of treatment of the 21 patients, 16 (76.2%) had greater than 50% improvement in symptoms after one treatment with 200 units of onabotulinumtoxinA. The mean duration of efficacy, defined as the interval until symptoms were greater than 50% of the pre-treatment baseline, was 7.12 months. There was no reported urinary retention.

Otherwise, community dwelling older persons have been included in clinical trials but results have not been reported separately. [104] The main concern with the use of this therapeutic modality in frailer older people is the risk of ineffective voiding post-procedure and the need for the patient to undertake clean intermittent self-catheterization until the effect of the botulinum toxin has worn off. Older people with detrusor overactivity have a true reduction in detrusor contractility, in addition to the impaired bladder emptying seen in association with later life, probably due to the accumulation of connective tissue in the bladder wall and its "damping effect." [105–107] The lower, 100 unit, doses of botulinum toxin used more recently for idiopathic overactive bladder may, in fact, lend its use to managing the condition in older people, without an observed increase in impaired emptying. There are certain groups for whom botulinum may be of benefit, particularly those with degenerative neurological disease such as Parkinson's disease, [108] who are sensitive to adverse events with anticholinergic medications, but the value of this intervention must be balanced against the problems of impaired dexterity should urinary retention be precipitated.

Summary

Overactive bladder is a significant problem for many robust and frail older people. There are distinct alterations in the pathophysiology of OAB in older people about which knowledge is slowly accumulating, which aids our understanding of the condition and may, in future, shed light on targets for prevention. Although there continues to be a paucity of clinical intervention evidence relating to the frail elderly, there is no reason to assume that interventions which are proven to be effective in community dwelling older people might not be effective for them. Robust and frail older people tend to have multi-morbidity and polypharmacy, both factors which need to be taken into account when managing their OAB.

References

1 Sexton CC, Coyne KS, Thompson C, et al. Prevalence and effect on health–related quality of life of overactive bladder in older americans: results from the epidemiology of lower urinary tract symptoms study. *J Am Geriatr Soc.* Aug 2011;**59**(8):1465–1470.

2 Cacioppo JT, Hawkley LC, Norman GJ, Berntson GG. Social isolation. *Ann N Y Acad Sci.* Aug 2011;**1231**(1):17–22.

3 Milsom I, Abrams P, Cardozo L, et al. How widespread are the symptoms of an overactive bladder and how are they managed? A population-based prevalence study. *BJU Int.* Jun 2001; **87**(9):760–766.

4 Irwin DE, Milsom I, Hunskaar S, et al. Population–based survey of urinary incontinence, overactive bladder, and other lower urinary tract symptoms in five countries: results of the EPIC study. *Eur Urol.* Dec 2006;**50**(6):1306–1314; discussion 1314–1305.

5 Stewart WF, Van Rooyen JB, Cundiff GW, et al. Prevalence and burden of overactive bladder in the United States. *World J Urol.* May 2003;**20**(6):327–336.

6 Malmsten UG, Molander U, Peeker R, et al. Urinary incontinence, overactive bladder, and other lower urinary tract symptoms: a longitudinal population–based survey in men aged 45–103 years. *Eur Urol.* Jul 2010;**58**(1): 149–156.

7 Wennberg AL, Molander U, Fall M, et al. a longitudinal population-based survey of urinary incontinence, overactive bladder, and other lower urinary tract symptoms in women. *Eur Urol.* Jan;**55**(4):783–791.

8 Milsom I, Kaplan SA, Coyne KS, et al. Effect of bothersome overactive bladder symptoms on health–related quality of life, anxiety, depression, and treatment seeking in the United States: results from EpiLUTS. *Urology* Jul 2012; **80**(1):90–96.

9 Coyne KS, Kvasz M, Ireland AM, et al. Urinary incontinence and its relationship to mental health and health–related quality of life in men and women in Sweden, the United Kingdom, and the United States. *Eur Urol.* Jan 2012;**61**(1):88–95.

10 Brown JS, McGhan WF, Chokroverty S. Comorbidities associated with overactive bladder. *Am J Manag Care* Jul 2000;**6**(11 Suppl):S574–579.

11 Thom DH, Haan MN, Van Den Eeden SK. Medically recognized urinary incontinence and risks of hospitalization, nursing home admission and mortality. *Age Ageing* Sep 1997;**26**(5):367–374.

12 Kirkwood TBL. The evolution of ageing. *Rev Clin Gerontol.* 1995;**5**:3–9.

13 Martin LG, Schoeni RF, Andreski PM. Trends in health of older adults in the United States: past, present, future. *Demography* 2010;**47** Suppl:S17–40.

14 Ferrucci L, Guralnik JM, Studenski S, et al. Designing randomized, controlled trials aimed at preventing or delaying functional decline and disability in frail, older persons: a consensus report. *J Am Geriatr Soc.* Apr 2004; **52**(4):625–634.

15 Fried L, Tangen C, Walston J, et al. Frailty in older adults: evidence for a phenotype. *J Gerontol A Biol Sci Med Sci.* Mar 2001;**56**(3):M146–156.

16 Centers for Disease Control National Center for Health Statistics. Health, United States, 2003 With Chartbook on Trends in the Health of Americans. http://www.cdc.gov/nchs/products/pubs/pubd/hus/highlits.pdf. Accessed June 11, 2004.

17 Lacas A, Rockwood K. Frailty in primary care: a review of its conceptualization and implications for practice. *BMC Med.* 2012;**10**:4.

18 Malone-Lee J, Wahedna, I. Characterisation of detrusor contractile function in relation to old-age. *Br J Urol* 1993;**72**:873–880.

19 Collas D, Malone-Lee, JG. Age associated changes in detrusor sensory function in patients with lower urinary tract symptoms. *Int Urogynecol J Pelvic Floor Dysfunct.* 1996;**7**:24–29.

20 Pfisterer MH, Griffiths DJ, Schaefer W, Resnick NM. The effect of age on lower urinary tract function: a study in women. *J Am Geriatr Soc.* Mar 2006;**54**(3):405–412.

21 Pfisterer MH, Griffiths DJ, Rosenberg L, et al. The impact of detrusor overactivity on bladder function in younger and older women. *J Urol.* May 2006;**175**(5):1777–1783; discussion 1783.

22 Resnick NM, Yalla SV, Laurino E. The pathophysiology of urinary incontinence among institutionalized elderly persons. *N Engl J Med.* Jan 5 1989;**320**(1):1–7.

23 Resnick NM, Yalla SV. Detrusor hyperactivity with impaired contractile function. An unrecognized but common cause of incontinence in elderly patients. *JAMA* Jun 12 1987;**257** (22):3076–3081.

24 Taylor JA 3rd, Kuchel GA. Detrusor underactivity: Clinical features and pathogenesis of an underdiagnosed geriatric condition. *J Am Geriatr Soc.* Dec 2006;**54**(12):1920–1932.

25 Elbadawi A, Yalla SV, Resnick NM. Structural basis of geriatric voiding dysfunction. II. Aging detrusor: normal versus impaired contractility. *J Urol.* Nov 1993;**150**(5 Pt 2):1657–1667.

26 Elbadawi A, Yalla SV, Resnick NM. Structural basis of geriatric voiding dysfunction. I. Methods of a prospective ultrastructural/urodynamic study and an overview of the findings. *J Urol.* Nov 1993;**150**(5 Pt 2): 1650–1656.

27 Elbadawi A, Yalla SV, Resnick NM. Structural basis of geriatric voiding dysfunction. IV. Bladder outlet obstruction. *J Urol.* Nov 1993;**150**(5 Pt 2):1681–1695.

28 Elbadawi A, Yalla SV, Resnick NM. Structural basis of geriatric voiding dysfunction. III. Detrusor overactivity. *J Urol.* Nov 1993;**150**(5 Pt 2):1668–1680.

29 Elbadawi A, Hailemariam S, Yalla SV, Resnick NM. Structural basis of geriatric voiding dysfunction. VII. Prospective ultrastructural/urodynamic evaluation of its natural evolution. *J Urol.* May 1997;**157**(5):1814–1822.

30 Elbadawi A, Hailemariam S, Yalla SV, Resnick NM. Structural basis of geriatric voiding dysfunction. VI. Validation and update of diagnostic criteria in 71 detrusor biopsies. *J Urol.* May 1997;**157**(5):1802–1813.

31 Carey MP, De Jong S, Friedhuber A, et al. A prospective evaluation of the pathogenesis of detrusor instability in women, using electron microscopy and immunohistochemistry. *BJU Int.* Dec 2000;**86**(9):970–976.

32 Matsuura S, Kakizaki H, Mitsui T, et al. Human brain region response to distention or cold stimulation of the bladder: a positron emission tomography study. *J Urol*. Nov 2002;**168**(5): 2035–2039.

33 Griffiths D, Tadic SD, Schaefer W, Resnick NM. Cerebral control of the bladder in normal and urge–incontinent women. *Neuroimage*. Aug 1 2007;**37**(1):1–7.

34 Linnman C, Moulton EA, Barmettler G, et al. Neuroimaging of the periaqueductal gray: state of the field. *Neuroimage*. Mar 2012;**60**(1):505–522.

35 Ponholzer A, Temml C, Wehrberger C, et al. The association between vascular risk factors and lower urinary tract symptoms in both sexes. *Eur Urol*. Sep 2006;**50**(3):581–586.

36 Kuchel GA, Moscufo N, Guttmann CR, et al. Localization of brain white matter hyperintensities and urinary incontinence in community–dwelling older adults. *J Gerontol A Biol Sci Med Sci*. Aug 2009;**64**(8):902–909.

37 Kuo HK, Lipsitz LA. Cerebral white matter changes and geriatric syndromes: is there a link? *J Gerontol A Biol Sci Med Sci*. Aug 2004;**59**(8):818–826.

38 Griffiths D, Derbyshire S, Stenger A, Resnick N. Brain control of normal and overactive bladder. *J Urol*. Nov 2005;**174**(5):1862–1867.

39 Monsuez JJ, Gesquiere-Dando A, Rivera S. Cardiovascular prevention of cognitive decline. *Cardiol Res Pract*. 2011;**2011**:250970.

40 Cigolle CT, Langa KM, Kabeto MU et al. Geriatric conditions and disability: the Health and Retirement Study. *Ann Intern Med*. Aug 7 2007;**147**(3):156–164.

41 van Houten P, Achterberg W, Ribbe M. Urinary incontinence in disabled elderly women: a randomized clinical trial on the effect of training mobility and toileting skills to achieve independent toileting. *Gerontology* 2007;**53**(4):205–210.

42 Kim H, Suzuki T, Yoshida Y, Yoshida H. Effectiveness of multidimensional exercises for the treatment of stress urinary incontinence in elderly community–dwelling Japanese women: a randomized, controlled, crossover trial. *J Am Geriatr Soc*. Dec 2007;**55**(12):1932–1939.

43 Arnett RH 3rd, Blank LA, Brown AP, et al. National health expenditures, 1988. Office of National Cost Estimates. *Health Care Financ Rev*. Summer 1990;**11**(4):1–41.

44 Gupta S, Rappaport HM, Bennett LT. Inappropriate drug prescribing and related outcomes for elderly medicaid beneficiaries residing in nursing homes. *Clinical Ther*. Jan–Feb 1996;**18**(1):183–196.

45 Golden AG, Preston RA, Barnett SD, et al. Inappropriate medication prescribing in home-bound older adults. *J Am Geriatr Soc*. Aug 1999;**47**(8):948–953.

46 Kennerfalk A, Ruigomez A, Wallander MA, et al. Geriatric drug therapy and healthcare utilization in the United Kingdom. *Ann Pharmacother*. May 2002;**36**(5):797–803.

47 Ruby CM, Hanlon JT, Boudreau RM, et al. Aging and body composition study. THe effect of medication use on urinary incontinence in community dwelling elderly women. *J Am Geriatr Soc*. 2010;**58**(9): 1715–1720.

48 Gill SS, Mamdani M, Naglie G, et al. A prescribing cascade involving cholinesterase inhibitors and anticholinergic drugs. *Archives Intern Med*. Apr 11 2005;**165**(7):808–813.

49 Starr JM. Cholinesterase inhibitor treatment and urinary incontinence in Alzheimer's disease. *J Am Geriatr Soc*. May 2007;**55**(5): 800–801.

50 Alzheimer's disease: beware of interactions with cholinesterase inhibitors. *Prescrire Int*. Jun 2006;**15**(83):103–106.

51 Siegler EL, Reidenberg M. Treatment of urinary incontinence with anticholinergics in patients taking cholinesterase inhibitors for dementia. *Clin Pharmacol Ther*. May 2004; **75**(5):484–488.

52 Sink KM, Thomas J 3rd, Xu H, et al. Dual use of bladder anticholinergics and cholinesterase inhibitors: long–term functional and cognitive outcomes. *J Am Ger Soc*. May 2008;**56**(5): 847–853.

53 Isik AT, Celik T, Bozoglu E, Doruk H. Trospium and cognition in patients with late onset Alzheimer disease. *J Nutr Health Aging* Aug 2009;**13**(8):672–676.

54 Sakakibara R, Ogata T, Uchiyama T, et al. How to manage overactive bladder in elderly individuals with dementia? A combined use of donepezil, a central acetylcholinesterase inhibitor, and propiverine, a peripheral muscarine receptor antagonist. *J Am Geriatr Soc*. Aug 2009;**57**(8):1515–1517.

55 Kincade JE, Dougherty MC, Carlson JR, et al. Randomized clinical trial of efficacy of self–monitoring techniques to treat urinary incontinence in women. *Neurourol Urodyn.* 2007;**26**(4):507–511.

56 Landefeld CS. Pragmatic approaches that improve care for geriatric conditions: balancing the promise and the peril of quality indicators. *J Am Geriatr Soc.* Mar 2009; **57**(3):556–558.

57 Bryant CM, Dowell CJ, Fairbrother G. Caffeine reduction education to improve urinary symptoms. *Br J Nurs.* Apr 25–May 8 2002;**11**(8): 560–565.

58 Schnelle JF, Leung FW, Rao SS, et al. A controlled trial of an intervention to improve urinary and fecal incontinence and constipation. *J Am Geriatr Soc.* Aug 2010;**58**(8): 1504–1511.

59 Dowd TT, Campbell JM, Jones JA. Fluid intake and urinary incontinence in older community–dwelling women. *J Community Health Nurs.* 1996;**13**(3):179–186.

60 Spangler PF, Risley TR, Bilyew DD. The management of dehydration and incontinence in nonambulatory geriatric patients. *J Appl Behav Anal.* Fall 1984;**17**(3):397–401.

61 Wallace SA, Roe B, Williams K, Palmer M. Bladder training for urinary incontinence in adults. *Cochrane Database Syst Rev.* 2004(**1**):CD001308.

62 Ouslander JG, Schnelle JF, Uman G, et al. Predictors of successful prompted voiding among incontinent nursing home residents. *JAMA* May 3 1995;**273**(17):1366–1370.

63 Schnelle JF, Sowell VA, Hu TW, Traughber B. Reduction of urinary incontinence in nursing homes: does it reduce or increase costs? *J Am Geriatr Soc.* Jan 1988;**36**(1):34–39.

64 Palmer MH. Effectiveness of prompted voiding for incontinent nursing home residents. In: B. M. Melnyk EF-O, ed. *Evidence-Based Practice in Nursing and Healthcare: A Guide to the Best Practice.* Lippincott Williams & Wilkins, 2005: 20–30.

65 Roe B, Ostaszkiewicz J, Milne J, Wallace S. Systematic reviews of bladder training and voiding programmes in adults: a synopsis of findings from data analysis and outcomes using metastudy techniques. *J Adv Nurs.* Jan 2007;**57**(1):15–31.

66 Ostaszkiewicz J, Roe B, Johnston L. Effects of timed voiding for the management of urinary incontinence in adults: systematic review. *J Adv Nurs.* Nov 2005;**52**(4):420–431.

67 Perry S, Shaw C, Assassa P, et al. An epidemiological study to establish the prevalence of urinary symptoms and felt need in the community: the Leicestershire MRC Incontinence Study. Leicestershire MRC Incontinence Study Team. *J Public Health Med.* Sep 2000;**22**(3):427–434.

68 Wagg AS, Cardozo L, Chapple C, et al. Overactive bladder syndrome in older people. *BJU Int.* Mar 2007;**99**(3):502–509.

69 Wagg A, Wyndaele JJ, Sieber P. Efficacy and tolerability of solifenacin in elderly subjects with overactive bladder syndrome: a pooled analysis. *Am J Geriatr Pharmacother.* Mar 2006;**4**(1):14–24.

70 Kraus SR, Ruiz-Cerda JL, Martire D, et al. Efficacy and tolerability of fesoterodine in older and younger subjects with overactive bladder. *Urology* Dec 2010;**76**(6): 1350–1357.

71 Campanelli C.American Geriatrics Society Updated Beers Criteria for potentially inappropriate medication use in older adults. *J Am Geriatr Soc.* Apr 2012;**60**(4):616–631.

72 Gomes T, Juurlink DN, Ho JM, et al. Risk of serious falls associated with oxybutynin and tolterodine: a population based study. *J Urol.* Oct 2011;**186**(4):1340–1344.

73 Lackner TE, Wyman JF, McCarthy TC, et al. Randomized, placebo–controlled trial of the cognitive effect, safety, and tolerability of oral extended–release oxybutynin in cognitively impaired nursing home residents with urge urinary incontinence. *J Am Geriatr Soc.* May 2008;**56**(5):862–870.

74 Ouslander JG, Schnelle JF, Uman G, et al. Does oxybutynin add to the effectiveness of prompted voiding for urinary incontinence among nursing home residents? A placebo–controlled trial. *J Am Geriatr Soc.* Jun 1995;**43**(6):610–617.

75 Minassian VA, Ross S, Sumabat O, et al. Randomized trial of oxybutynin extended versus immediate release for women aged 65 and older with overactive bladder: lessons learned from conducting a trial. *J Obstet Gynaecol Can.* Sep 2007;**29**(9):726–732.

76 DuBeau CE, Kraus SR, Griebling TL, et al. Effect of fesoterodine in vulnerable elderly subjects with urgency incontinence: a double-blind, placebo-controlled trial. *J Urol.* 2013;JURO 10640.

77 Szonyi G, Collas DM, Ding YY, Malone-Lee JG. Oxybutynin with bladder retraining for detrusor instability in elderly people: a randomized controlled trial. *Age Ageing* Jul 1995;**24**(4): 287–291.

78 Bemelmans BL, Kiemeney LA, Debruyne FM. Low-dose oxybutynin for the treatment of urge incontinence: good efficacy and few side effects. *Eur Urol.* Jun 2000;**37**(6):709–713.

79 Buser N, Ivic S, Kessler TM, et al. Efficacy and adverse events of antimuscarinics for treating overactive bladder: network meta-analyses. *Eur Urol.* 2012 Dec;**62**(6):1040–1060.

80 Zinner NR, Mattiasson A, Stanton SL. Efficacy, safety, and tolerability of extended–release once–daily tolterodine treatment for overactive bladder in older versus younger patients. *J Am Geriatr Soc.* May 2002;**50**(5):799–807.

81 Millard R, Tuttle J, Moore K, et al. Clinical efficacy and safety of tolterodine compared to placebo in detrusor overactivity. *J Urol.* May 1999;**161**(5):1551–1555.

82 Drutz HP, Appell RA, Gleason D, et al. Clinical efficacy and safety of tolterodine compared to oxybutynin and placebo in patients with overactive bladder. *Int Urogynecol J Pelvic Floor Dysfunct.* 1999;**10**(5):283–289.

83 Michel MC, Schneider T, Krege S, Goepel M. Does gender or age affect the efficacy and safety of tolterodine? *J Urol.* Sep 2002;**168**(3): 1027–1031.

84 Chung SD, Chang HC, Chiu B, et al. The efficacy of additive tolterodine extended release for 1–year in older men with storage symptoms and clinical benign proastatic hyperplasia. *Neurourol Urodyn.* Apr 2011;**30**(4): 568–571.

85 Chapple C, DuBeau C, Ebinger U, et al. Darifenacin treatment of patients > or = 65 years with overactive bladder: results of a randomized, controlled, 12-week trial. *Curr Med Res Opin.* Oct 2007;**23**(10):2347–2358.

86 Hill S, Elhilali M, Millard RJ, et al. Long–term darifenacin treatment for overactive bladder in patients aged 65 years and older: analysis of results from a 2-year, open-label extension study. *Curr Med Res Opin.* Nov 2007;**23**(11):2697–2704.

87 Lipton RB, Kolodner K, Wesnes K. Assessment of cognitive function of the elderly population: effects of darifenacin. *J Urol.* Feb 2005;**173**(2): 493–498.

88 Kay G, Crook T, Rekeda L, et al. Differential effects of the antimuscarinic agents darifenacin and oxybutynin ER on memory in older subjects. *Eur Urol.* Aug 2006;**50**(2):317–326.

89 Malhotra BK, Wood N, Sachse R. Influence of age, gender, and race on pharmacokinetics, pharmacodynamics, and safety of fesoterodine. *Int J Clin Pharmacol Ther.* Sep 2009;**47**(9): 570–578.

90 Wagg A, Khullar V, Marschall-Kehrel D, et al. Flexible-dose fesoterodine in elderly adults with overactive bladder: results of the randomized, double–blind, placebo–controlled study of fesoterodine in an aging population trial. *J Am Geriatr Soc.* Feb 2013;**61**(2): 185–193.

91 Wagg A, Khullar V, Michel MC, et al.. Long–term safety, tolerability and efficacy of flex-ible–dose fesoterodine in elderly patients with overactive bladder: Open–label extension of the SOFIA trial. *Neurourol Urodyn.* Jan 2014;**33**(1):106–114.

92 Saliba D, Elliott M, Rubenstein LZ, et al. The Vulnerable Elders Survey: a tool for identifying vulnerable older people in the community. *J Am Geriatr Soc.* Dec 2001;**49**(12): 1691–1699.

93 Kay GG, Maruff P, Scholfield D, et al. Evaluation of cognitive function in healthy older subjects treated with fesoterodine. *Postgrad Med.* May 2012;**124**(3):7–15.

94 Herschorn S, Pommerville P, Stothers L, et al. Tolerability of solifenacin and oxybutynin immediate release in older (>65 years) and younger (</=65 years) patients with overactive bladder: sub–analysis from a Canadian, randomized, double-blind study. *Curr Med Res Opin.* Feb 2011;**27**(2):375–382.

95 Wagg A, Dale M, Tretter R, Stow B, Compion G. Randomised, multicentre, placebo–controlled, double-blind crossover study investigating the effect of solifenacin and oxybutynin in elderly people with mild cognitive impairment: the SENIOR study. *Eur Urol.* Jul 2013;**64**(1):74–81.

96 Dmochowski RR, Sand PK, Zinner NR, Staskin DR. Trospium 60 mg once daily (QD) for overactive bladder syndrome: results from a placebo–controlled interventional study. *Urology.* Mar 2008;**71**(3):449–454.

97 Staskin D, Kay G, Tannenbaum C, et al. Trospium chloride has no effect on memory testing and is assay undetectable in the central nervous system of older patients with overactive bladder. *IntJ Clin Pract.* 2010;**64**(9):1294–1300.

98 Madersbacher H, Murtz G. Efficacy, tolerability and safety profile of propiverine in the treatment of the overactive bladder (non-neurogenic and neurogenic). *World J Urol.* Nov 2001;**19**(5):324–335.

99 Mori S, Kojima M, Sakai Y, Nakajima K. Bladder dysfunction in dementia patients showing urinary incontinence: evaluation with cystometry and treatment with propiverine hydrochloride. *Nippon Ronen Igakkai Zasshi.* Jul 1999;**36**(7):489–494.

100 Dorschner W, Stolzenburg JU, Griebenow R, et al. The elderly patient with urge incontinence or urge–stress incontinence – efficacy and cardiac safety of propiverine. *Aktuelle Urol.* Mar 2003;**34**(2):102–108.

101 Oelke M, Murgas S, Schneider T, Heßdörfer E. Influence of Propiverine ER 30 mg once daily on cognitive function in elderly female and male patients with overactive bladder: A non-interventional study to assess real life data. *Neurourol Urodyn.* 2013;**32**(6):800–802.

102 Wagg A, Cardozo L, Nitti VW, et al. The efficacy and tolerability of the beta–3 adrenoreceptor agonist mirabegron for the treatment of symptoms of overactive bladder in older patients. *Age Ageing* Sep 2014;**43**(5):666–675. Epub 2014 Mar 6.

103 White WM, Pickens RB, Doggweiler R, Klein FA. Short–term efficacy of botulinum toxin a for refractory overactive bladder in the elderly population. *J Urol.* Dec 2008;**180**(6):2522–2526.

104 Nitti VW, Dmochowski R, Herschorn S, et al. OnabotulinumtoxinA for the treatment of patients with overactive bladder and urinary incontinence: results of a phase 3, randomized, placebo controlled trial. *J Urol.* Jun 2013;**189**(6):2186–2193.

105 Bonde HV, Sejr T, Erdmann L, et al. Residual urine in 75-year-old men and women. A normative population study. *Scandinavian J Urol Nephrol.* Apr 1996;**30**(2):89–91.

106 Susset JG, Servot-Viguier D, Lamy F, et al. Collagen in 155 human bladders. *Invest Urol.* Nov 1978;**16**(3):204–206.

107 Fry CH, Bayliss M, Young JS, Hussain M. Influence of age and bladder dysfunction on the contractile properties of isolated human detrusor smooth muscle. *BJU Int.* Jul 2011;**108**(2 Pt 2):E91–96.

108 Giannantoni A, Conte A, Proietti S, et al. Botulinum toxin type A in patients with Parkinson's disease and refractory overactive bladder. *J Urol.* Sep 2011;**186**(3):960–964.

CHAPTER 19

Bladder outlet obstruction and the overactive bladder

Nadir I. Osman and Christopher R. Chapple

Department of Urology, Royal Hallamshire Hospital, Sheffield, UK

KEY POINTS

- Overactive bladder (OAB) frequently co-exists with bladder outlet obstruction due to benign prostatic hyperplasia in men.

- OAB, detrusor overactivity, and bladder outlet obstruction all increase in frequency with aging.

- Bladder outlet obstruction may induce OAB through morphological and functional changes in the bladder wall induced by ischemia.

- TURP may improve OAB symptoms by de-afferentiation of prostatic neurons rather than de-obstruction.

- OAB symptoms and detrusor overactivity fail to resolve in approximately one third of patients after transurethral resection of the prostate (TURP), despite resolution of BOO.

- Persistent OAB symptoms after bladder outlet surgery are associated with an unfavorable outcome.

- If OAB symptoms do not resolve with conservative management, a urodynamic study is recommended before any invasive therapy is considered due to the wide range of possible underlying abnormalities.

Introduction

Lower urinary tract symptom (LUTS) are highly frequent in the male population, [1] affecting around 30% of older men, 8% of whom require surgical treatment for bladder outlet obstruction (BOO). [2] Most commonly, BOO occurs as a consequence of encroachment onto the urethral lumen by an enlarged prostate gland due to benign prostatic hyperplasia (BPH). [3] Usually this manifests as voiding LUTS such as weak flow and intermittency. Many patients also complain of storage LUTS such as urinary urgency, frequency, nocturia, and urgency urinary incontinence (UUI) which are often more bothersome. [4] When urgency with or without UUI is present, these symptoms are termed Overactive Bladder (OAB), an important subset of storage LUTS that is

---

Overactive Bladder: Practical Management, First Edition. Edited by Jacques Corcos, Scott MacDiarmid and John Heesakkers.

© 2015 John Wiley & Sons, Ltd. Published 2015 by John Wiley & Sons, Ltd.

highly correlated with another principle urodynamic diagnosis in men: detrusor overactivity (DOA). [5] Although it has long been a tenant of urological teaching that OAB symptoms in men arise as a result of BOO caused by BPH, it is apparent that the presence of OAB/DO cannot always be explained by BOO. In this chapter we discuss the relationship between BOO and OAB/DOA, in light of the epidemiological, animal, and clinical data, and its relevance to the evaluation and treatment of patients with OAB.

Bladder outlet obstruction

Male BOO is a common, well-studied and characterized phenomenon. Its accurate diagnosis requires a pressure–flow study as a low flow rate and raised post-voiding residual could equally arise from an under-active detrusor in the absence of BOO. In men undergoing urodynamic studies for non-neurogenic LUTS, BOO is found in approximately one third. [6, 7] The finding of a high-pressure low-flow pattern is diagnostic (Figure 19.1). From historical series of men undergoing bladder outlet surgery, standardized nomograms have been developed which allow the determination of whether a patient's pressure–flow study shows obstruction. Of these, the international continence society (ICS) nomogram is the most widely accepted. [8] By plotting the maximal flow rate (Qmax) against the detrusor pressure at maximal flow (PdetQmax), a given void can be classed into one of three categories; unobstructed, equivocal, and obstructed (Figure 19.2).

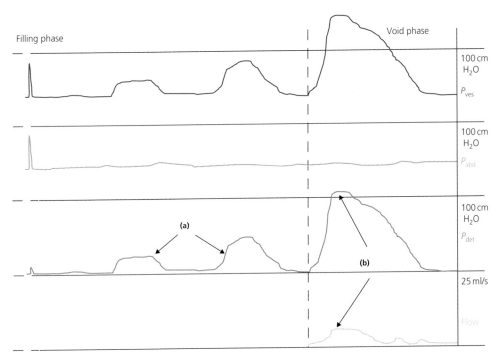

Figure 19.1 Typical Pressure-flow study of an elderly male with OAB and voiding LUTS demonstrating (a) phasic systolic DO and (b) high pressure low flow voiding.

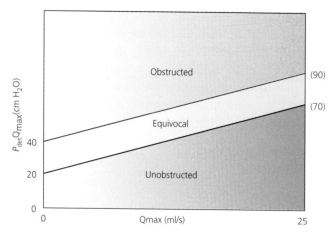

Figure 19.2 The ICS nomogram By plotting the maximal flow rate (Q_{max}) against the detrusor pressure at maximal flow ($P_{det}Q_{max}$), a given void can be classed as unobstructed, equivocal or obstructed. Source: Modified from Abrams 1999 [8].

The most frequent cause of BOO in men is BPH; the non-malignant histological expansion of the stromal and epithelial components of the prostate gland. BOO arising due to BPH has been conceptualized as consisting of two components: static (due to the bulk effect of the prostatic tissue) and dynamic (due to the tension exerted by smooth muscle).

BOO due to BPH is considered a compressive (flexible) obstruction according to Schafers description of the passive urethral resistance relation (PURR) curve. [9] In this type of obstruction the detrusor opening pressure, the detrusor pressure at the very start of flow, is raised but then subsequently little further pressure is needed to increase the flow rate. In the alternative type of obstruction, termed constrictive, the opening pressure is normal but then increasing pressure is required to increase the flow rate. This is seen with fixed anatomical obstructions, such as urethral stricture, meatal stenosis, and the tight fibrotic prostate.

The relationship between bladder outlet obstruction and overactive bladder

OAB/DO has long been assumed to arise as a consequence of BOO. Hunter, writing in the eighteenth century, noted that "the diseases of the bladder arising from obstruction and its consequence is an increase irritability, by which the bladder admits of little distention because quick its action ..." This supposition was supported by a range of animal models demonstrating DOA after experimental BOO, yet the epidemiological, clinical, and empirical data suggests that the relationship between BOO and OAB is more complex.

A multitude of studies in a range of non-primate mammals have consistently demonstrated non-voiding detrusor contractions following experimental BOO. However, there are several important factors that limit the extrapolation of such data to the human situation. The methods of inducing BOO commonly entail implanting a ring around the animal's urethra which, as the animal grows, causes a constriction and urethral obstruction. This contrasts to the common scenario in man, which is a compressive prostatic obstruction. Moreover, the obstruction often occurs rather acutely, whereas BPH and urethral stricture presumably cause a gradual obstruction over months to years. Additionally, young female animals are often studied rather than older males. Finally, in most non-primate mammalian species, particularly rodents, there is a considerable non-cholinergic non-adrenergic component to the functional innervation of the bladder as contrasted to the predominant cholinergic innervation in man.

In men, both OAB and BPH increase in prevalence with aging. [10, 11] Large population studies have shown that OAB is equally as common in women and shows an almost identical age-related increase in prevalence. [10] Whereas in men the increase could be explained by the effect of BPH, the absence of an analogous cause of BOO in women suggests a pathogenesis related to the aging process. Indeed aging was found to be an independent predictor of DOA in men with LUTS due to BOO suggesting it is an important etiological factor in both sexes. [12] Urodynamic data also show that DOA commonly occurs in men with BOO due to BPH (present in 52–80%). [13] Some series have found that BOO is a predictor of DOA with increasing severity of obstruction correlating to an increasing probability of DOA. [12, 14] Meanwhile, others failed to demonstrate such a relationship suggesting the co-existence of BOO and DOA may be circumstantial. [15, 16]

Empirical clinical evidence also suggests OAB is not a necessary consequence of BOO. Whilst OAB/DOA is often seen in men with enlarged prostates, men with urethral stricture disease, a constrictive obstruction, rarely complain of urgency suggesting the development of OAB may depend on the type of obstruction. A further relevant observation is the persistence of OAB after bladder outlet surgery in approximately one third of men [17] and the persistence of DOA in a similar proportion; [18] suggesting that in some individuals OAB/DO has an etiopathogenesis unrelated to obstruction. Further evidence of this is provided by the work of Chalfin and Bradley, who demonstrated the resolution of OAB symptoms and DOA in 10 out of 11 patients with urodynamically confirmed BOO after transperineal injection of lidocaine into the prostate despite the persistence of BOO. [19]

In summary, it would appear that BOO almost certainly causes OAB/DOA in some individuals whereas in others OAB/DOA is an entirely coincidental finding due its high prevalence, particularly in older individuals.

Pathogenesis of OAB in patients with bladder outlet obstruction

Several theories for the development of OAB/DO have been proposed and are the subject of academic discourse; these have been discussed in detail elsewhere in this book and in the literature. [20] In terms of OAB caused by BOO, morphological bladder wall changes (e.g., detrusor wall thickening, increased collagen content, changes in neuronal density, increase and alteration of adrenoceptors) and functional bladder wall changes (e.g., partial denervation, hypersensitivity of muscarinic receptors to acetylcholine, neurotransmitter imbalance, changes in electrical properties of detrusor smooth muscle cells, reorganization of the spinal micturition reflex) are thought to contribute to the development of DO and/or a reduction in bladder capacity.

Brading's theory of "Denervation hypersensitivity," [21] based upon a series of landmark studies conducted in pigs, [22–24] is the most established explanation for the development of DOA after BOO. The cholinergic innervation of pig bladders has a significant functional role that is more analogous to the human bladder than other non-primate mammals. BOO was created by tying a silk suture or placing a metal ring around the proximal urethra. The response of bladder muscle strips to acetylcholine, muscarinic receptor agonists, and intramural nerve stimulation was then compared to unobstructed controls. An increased response to cholinergic stimulation but a reduced response to nerve stimulation was observed in the obstructed animals compared to the controls. These findings were suggested as signifying partial denervation of the bladder consequent upon obstruction with a resulting post-junctional hypersensitivity of the detrusor. This was postulated as the reason DOA occurred in men with BOO. Studies of blood flow in this model showed evidence of prolonged episodes of detrusor ischemia which may explain the neuronal and biochemical changes. [25]

The findings of this work have not been consistently reproduced by other groups and in other mammals. In some cases, no change in cholinergic responses occurred or reduced responses were seen particularly in the context of long standing or severe BOO. [26] Therefore it may be the case that DO occurring in early/mild obstruction is related to denervation and increased responses to cholinergic stimulation whereas in later or more severe obstruction there is an alternative mechanism for the development of DO. [27]

The observation that in most patients OAB/DOA resolves after transurethral resection of the prostate (TURP) supports the notion that BOO is the cause of OAB/DOA. However, the work of Chalfin and Bradley would suggest a sensory mechanism is also plausible. In TURP the first part of the operation involves destruction of the urothelium and submucosal structures of the prostate and bladder neck, certain to include afferent nerve endings. TURP may therefore resolve OAB/DO not by de-obstruction but by de-afferentiation. Data from the CLaSP (Conservative management Laser therapy transurethral resection of the Prostate) study would support this possibility. [28] Side fire laser treatment, although being significantly worse than TURP at reducing BOO, was equally as effective in reducing OAB and DOA. Thus, it may be the case, as Chalfin and Bradley had originally proposed, that it is an abnormal sensory stimulus from a hyperplastic prostate that leads to OAB/DO in men with BOO. A summary of the possible mechanism leading to the development of OAB/DOA is provided in Figure 19.3.

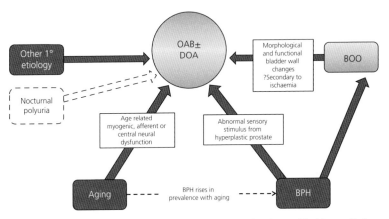

Figure 19.3 The aetio-pathogenesis of OAB in men. OAB may arise due to bladder wall changes induced by BOO or due a sensory mechanism related to the hyperplastic prostate. Alternatively OAB may be caused by changes associated with aging or a separate primary etiology. Nocturnal polyuria is an important contributory factor to nocturia, particularly in older patients.

OAB and the treatment of male BOO

Alpha-blockers

Alpha-blockers (AB) are the most frequently used pharmacotherapy in the treatment of men with LUTS/BPH. AB lead to both an improvement in voiding and storage LUTS in addition to urinary flow rates. [29] The overarching view is that AB work by inducing smooth muscle relaxation in the prostate and bladder neck by antagonism of the α-1 adrenoreceptors. [30] The implication is that the mechanism for their efficacy is the amelioration the dynamic component of BOO due to BPH. Yet it is apparent that BOO is not present in all patients who derive benefit from AB treatment and it is often the case that patients show considerable symptomatic improvement with only minimal (often not significant) changes in detrusor voiding pressures. [31–33] In addition, the finding of BOO on pre-treatment urodynamics was shown to have no impact upon the chance

of treatment success. [31] Consequently, it has been suggested that AB may work through an alternative mechanism that improves OAB/DOA through central or peripheral antagonism of α-adrenorecep-tors. [34] In particular, the α-1d adrenoreceptor that is present in the bladder body and spinal cord has been mooted as having an important role in the pathogenesis of storage LUTS in men. Studies in obstructed animals appear to support this, where intrathecal administration of an α-1 type selective AB led to reductions in urinary frequency and DO suggesting an inhibition of spinal reflexes. [34, 35]

Surgery for BOO

Surgery for BOO due to BPH is often performed. The estimated lifetime risk for a man to require outlet surgery is 29%. [36] Longitudinal data from the Veteran's Affairs study in the USA has demonstrated that 36% of men with LUTS due to BPH randomized to watchful waiting switched to invasive therapy within five years of enrolment, [37] whilst in an observational study of men with LUTS due to BPH 10, 24, and 39% of men with mild, moderate, and severe baseline symptoms respectively required surgery over a four-year period. [38] TURP is widely considered as the gold standard surgical treatment for LUTS due to BPH. [39] A seminal multi-center randomized trial comparing TURP with watchful waiting (WW) demonstrated a 52% reduction in risk of treatment failure with TURP compared to WW whilst there was a 1% risk of urinary incontinence, similar to the WW group. [40]

DOA is present in 31–68% of men who had urodynamic evaluation prior to TURP. [17, 41, 42] At six months follow-up after TURP, DOA resolves in 41–69% of patients, which is sustained through to medium term follow-up (1–5 yrs). A unique study from Bristol (UK) assessing 10-year outcomes of TURP showed an increase in DOA from 40 to 60% despite patients remaining unobstructed. [43] Another study by the same group, reporting long-term follow-up of patients with untreated BOO, showed a similar increase. [44] Taken together, this data can be interpreted as indicating that the recurrence of DOA is either due to the aging process or a degree of re-innervation of the prostatic urethra and bladder neck with time.

TURP has an unsatisfactory result in around 25–30% of patients. [45] Poor outcomes are often attributed to the persistence of storage LUTS/OAB which are typically the ones that the patient found most bothersome pre-operatively. [45] It should be noted that nocturia in particular is highly bothersome as it may impact upon quality of sleep leading to daytime somnolence and a reduction in quality of life. [46] In men with persistent symptoms

after TURP a range of urodynamic diagnoses are found. An analysis of 185 patients showed DOA in 19.6%, low detrusor contractility in 18.7%, detrusor hyperactivity with impaired contractility (DHIC) in 14.4%, poor relaxation of the urethral sphincter in 19.3%, and BOO in 27.8% whilst 10% had a normal study. [47] A further study showed DOA in 50% of patients, finding no difference in total, voiding, and storage symptom scores between patients with and without DOA. [48] This emphasizes the need for a repeat urodynamic assessment before any further invasive therapy is considered.

Whether the presence of OAB/DOA pre-operatively predicts a poorer outcome of TURP is unclear. In a study of 127 men followed up with urodynamics at three months post-operatively, there was no difference in pre-operative International prostate symptom storage scores between patients who had improved and those who had not. The authors did note a tendency to "more bladder irritability" and slightly less obstruction in those not improving. [49] A smaller study, including 37 patients, found pre-operative DOA did not impact on the rate of re-operation whilst BOO co-existent with DO did not lead to a decrease in the efficacy of surgery. [50] Another study assessed the impact of type of DOA on treatment outcome in 19 men who had undergone TURP, finding that patients in whom DOA manifested as single large terminal contraction were more likely to show resolution of DOA at six months post-operatively compared to those with phasic systolic contractions and poor compliance. [51]

In practice, persisting symptoms after a TURP will resolve spontaneously in most patients. It should be emphasized that this can take anywhere from a few weeks to a year. Apart from residual BOO and DOA, such symptoms could also be attributable to prolonged wound healing, infection, and bladder neck irritation. [49] In patients in whom OAB symptoms do not resolve, an antimuscarinic (anti-M) can be trialed. A urodynamic study should be repeated before consideration is given to any further invasive intervention. If persistent DOA is found, intravesical botulinum toxin may be considered. If there is strong evidence that the patient remains obstructed due to BPH, re-operation may be contemplated taking into careful consideration other important factors such as the severity of voiding symptoms. Certainly repeat surgery should not be rushed into. There is a need for further studies investigating the management of persistent OAB/DOA after TURP.

BOO and antimuscarinics

Anti-Ms were traditionally contraindicated in men due to the fear of precipitating urinary retention. A large number of well-designed, randomized controlled trials have now demonstrated the safety and efficacy of anti-Ms as a single agent or in combination with an AB in the treatment of storage LUTS in men. [52] Relatively fewer studies have assessed the use of anti-Ms in men with urodynamically confirmed BOO, as in practice pharmacotherapy is usually commenced on the basis of symptoms before a urodynamic assessment is undertaken. Abrams et al. conducted one of the first such studies, assessing tolterodine 2 mg BD in a small randomized trial in men over 40 years with BOO and DOA. [53] A total of 149 and 72 men were randomized to tolterodine and placebo respectively. Urodynamic studies were performed at baseline and at 12 weeks. There was no significant difference in terms of Qmax and pdet@Qmax between the groups at baseline. At 12 weeks, tolterodine caused a reduction in the bladder contractility index (BCI) (-5 vs. +5, $p = .0045$) and an increase in PVR compared to placebo (25 ml vs. 0 ml, $p \leq .004$). Urinary retention was reported in only one patient who had received placebo. The incidence of adverse events was similar between the groups. A further eight-week study by Lee demonstrated a similar small rise in PVR with the anti-M propiverine (in combination with doxazosin) and no increased risk of urinary retention. [54] Although longer term studies are needed, these data suggest anti-Ms have little impact on risk of urinary retention in men with BOO. Most national and international guidelines now make recommendations on the institution of anti-M therapy in men; readers should refer to their local guidance.

Conclusions

The relationship between OAB and BOO is complex and incompletely understood. In some individuals it would appear that OAB is a direct consequence of BOO, witnessed by the prompt resolution of symptoms after medical or surgical therapies. This supposition is supported by animal studies which demonstrate DOA following after BOO is induced by ligation of the urethra. In other individuals, OAB symptoms and DOA may have a separate etiology or occur as part of the aging process. The mechanism by which therapies targeting the bladder outlet, such as AB or TURP, work may not be as simple as previously thought. It is probable that TURP improves OAB by de-affrentiation of the prostatic neurons whilst AB may inhibit bladder reflexes through a central mechanism. A better understanding of the genesis of OAB symptoms and DOA in the context of BOO will help to better delineate which patients are likely to respond to de-obstructive surgery. There is need for further studies addressing the management of persistent OAB/DOA after TURP.

References

1 Kupelian V, Wei JT, O'Leary MP, et al. Prevalence of lower urinary tract symptoms and effect on quality of life in a racially and ethnically diverse random sample: the Boston Area Community Health (BACH) Survey. *Arch Intern Med.* 2006 Nov 27;**166**:2381–2387.

2 Madersbacher S, Haidinger G, Temml C, Schmidbauer CP. Prevalence of lower urinary tract symptoms in Austria as assessed by an open survey of 2,096 men. *Eur Urol.* 1998 Aug;**34**:136–141.

3 [3]C C. Medical treatment for benign prostatic hyperplasia. *BMJ.* 1992 May 9; **304**:1198–1199.

4 Coyne KS, Sexton CC, Kopp ZS, et al. The impact of overactive bladder on mental health, work productivity and health–related quality of life in the UK and Sweden: results from EpiLUTS. *BJU Int.* 2011 Nov;**108**:1459–1471.

5 Hashim H, Abrams P. Is the bladder a reliable witness for predicting detrusor overactivity? J Urol. 2006 Jan;**175**:191–194; discussion 4–5.

6 Jeong SJ, Kim HJ, Lee YJ, et al. Prevalence and clinical features of detrusor underactivity among elderly with lower urinary tract symptoms: a comparison between men and women. *Korean J Urol.* 2012 May;**53**:342–348.

7 Abarbanel J, Marcus EL. Impaired detrusor contractility in community–dwelling elderly presenting with lower urinary tract symptoms. *Urology* 2007 Mar;**69**:436–440.

8 Abrams P. Bladder outlet obstruction index, bladder contractility index and bladder voiding efficiency: three simple indices to define bladder voiding function. *BJU Int.* 1999 Jul;**84**:14–15.

9 Schäfer W. Urodynamics of micturition. *Curr Opin Urol.* 1992;**2**:252–256.

10 Irwin DE, Milsom I, Hunskaar S, et al. Population-based survey of urinary incontinence, overactive bladder, and other lower urinary tract symptoms in five countries: results of the EPIC study. *Eur Urol.* 2006 Dec;**50**:1306–1314; discussion 14–15.

11 Berry SJ, Coffey DS, Walsh PC, Ewing LL. The development of human benign prostatic hyperplasia with age. *J Urol.* 1984 Sep;**132**:474–479.

12 Oelke M, Baard J, Wijkstra H, et al. Age and bladder outlet obstruction are independently associated with detrusor overactivity in patients with benign prostatic hyperplasia. *Eur Urol.* 2008 Aug;**54**:419–426.

13 Chapple CR, Smith D. The pathophysiological changes in the bladder obstructed by benign prostatic hyperplasia. *Br J Urol.* 1994 Feb;**73**: 117–123.

14 Vesely S, Knutson T, Fall M, et al. Clinical diagnosis of bladder outlet obstruction in men with lower urinary tract symptoms: reliability of commonly measured parameters and the role of idiopathic detrusor overactivity. *Neurourol Urodyn.* 2003;**22**:301–305.

15 Rosier PF, de la Rosette JJ, Wijkstra H, et al. Is detrusor instability in elderly males related to the grade of obstruction? *Neurourol Urodyn.* 1995; **14**:625–633.

16 Abrams P. Detrusor instability and bladder outlet obstruction. *N Neurourol Urodyn.* 1985;**4**:317–328.

17 Abrams PH, Farrar DJ, Turner–Warwick RT, et al. The results of prostatectomy: a symptomatic and urodynamic analysis of 152 patients. *J Urol.* 1979 May;**121**:640–642.

18 Machino R, Kakizaki H, Ameda K, et al. Detrusor instability with equivocal obstruction: A predictor of unfavorable symptomatic outcomes after transurethral prostatectomy. *Neurourol Urodyn.* 2002;**21**:444–449.

19 Chalfin SA, Bradley WE. The etiology of detrusor hyperreflexia in patients with infravesical obstruction. *J Urol.* 1982 May: **127**;938–942.

20 Roosen A, Chapple CR, Dmochowski RR, et al. A refocus on the bladder as the originator of storage lower urinary tract symptoms: a systematic review of the latest literature. *EurUrol.* 2009 Nov;**56**:810–819.

21 Brading AF. A myogenic basis for the overactive bladder. *Urology* 1997 Dec;**50**:57–67; discussion 8–73.

22 Sibley GN. An experimental model of detrusor instability in the obstructed pig. *Br J Urol.* 1985 Jun;**57**:292–298.

23 Sibley GN. The physiological response of the detrusor muscle to experimental bladder outflow obstruction in the pig. *Br J Urol.* 1987 Oct;**60**:332–336.

24 Speakman MJ, Brading AF, Gilpin CJ, Dixon JS, Gilpin SA, Gosling JA. Bladder outflow obstruction—a cause of denervation supersensitivity. *J Urol.* 1987 Dec;**138**:1461–1466.

25 Greenland JE, Brading AF. The effect of bladder outflow obstruction on detrusor blood flow changes during the voiding cycle in conscious pigs. *J Urol.* 2001 Jan;**165**:245–248.

26 Michel MC, Barendrecht MM. Physiological and pathological regulation of the autonomic control of urinary bladder contractility. *Pharmthera.* 2008 Mar;**117**:297–312.

27 Michel MC, Chapple CR. Basic mechanisms of urgency: preclinical and clinical evidence. *Eur Urol.* 2009 Aug;**56**:298–307.

28 Donovan JL, Peters TJ, Neal DE, et al. A randomized trial comparing transurethral resection of the prostate, laser therapy and conservative treatment of men with symptoms associated with benign prostatic enlargement: The CLasP study. *J Urol.* 2000: **164**.

29 Djavan B, Marberger M. A meta–analysis on the efficacy and tolerability of alpha1–adrenoceptor antagonists in patients with lower urinary tract symptoms suggestive of benign prostatic obstruction. *Euro Urol.* 1999;**36**:1–13.

30 Andersson KE, Lepor H, Wyllie MG. Prostatic alpha 1–adrenoceptors and uroselectivity. *Prostate* 1997 Feb 15;**30**:202–215.

31 Gerber GS, Kim JH, Contreras BA et al. An observational urodynamic evaluation of men with lower urinary tract symptoms treated with doxazosin. *Urology* 1996 Jun;**47**:840–84.

32 Chapple CR, Carter P, Christmas TJ, et al. A three month double–blind study of doxazosin as treatment for benign prostatic bladder outlet obstruction. *Br J Urol.* 1994 Jul;**74**:50–56.

33 Kirby RS, Coppinger SW, Corcoran MO et al. Prazosin in the treatment of prostatic obstruction. A placebo-controlled study. *Br J Urol.* 1987 Aug;**60**:136–142.

34 Andersson K. Alpha1–adrenoceptors and bladder function. *Eur Urol.* 1999;**36** Suppl 1:96–102.

35 Fullhase C, Soler R, Gratzke C, et al. Spinal effects of the fesoterodine metabolite 5–hydroxymethyl tolterodine and/or doxazosin in rats with or without partial urethral obstruction. *J Urol.* 2010 Aug;**184**:783–789.

36 Glynn RJ, Campion EW, Bouchard GR, Silbert JE. The development of benign prostatic hyperplasia among volunteers in the Normative Aging Study. *Am J Epidemiol.* 1985 Jan;**121**:78–90.

37 Flanigan RC, Reda DJ, Wasson JH, et al. 5–year outcome of surgical resection and watchful waiting for men with moderately symptomatic benign prostatic hyperplasia: a Department of Veterans Affairs cooperative study. *J Urol.* 1998 Jul;**160**:12–16; discussion 6–7.

38 Barry MJ, Fowler FJ Jr., Bin L, et al. The natural history of patients with benign prostatic hyperplasia as diagnosed by North American urologists. *J Urol.* 1997 Jan;**157**:10–14; discussion 4–5.

39 Kaplan SA. Transurethral resection of the prostate– is our gold standard still a precious commodity? *J Urol.* 2008 Jul;**180**:15–16.

40 Wasson JH, Reda DJ, Bruskewitz RC, et al. A comparison of transurethral surgery with watchful waiting for moderate symptoms of benign prostatic hyperplasia. The Veterans Affairs Cooperative Study Group on Transurethral Resection of the Prostate. *N Engl J Med.* 1995 Jan 12;**332**:75–79.

41 Van Venrooij GE, Van Melick HH, Eckhardt MD, Boon TA. Correlations of urodynamic changes with changes in symptoms and well–being after transurethral resection of the prostate. *J Urol.* 2002 Aug;**168**:605–609.

42 Seki N, Kai N, Seguchi H, Takei M, et al. Predictives regarding outcome after transurethral resection for prostatic adenoma associated with detrusor underactivity. *Urology* 2006 Feb;**67**:306–310.

43 Thomas AW, Cannon A, Bartlett E, et al. The natural history of lower urinary tract dysfunction in men: minimum 10–year urodynamic followup of transurethral resection of prostate for bladder outlet obstruction. *J Urol.* 2005 Nov;**174**:1887–1891.

44 Thomas AW, Cannon A, Bartlett E et al. The natural history of lower urinary tract

dysfunction in men: minimum 10-year urodynamic follow–up of untreated bladder outlet obstruction. *BJU Int.* 2005 Dec;**96**:1301–1306.

45 Emberton M, Neal DE, Black N, et al. The effect of prostatectomy on symptom severity and quality of life. *Br J Urol.* 1996 Feb;**77**:233–247.

46 Osman NI, Chapple CR, Wein AJ. Nocturia: current concepts and future perspectives. *Acta Physiol (Oxf).* 2013 Jan;**207**:53–65.

47 Kuo HC. Analysis of the pathophysiology of lower urinary tract symptoms in patients after prostatectomy. *Urologia Internationalis* 2002;**68**: 99–104.

48 Nitti VW, Kim Y, Combs AJ. Voiding dysfunction following transurethral resection of the prostate: symptoms and urodynamic findings. *J Urol.* 1997 Feb; **157**:600–603.

49 Hakenberg OW, Pinnock CB, Marshall VR. The follow–up of patients with unfavourable early results of transurethral prostatectomy. *BJU Int.* 1999 Nov; **84**:799–804.

50 Knutson T, Schafer W, Fall M, et al. Can urodynamic assessment of outflow obstruction predict outcome from watchful waiting?—A four–year follow–up study. *Scand J Urol Nephrol.* 2001 Dec;**35**:463–469.

51 Kageyama S, Watanabe T, Kurita Y, et al. Can persisting detrusor hyperreflexia be predicted after transurethral prostatectomy for benign prostatic hypertrophy? *Neurourol Urodyn.* 2000;**19**:233–240.

52 Athanasopoulos A, Chapple C, Fowler C, et al. The role of antimuscarinics in the management of men with symptoms of overactive bladder associated with concomitant bladder outlet obstruction: an update. *Eur Urol.* 2011 Jul;**60**: 94–105.

53 Abrams P, Kaplan S, De Koning Gans HJ, Millard R. Safety and tolerability of tolterodine for the treatment of overactive bladder in men with bladder outlet obstruction. *J Urol.* 2006 Mar;**175**:999–1004; discussion.

54 Lee KS, Choo MS, Kim DY, et al. Combination treatment with propiverine hydrochloride plus doxazosin controlled release gastrointestinal therapeutic system formulation for overactive bladder and coexisting benign prostatic obstruction: a prospective, randomized, controlled multicenter study. *J Urol.* 2005 Oct;**174**:1334–1338.

CHAPTER 20

Synthesis of practical approaches to overactive bladder

Jacques Corcos

Department of Urology, McGill University, Montreal, Canada

> **KEY POINTS**
>
> - Take the time to conduct a thorough interview and include validated questionnaires.
> - Rule out secondary causes of OAB (neurogenic, obstruction, localized disease).
> - Behavioral therapy and physiotherapy are the first-line treatments.
> - Pharmacotherapy has evolved and should be well monitored.
> - Intractable OAB is a major challenge, requiring well-defined, step-by-step management.
> - A significant number of patients find that the results of the treatment do not correspond with personal expectations.

Two groups of patients with OAB symptoms are usually encountered in physician practice: the more predominant group comprises "naïve" patients consulting, for the first time, for bothersome symptoms; and the second group is referred by other physicians after failed OAB management.

Initial management of "naïve" patients with OAB symptoms

The first visit by patients complaining of frequency, urgency with or without incontinence, and nocturia has to be complete and detailed to identify the cause(s) of these symptoms and how bothersome they are.

Current medication, allergies, past medical and surgical history have to be considered in detail. History of symptoms, their onset, progression, and impact on daily life, social and personal activities are recorded. Several validated questionnaires can be administered in this evaluation. Initially used questionnaires can be repeated at each visit and become excellent treatment-surveillance tools. These specific questionnaires are relatively easy to administer in specialized practice where most patients are consulting for voiding dysfunction and fill in the same questionnaire before seeing

Overactive Bladder: Practical Management, First Edition. Edited by Jacques Corcos, Scott MacDiarmid and John Heesakkers.
© 2015 John Wiley & Sons, Ltd. Published 2015 by John Wiley & Sons, Ltd.

physicians. They are obviously more difficult to integrate in more general practice and are then usually completed after having seen practitioners, limiting their utility.

Physical examination comprises complete pelvic assessment, obviously including digital rectal examination in men and vaginal examination in women. Post-void residual evaluation by bladder scan is mandatory to complete this examination.

Basic blood work-up with creatinine and glucose evaluation as well as urine analysis is usually suggested at the first visit.

This initial clinical evaluation, which is much more detailed and referenced in Chapters 5 and 6, will give a good idea of possible symptom origin. The symptoms could be "primary," with no obvious cause, or "secondary" to obstruction, neurogenic conditions, and so on. This practical guide focuses on primary OAB.

Behavioral modification, also called lifestyle change, involves the elimination of dietary irritants, management of fluid intake, weight control, bowel regularity, and smoking cessation. It has been shown that independently and, if well done, these changes alone can make a real difference in patients' symptoms. In Chapter 7, D. Newman reviews all evidence and techniques to implement such measures in clinical practice.

Physiotherapy is widely used in Europe for various pelvic floor dysfunctions, as developed by K. Bo in Chapter 8. In North America, physiotherapy is not yet part of the OAB treatment algorithm, but will probably find its place in the future based on evidence coming from Europe.

Practically speaking, and to avoid too frequent visits to the patient, it is usual to suggest lifestyle changes and to give first-line medication at the first consultation. Medication is mainly in the form of anticholinergics and/or β3-agonists. The dosages of these drugs have to be tailored to the age, gender, and body mass index of each patient, to avoid discontinuation because of poor tolerance. Patients have to be informed of side-effects and educated on how to prevent/minimize them. This information to patients is an important part of prescriptions, and a nurse continence advisor (NCA) can often be helpful in this respect.

Details of different drugs, their mechanism of action, medication interaction, dosage and "best use" appear in Chapters 9 and 10 by Dmochowski and Davila, respectively. New pharmacological avenues are in the industry's pipeline and promise better efficacy and side-effect profiles than existing therapies. Chapple et al. explore medication combinations in Chapter 12. K.E. Anderson develops the future of pharmacological manipulations in Chapter 11.

Either physicians or NCAs must see patients again, four to six weeks after treatment initiation, to review progress with lifestyle change and response to medication. Some patients will respond better and tolerate one anticholinergic rather than another; this is why, in case of intolerance or inefficacy, alternative drug(s) can be offered. The recent availability of β3-agonists represents a new, interesting treatment avenue, as first- or second-line modalities, or even associated with anticholinergics. More data are presently needed to better understand their best place in the OAB treatment algorithm.

If patients respond well to first-line treatment, continuation of treatment for six months and stoppage are usually proposed. Some patients will see their symptoms disappear after just a few months of treatment; others will have to continue to take the same medication for a longer time period. In these cases, stopping medication has to be suggested from time to time.

Patients failing initial management

These patients have usually taken their medication properly and completed their lifestyle change program without experiencing real improvement of their OAB symptoms. Often, they will be referred to a specialized center and, for some physicians, they constitute the type of OAB patients who are seen most often.

These patients will report that their physician(s) have tried everything and that nothing worked! They are considered to have an "intractable bladder" or, more precisely, "oral drug-resistant OAB." These patients are frequently desperate, and happy to be referred to a "specialized" center.

In our specialized practice, we propose a seven-step approach to their management:

Step 1: Reassess patients

We consider the entire medical history to precisely ensure that previous physician(s) did not miss any detail that may have related the condition to existing disease. Symptoms of neurological disease, obstruction, or medication with anticholinergic or diuretic effects are examples of often-missed conditions.

Physical examination will include neurological assessment and evaluation of sphincter function with full bladder (stress test) to eliminate mixed urinary incontinence (MUI). Patients with MUI will not be fully satisfied, most of the time, if OAB symptoms are treated alone, leaving the stress incontinence component untreated.

Urodynamic study is mandatory in these intractable OAB cases, as it often reveals significant uninhibited detrusor contractions not usual in primary OAB and more compatible with a neurological condition.

Imaging techniques, and particularly spine magnetic resonance imaging, are often requested to eliminate a neurological explanation of the condition.

Rule 2: Understand exactly what is bothering them

Most of the time, patients will consult for a specific reason that is impairing their quality of life. We should not set their expectations too high. To return to completely normal bladder function is often an illusion. If patients are mainly bothered by their nocturia not allowing them to rest properly, by frequency not allowing them to play cards, by incontinence not allowing them to sleep at their children's' or friends' homes, and so on, our objective must be to correct such specific problems. Setting treatment objectives increases chances of success.

Rule 3: Review lifestyle changes

Behavioral changes are reviewed in detail to ensure that patients understand them and try them. Once again, NCAs can be extremely helpful not only in implementing such measures, but also in patient follow-up and continuous motivation.

Rule 4: Review past/current medications

An exact list of already-tried OAB medications should be compiled along with the exact reason(s) why they were stopped. Often, the starting dose is not adjusted for each patient, and the prescribed dose is too high. Re-starting these drugs with the proper initial dosage and increasing them progressively under NCA supervision are often the best approach. Help and recommendations to improve dry mouth and/or constipation also improve tolerability and compliance with anticholinergics.

Step 5: Consider adding medication

The unclear place of β3-agonists has already been discussed and will become apparent "*au fur et à mesure*" when research studies have been completed and their results published. Drugs, such as DDAVP, with their various presentations, could be extremely useful in patients complaining mainly of nocturia.

Step 6: Intensify follow-up

Such cases, which are difficult to manage, need much more attention than simple OAB patients. These subjects are frustrated, and good telephone follow-up by NCAs, in association with regular physician visits, is often necessary to adjust/change medication.

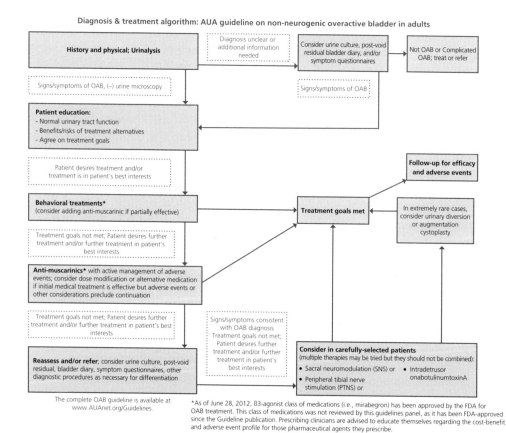

Figure 20.1 OAB algorithm of care.

Step 7: Take the time to explain alternative treatments in detail to patients who fail all these measures

Botulinum toxin injections, neuromodulation by tibial nerve stimulation or sacral root neuromodulation, and, ultimately, surgery have to be offered rationally to each patient, depending on availability, cost, patient choices, and expectations. All these techniques are covered in detail in Chapters 15 to 19.

If well applied, this stepwise approach to primary OAB will give the best results.

Specialized centers must be able to offer the whole spectrum of treatment. Lifestyle changes are always necessary, whatever other approaches are proposed. Oral medication remains the simplest treatment and the one given in proportion to the best results obtained. Others are much more invasive and costly, and should be reserved for use in expert centers after each of these steps has been attempted.

The American Urological Association guideline algorithm for OAB management is appended for a more visual understanding of this approach Figure 20.1.

Index

Page numbers in *italics* refer to illustrations; those in **bold** refer to tables

---

Overactive Bladder: Practical Management, First Edition. Edited by Jacques Corcos, Scott MacDiarmid
and John Heesakkers.
© 2015 John Wiley & Sons, Ltd. Published 2015 by John Wiley & Sons, Ltd.